T0331004

Explorations in Baltic Medical History, 1850–2015

Rochester Studies in Medical History

Christopher Crenner, Series Editor
Hudson and Ralph Major Professor and Chair
Department of History and Philosophy of Medicine
University of Kansas School of Medicine

Additional Titles of Interest

A complete list of titles in the Rochester Studies in Medical History series
may be found on our website, www.urpress.com.

Explorations in Baltic Medical History, 1850–2015

EDITED BY
NILS HANSSON AND JONATAN WISTRAND

UNIVERSITY OF ROCHESTER PRESS

The University of Rochester Press gratefully acknowledges generous support from
the Marcus Wallenberg Foundation for International Scientific Collaboration and
the Philip and Grace Sandblom Foundation.

First published 2019

University of Rochester Press
668 Mt. Hope Avenue, Rochester, NY 14620, USA
www.urpress.com
and Boydell & Brewer Limited
PO Box 9, Woodbridge, Suffolk IP12 3DF, UK
www.boydellandbrewer.com

ISBN-13: 978-1-58046-940-1
ISSN: 1526-2715

Library of Congress Cataloging-in-Publication Data

Names: Hansson, Nils, 1983– editor. | Wistrand, Jonatan, 1981– editor.
Title: Explorations in Baltic medical history, 1850–2015 / edited by Nils Hansson
    and Jonatan Wistrand.
Description: Rochester, NY : University of Rochester Press, 2019. | Series: Rochester
    studies in medical history, ISSN 1526-2715 ; v. 44 | Includes bibliographical
    references and index.
Identifiers: LCCN 2018059863 | ISBN 9781580469401 (hardcover : alk. paper)
Subjects: LCSH: Medicine—Baltic States—History.
Classification: LCC R131 .E97 2019 | DDC 610.9479—dc23 LC record available at
    https://lccn.loc.gov/2018059863

This publication is printed on acid-free paper.
Printed in the United States of America.

Contents

Part Two:
Bridging the Baltic: Comparative Studies

Foreword

The conference "Explorations in Medical History in the Baltic Sea Region 1850–2015" in 2014 took place at the Lund University in Sweden, financially supported by the Department for the History of Medicine at the Faculty of Medicine belonging to the Lund University. As the current head of this department (founded in 1981) I am glad that two young researchers, Nils Hansson and Jonatan Wistrand, organized and documented this successful conference. I am grateful for their work and would like to thank them both on behalf of the department. The Department for the History of Medicine in Lund works at the interface of medicine, culture, and society, and has a keen ambition to bring the more overarching theme of medical humanities into our discipline. This manifests in, for example, a close collaboration with scholars of art and literature as well as other areas of the humanistic sciences at Lund University and abroad.

It is noteworthy that our Lund University of today is 350 years old and located closer to the continent than other contemporary Swedish universities. This has influenced us through many and rich contacts with the countries bordering the southern shores of the Baltic Sea. Ever since Hanseatic times this region has been vibrant in culture, commerce, and science. We have therefore in contemporary times tried to develop our contacts with especially Denmark and Germany, but also with Poland and the Baltic states. We believe that we have benefited from strong historical contacts with our neighbors and this is also relevant for the history of medicine from the perspective of the conference.

I welcome the reader to this collection of some of the most interesting papers presented during the conference, carefully edited by Nils Hansson and Jonatan Wistrand.

Peter M. Nilsson
Head of the Department for History of Medicine
Lund University, Sweden

Preface

Almost ninety years ago, in 1931, the Romanian historian of medicine Valeriu Bologa wrote an essay about the value of national historiographies. He rejected nationalistic approaches as unscientific but strongly argued for a national standpoint to allow for "optimum" and "maximum" results from researchers who are familiar with a specific context. However, for him the national perspective was only a start. He pursued a broader objective: he followed the idea that national perspectives should contribute brick by brick to a larger general understanding of the history of medicine. Consequently, he argued for international cooperation and syntheses.

Bologa's focus was the history of medicine in Eastern Europe, and he wrote in an era of nationalistic thinking. Thus, he is quite remote from the historiography of medicine focusing the Baltic between 1850 and 2015. Nevertheless, it is striking that even today Bologa's basic idea of the history of medicine as an international endeavor still seems to be an unachieved goal rather worth striving for.

Shifting time (away from 1931 to today) and space (from Eastern Europe to the Baltic Sea) in a historiographic approach illustrates the strength of comparative transnational perspectives: a whole national, cultural, political, and geographical background changes. The connotations of the collective terms Eastern Europe and the Baltic transport completely different ideas of lands, people, lives, languages, and cities. However, some features, like social inequalities in health or in the provision of care, seem to persist over time and space. In this tension lies the great benefit of transnational perspectives on the history of medicine. It is an immense task to investigate international networks of doctors; the movement of knowledge across borders; and the appropriation, change, and adaptation of ideas and practices in different political and cultural contexts in order to reconstruct and understand, for example, the triumph of physicochemical approaches in medicine all over Europe.

This book is just such a collaborative work that transgresses the national boundaries of medical history. These international historians of medicine contribute to an international perspective on their field by comparatively traversing the borders of states and minds located on and shaped by the

Baltic Sea. The different meanings of the Baltic are taken seriously and productively used to reconstruct networks of people and ideas in order to show that medicine as an "art and science," with its practical and theoretical elements, truly is traveling across borders. The case studies collected in this volume will help to create a wider picture of what the circulation of medical knowledge in the Baltic Sea region meant during the nineteenth and twentieth centuries.

Medicine as a science and practice has always transgressed borders; the same is true for the historiography of medicine. I hope that this collection of essays is a starting point for further works on the European history of medicine that on the one hand comprehensively combine studies on local medical knowledge and its relation to international science and on the other hand take regional, geographical, political, and cultural aspects as comparative elements into account.

Heiner Fangerau
President of the European Association for the
History of Medicine and Health
2013–2015

Note

1. Valeriu Lucian Bologa, "Nationale oder nationalistische Medizingeschichtsschreibung? Randbemerkungen zu einer Kritik," Archeion 13 (1931): 449–59.

Circulation of Knowledge in the Baltic Sea Region: An Introduction

Nils Hansson and Jonatan Wistrand

> There are days when the Baltic is a calm endless roof.
> Dream your naive dreams then about someone coming crawling on the
> roof trying to sort out the flag-lines, trying to hoist the rag-
>
> the flag which is so eroded by the wind and blackened by the funnels
> and bleached by the sun it can be everyone's.
>
> —Tomas Tranströmer, "Östersjöar" (1974)

Mare Balticum, a term coined one thousand years ago by the German chronicler Adam von Bremen, is a sea between central and northern Europe that stretches from latitude 53°N to 66°N and from longitude 10°E to 30°E. Located between Sweden, Finland, Russia, Estonia, Latvia, Lithuania, Poland, Germany, and Denmark, it is linked with the North Sea and the Øresund channel. Although today most commonly known as the Baltic Sea, it is—depending on the viewpoint—also referred to as the East Sea or the West Sea. The definition of the Baltic Sea *region* is not as clear cut. Its boundaries have been described as "fuzzy, vague and contingent."[1] Baltoscandia, northeastern Europe, northern Europe, the Baltic World, or the German Ostseeraum appear at first glance to be synonyms, but they carry different ideological connotations and political assumptions of constructed communities.[2] As hinted in Tranströmer's poem, "Östersjöar" (The Baltic Seas), this "European macro region"[3] is multicultural, multilingual, and characterized by a plurality of identities that have intermingled and separated to a higher or lower extent in different eras throughout history. Partly because of these crossroads of several cultures and peoples, the region has attracted—and still attracts—broad scholarly interest, not least in the field of *area studies*.[4] Several research programs in Baltic studies have been

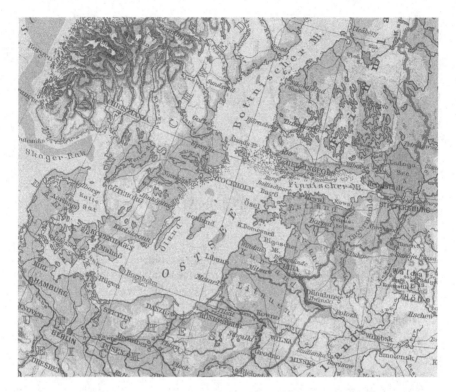

Figure I.1. Map of the Baltic Sea region from 1920. Source: Carl Diercke, *Skolatlas: Kartorna över Norden utarbetade av N. Rönnholm* (Stockholm: Norstedt, 1920).

established throughout Europe and beyond, as well as scientific journals to foster research on this territory.[5]

Time and space are the two main categories every historian has to take into account. For a long time, however, historiography has marginalized the spatial dimension of human experience by paying considerably more attention to the different temporalities of historical change. Since the 1990s, this disproportionate emphasis on time over space has been steadily altered, following political geographer Edward Soja's demand "to spatialize the historical narrative"[6] and to open historical science to a geographical imagination including a spatial organization of human society. One of the most influential thinkers on this topic was the French historian Fernand Braudel. In his book *The Mediterranean in the Age of Philip II* (first published in 1949 and revised several times in succeeding years),[7] Braudel demonstrated a close link between a geographically determined and socially constructed area. The Braudelian philosophy of history can be imagined in the metaphorical framework of an ocean itself: the foam on the crests of the waves (by which he meant the historical events) are nothing but superficial layers hiding more powerful currents, conjunctures, or structures. The sea has unifying functions but also set up natural boundaries. Today, Braudel's considerations continue to raise exciting questions about how to write about scientific exchange within certain spaces, especially when combined with current analytical approaches such as network theory and transnational history.[8] During recent decades, interest in comparative, transfer, center versus periphery, transnational, and global history, or even microhistory, has challenged the traditional historiography of nation-states. Several approaches have thus been combined to shed light on "space" as a category of analysis and the interaction of historical and current phenomena in different countries, regions, and continents.[9]

Studying the development and transfer of scientific theories in a given area is not a novel approach. As James Secord points out, "Every academic conference ever held could well be said to exemplify the theme of knowledge in circulation."[10] Over the past decades however, "circulation" and "transfer" have become explicit labels, or themes, classifying research projects into categories. Topics such as knowledge exchange between Asia and Europe during the Hellenistic period, transfers in pre-Columbian America, and the export of science during colonialism have received much attention from historians of science. A common narrative has been the portrayal of European scientists as heroes who travel to exotic lands and "revolutionize" science and societies. This European perspective has been questioned by postcolonial theorists since the 1960s, and, among historians of medicine, a stronger emphasis on looking "beyond the great doctors"[11] has emerged.[12] Since then, the number of research projects investigating historical transfer processes within the fields of science and technology studies is steadily increasing.[13]

The idea for this book came about when we were preparing an introductory lecture for first-year medical students at Lund University about medical history in Scandinavia during the twentieth century. In reviewing the literature, we found that an overview of medical history for the region was lacking. Whereas studies in the field of cultural transfer and cultural area studies within this time frame—for example, intercultural studies[14] between Sweden and Germany[15]—have been an area of investigation for decades, the production and spread of medical knowledge within the Baltic Sea region as a whole has not been systematically researched. Historians have proposed such studies of course—not least at the biannual Nordic Medical History Congresses—but not as a specific focus, it seems, and rarely with that multitude of approaches possible only when researchers from various corners of the Baltic Sea region are brought together to reflect upon one central question: How has the development and transfer of knowledge in the Baltic Sea region influenced medicine as a discipline, and illness as an experience, during the nineteenth and twentieth centuries? The Baltic Sea region, with its history of multiple cultural and social transformations, as well as mixture of national and regional scientific styles, is an excellent point of departure for case studies on such processes.

In October 2014, a three-day symposium gathering some thirty scholars from six countries was held in the University Main Building in Lund, Sweden.[16] This volume contains a selection of the papers presented at the symposium. The contributing authors are historians, physicians, geographers, ethnologists, and literary scholars. By presenting case studies of Baltic Medical history the contributors wish to shed light on how medical knowledge and devices[17] were and are developed in a multitude of different subcontexts, sometimes, but not necessarily, defined by national borders. Furthermore, by illuminating currents of ideas and traditions, contact zones, and areas of conflict, the anthology addresses technological, social, and economic aspects relevant to the circulation of medical knowledge across the Baltic Sea. In addition to studies of occupations, movements, and legislation in the region, the anthology also highlights the achievements of specific individuals within a medical framework. In such a person-centered approach, it deals with both the history of medical professionals as well as the history of patients and their illness experiences. By applying a "narrative medicine" stance to illness stories shared within and across the Baltic Sea region, the voice of the patient is sought for.[18] The primary objective guiding the editorial work has been to contribute to the understanding of adaption and transformation of knowledge in shaping medicine as a life science in northern Europe.

As illustrated by the ten chapters, we encouraged a multitude of suggestions and conceptions about what medicine is today and has been historically. Each author explores various aspects of how medicine has been envisioned by observers around the Baltic Sea. Through case studies of different historical actors (physicians, scientists, and—not least—patients), the dynamics in different medico-political debates, the impact of different ideological movements, and the spread of different scientific ideas, the anthology broadens our knowledge about how national and regional styles, or even "Nordic" patterns with common or diverging factors, have been constructed historically within the field(s) of medicine.[19] In that sense, these studies put us in a better position to evaluate where medicine is today and in which direction it might evolve. This book thus not only aims to improve our insufficient understanding of knowledge development in the Baltic Sea region, it also hopes to challenge national paradigms and not merely to provide an accumulated narrative of national histories. We deal with processes, which, as the following chapters show, are not linear and static but demonstrate complex reciprocal interactions. Each chapter constitutes a case study that ameliorates our understanding of a limited course of events taking place within the medical history of the Baltic Sea region. Rather than an encyclopedia of Baltic medical history, this anthology should thus be regarded as a contribution to such a larger concept, as well as a basis for further discussions.

The period covered stretches from the mid-nineteenth century up to 2015. As is always the case with historiographic start and end points, choice is in some sense arbitrary, constructed as it is from our present point of view. Still, the time span was not chosen by accident.

First of all, by the mid-nineteenth century, sometimes referred to as the first wave of globalization,[20] a remarkable development in the ability of scholars in northern Europe to communicate with one other took place. Railways were built in large parts of northern Europe, which, along with ferry lines, made it easier and cheaper to cross borders, resulting in a strong intensification of trade and human migration. In this era, a constant stream of goods, people, knowledge, and ideas crossed the Baltic Sea. Study trips across the Baltic Sea and between Baltic Sea countries gained increasing popularity. By the start of the twentieth century, it took less than a day to travel from one major city in Northern or Northeastern Europe to another.

Another important fact motivating the temporal point of departure of this anthology is that more and more specialized journals for various medical disciplines started to crop up in the second half of the nineteenth century, and scientific meetings like the ones organized by the Society of German Researchers and Physicians (Gesellschaft Deutscher Naturforscher und Ärzte, founded in 1822), or world exhibitions—with the first one taking place in London in 1851—became an arena for presenting new medical research. As a result, the dialogue between medical professionals and scientists was brought to a new level, with a continuous flow of theories, opinions, and newly discovered "facts" being exchanged to an extent never seen previously. In that sense, we *can* speak of a "globalization of science" during the second half of the nineteenth century in European medicine and the life sciences. For example, early medical journals like *Pflügers Archiv* (founded in 1868), one decade after Rudolf Virchow had founded the *Archiv für pathologische Anatomie und Physiologie und für klinische Medicin* (1858), among others, promoted contacts and collaboration across the Baltic Sea. This knowledge transfer of new scientific ideas within a specific professional setting is highlighted in, for example, the chapter by Anders Ottosson concerning the spread of Gustaf Zander's so-called medico-mechanical institutes (as the reader will see, they remind us of modern fitness studios today). They were introduced in Sweden in the early 1860s and soon spread to nearly all corners of the world. Zander gained such a strong reputation that he even became a prime candidate for the Nobel Prize in physiology or medicine in 1916. However, after the First World War, his devices quickly lost their appeal and disappeared as a social phenomenon, before a remarkable revival took place some five decades later. Another example of knowledge in motion is provided in the chapter by Michaela Malmberg on the Swedish physiotherapist Thure Brandt's practice of pelvic massage, a gynecological method that became hugely popular in Western medicine. Malmberg examines the discourses surrounding the massage in fin-de-siècle society, a phenomenon consisting of many threads, ranging from body, sexuality, and gender to specialization and competition between emerging occupational identities. Today, both Zander's machines and the practice of Brandt's pelvic massage are known to a wide international audience through blockbuster movies like *The Road to Wellville* (1994) and *Hysteria* (2001).

It is well known that German was the main scientific language in most parts of northern Europe from 1850 until it gradually changed to English during the first half of the twentieth century.[21] But this fact does not imply that German parts of the Baltic Sea were the scientific centers of this region at all times or that other coastal regions in that sense were regarded as being on the scientific peripheries. As Max Engman has shown, the constellation of centers in this region has undergone several shifts over time. If Lübeck, Visby, Riga, and Reval were major cities from the late Middle Ages and Hanseatic times[22] to the era of rising territorial states, they were subsequently followed by the preeminence of Stockholm, Amsterdam, and Danzig, which lasted until the Swedish defeat at Poltava in 1709. As suggested in this anthology, such shifts extend also to the leading centers for medicine and science. Whereas Halle an der Saale near Berlin, and Uppsala near Stockholm—where universities were founded in 1502 and 1477, respectively—were (and are) important sites for researchers traveling to Sweden or Germany, traditional travel routes changed when the Berliner Universität (1809) and the Karolinska Institute (1810) were founded and became new hubs at the turn of the nineteenth century. Also, because of the driving influence of steamships and ferries, port cities became crucial nodal points in the growing world market of this period.

The political scientist Bernd Henningsen argued in a publication on the construction of identities in the Baltic Sea region that "there is no unified history of the Baltic Sea Region, there is no central power, no overarching nation, person, or idea (religion!) that has left its imprint on the region in the long term—everything is plural: kings, cities, orders, ethnicities, ideas, languages."[23] Similarly, in terms of medical practice and ideas, the Baltic Sea region was not just invented, negotiated, or constructed once for all time; it is constantly being reinvented, renegotiated, and reconstructed.[24] One such renegotiation within a specific medical subcenter is explored by Joanna Nieznanowska in her chapter about the medical world of Stettin/Szczecin. This chapter also exemplifies the effects of World War II on identity and knowledge transfer between medical centers in the Baltic Sea region. Furthermore, Nieznanowska points out desiderata and evaluates the chances for different historical perspectives on the city.

Taking the city of Malmö in southern Sweden as example, the study by Motzi Eklöf also analyzes the tensions between the local and the global, here in terms of potential threats by sailors and foreigners to the national public health in general, and the strategies to combat a smallpox epidemic during the first half of the twentieth century in particular. Mapping these entanglements allows us to compare and contrast local strategies for dealing with the perceived health threats in the region and beyond.

Axel C. Hüntelmann's network analysis of Paul Ehrlich, Maike Rotzoll and Frank Grüner's approach to examining the changing concepts of melancholy with a focus on Emil Kraepelin, and Ken Kalling and Erki Tammiksaar's study on the abstinence movement in Estonia also demonstrate how the map of geographical medical melting pots, including leading scientists and their relationships to one another, have been transformed several times from the mid-nineteenth century to the present day. As, for example, Bruno Latour has shown, scientific activity is a collective action where people and things are entangled in a network of actors. Thus, "scientific facts" are constructed not in a vacuum but in a given time and space within a certain social, economic, and technological context.[25] In the Baltic Sea region several such contexts have in fact coexisted with more or less exchange throughout different decades of the twentieth century depending on how the political landscapes have changed.

Some concepts, devices, and practices relating to diagnosis, treatment, and prevention have received an enthusiastic reception immediately and have been adjusted to fit local customs or reinterpreted to fit local discourses, while others hardly spread at all. The personal motivation for recognition in the larger scientific community is undeniably a driving force behind some transfers. Illuminating a fragile network of basic researchers around the Salvarsan inventor and 1908 Nobel laureate in physiology or medicine Paul Ehrlich and his peers, Axel C. Hüntelmann investigates how contacts can develop from being informal and personal into more formal and fruitful networks in this region along the north-south axis across the Baltic Sea. Maike Rotzoll and Frank Grüner use psychiatrist Emil Kraepelin's "Estonian peasant" patient to explain the concept of melancholy with biographical sketches and to compare "Eastern" and "Western" concepts of psychiatry. In their chapter, Ken Kalling and Erki Tammiksaar evaluate the transnational influence of German racial hygiene in northern Europe by describing the formation and scientific layout of the anti-alcohol movement, analyzing the role of different indigenous groups and different classes in the context of the building and deconstruction of national identities.

During the chosen period, major changes also occurred in patient mobility, facilitating the transfer of patients' illness experience. The most obvious case of such large-scale travel among patients is the sanatorium, to which wealthy patients came from all over Europe in search of the most effective treatment. This increase in patient mobility and interaction during the time studied is exemplified in the chapter by Jonatan Wistrand on the sanatorium narrative by Swedish poet Harriet Löwenhjelm. This chapter contributes a more multifaceted understanding of medical history where the experience of illness and the psychological impact of illness at an individual level is highlighted.[26] Through narrative analysis of the stories provided by patients from the past, complementary ways of understanding medical history as something more than scientific discoveries, classifications, and debates is sought. [27]

As the time frame of the anthology stretches up to, and even beyond, the turn of the millennium, the reader is also provided with analyses of medico-political debates from our more recent history with comparative approaches. This is represented in two chapters with two different ways of exploring contemporary Baltic medicine. Katharina Beier, on the one hand, studies the policies and outcome of biobanking activities in Estonia, Germany, and Sweden on a state and population level: Is there a "Nordic unity" regarding these questions? She compares the ethical, economic, juridical, and political discourses linked to the collection of biological data in these countries, reflecting the Islandic genome project, and explains the differences between national attitudes and the European settings. Martin Gunnarson, on the other hand, takes an ethnological perspective and investigates the standpoints of individual patients undergoing hemodialysis in Riga and Stockholm. He poses questions to find deeper information on the very different cultures of patient-doctor and patient-patient interactions. These two chapters illustrate that similarities and differences in the medical debates of today are grounded in the history of the region. Furthermore, they exemplify how the anthology embraces a wide spectrum of methodological approaches, each providing an important piece for the overall understanding of how medical knowledge has been carried across the Baltic Sea from the mid-nineteenth century to the present.

The following exploratory studies form a multifaceted picture that aims at expanding the traditions horizons of medical history. We consider it a particular strength that the authors look at transfers of medical knowledge and actors in medicine from different angles to make visible the multitude of medical voices, initiatives, thoughts, and expressions in the Baltic Sea region. The book is directed to a wide readership, including students, physicians, historians, teachers, and laypersons with an interest in medical humanities and Baltic studies. The anthology and the symposium were funded by the Marcus Wallenberg foundation for International Scientific Collaboration, Philip and Grace Sandblom's foundation, and Bengt I Lindskog's foundation. We are also indebted to Berndt Ehinger, Camilla Key, Peter M. Nilsson, and the Society for Medical History in Southern Sweden (SMHS) for their support.

Notes

Epigraph: Tomas Tranströmer, *New Collected Poems*, trans. Robin Fulton (Newcastle-upon-Tyne: Bloodaxe Books, 1997), 111.

Throughout the book, translations of non-English source material are by the author unless otherwise noted.

1. Marko Lehti, "Mapping the Study of the Baltic Sea Area: From Nation-Centric to Multinational History," *Journal of Baltic Studies* 33, no. 4 (2002): 431–46, 437.

2. Kazimierz Musial, "'Nordisch—Nordic—Nordisk': Die wandelbaren Topoi-Funktionen in den deutschen, anglo-amerikanischen und skandinavischen nationalen Diskursen," in *Die kulturelle Konstruktion von Gemeinschaften: Schweden und Deutschland im Modernisierungsprozeß*, ed. Alexandra Bänsch et al. (Baden-Baden: Nomos, 2001), 95–122.

3. Bernd Henningsen, *On Identity—No Identity: An Essay on the Constructions, Possibilities and Necessities for Understanding a European Macro Region; The Baltic Sea* (Copenhagen: Baltic Development Forum, 2011).

4. For example, the Nordic Experience book series and its second volume, Sverker Sörlin, ed., *Science, Geopolitics and Culture in the Polar Region. Norden Beyond Borders* (Farnham: Ashgate, 2013); the ongoing project Wissenschaftsbeziehungen im 19. Jahrhundert zwischen Deutschland und Russland auf den Gebieten Chemie, Pharmazie und Medizin, led by Ortrun Riha (Leipzig University); and the research program Baltic Borderlands: Shifting Boundaries of Mind and Culture in the Borderlands of the Baltic Sea Region (University of Greifswald). Lars Fredrik Stoecker, *Bridging the Baltic Sea: Networks of Resistance and Opposition during the Cold War Era* (London: Lexington Books, 2017); Björn Felder and Paul J. Weindling, eds., *Baltic Eugenics: Bio-politics, Race and Nation in Interwar Estonia, Latvia and Lithuania 1918–1940* (Amsterdam: Rodopi, 2013); Michael North, *Geschichte der Ostsee: Handel und Kulturen* (Munich: C. H. Beck, 2011); Gunnar Broberg and Nils Roll-Hansen, eds., *Eugenics and the Welfare State: Norway, Sweden, Denmark, and Finland* (Ann Arbor: Michigan State University Press, 2005); David Kirby, *The Baltic World 1772–1993: Europe's Northern Periphery in an Age of Change* (New York: Longman, 1995).

5. For example, the *Journal of Baltic Studies, Baltic Worlds, Nordeuropaforum*.

6. Edward W Soja, *Postmodern Geographies: The Reassertion of Space in Critical Social Theory* (London: Verso Press, 1989).

7. Fernand Braudel, *The Mediterranean and the Mediterranean World in the Age of Philip II* (Berkeley: University of California Press, 1996).

8. Lutz Sauerteig, "Vergleich: Ein Königsweg auch für die Medizingeschichte? Methodologische Fragen komparativen Forschens," in *Medizingeschichte, Aufgaben, Probleme, Perspektiven*, ed. Norbert Paul and Thomas Schlich (Frankfurt: Campus Verlag, 1998), 266–91; Klaus Bergdolt, "Medizin," in *Handbuch der Mediterranistik*, ed. Mihran Dabag, Dieter Haller, et al. (Paderborn: Ferdinand Schöning, 2015), 291–302; Heiner Fangerau and Irmgard Müller, "Scientific Exchange: Jacques Loeb (1859–1924) and Emil Godlewski (1875–1944) as Representatives of a Transatlantic Developmental Biology," *Studies in the History and Philosophy of Biological and Biomedical Sciences* 38 (2007): 608–17.

9. These aspects were discussed in detail by Susanne Michl in her lecture at the symposium, entitled "From Braudel's 'Méditérranée' to the Baltic area: Making and

Meaning of the 'Spatial Turn' in Historiography." We thank Susanne Michl for allowing us access to her manuscript.

10. James A. Secord, "Knowledge in Transit," *Isis* 95, no. 4 (2004): 654–72, 655.

11. Susan Reverby and David Rosner, "'Beyond the Great Doctors' Revisited: A Generation of the New Social History of Medicine," in *Locating Medical History: The Stories and Their Meaning*, ed. Frank Huisman and John Harley Warner (Baltimore: Johns Hopkins University Press, 2004), 167–93.

12. George Basalla, "The Spread of Western Science," *Science* 156 (1967): 3775.

13. Mitchell G Ash, "Wissens- und Wissenschaftstransfer—Einführende Bemerkungen," *Berichte zur Wissenschaftsgeschichte* 29 (2006): 181–89.

14. Johannes Paulmann, "Internationaler Vergleich und interkultureller Transfer: Zwei Forschungsansätze zur europäischen Geschichte des 18. bis 20. Jahrhunderts," *Historische Zeitschrift* 267, no. 3 (1998): 649–85; Greogory Paschalidis, "Exporting National Culture: Histories of Cultural Institutes Abroad," *International Journal of Cultural policy* 15, no. 3 (2009): 275–89.

15. Andreas Åkerlund, *Kulturtransfer och kulturpolitik: Sverige och Tyskland under det tjugonde århundradet* (Västerås: Opuscula Historica Upsaliensia 45. Edita Västra Aros, 2011); Helmut Müssener and Frank-Michael Kirsch, *Nachbarn im Ostseeraum unter sich: Vorurteile, Klischees und Stereotypen* (Stockholm: Almqvist & Wiksell, 2000); Birgitta Almgren, *Inte bara Stasi: Relationer Sverige-DDR 1949–1990* (Stockholm: Carlsson, 2009).

16. The following presenters attended: Louise Bergström, Tomas Bro, Nils Danielsen, Pieter Dhondt, Motzi Eklöf, Frank Grüner, Martin Gunnarson, Nils Hansson, Axel C. Hüntelmann, Ken Kalling, Guntis Kilkuts, Susanne Kreutzer, Øivind Larsen, Michaela Malmberg, Susanne Michl, Joanna Nieznanowska, Peter M Nilsson, Anders Ottosson, Anja K Peters, Maike Rotzoll, Nils-Otto Sjöberg, Ylva Söderfeldt, Matilda Svensson, Erki Tammiksaar, and Jonatan Wistrand.

17. Michel Espagne, "Der theoretische Stand der Kulturtransferforschung," in *Kulturelle Praxis im 16. Jahrhundert*, ed. Wolfgang Schmale (Vienna: 2. Studien Verlag, 2003), 63–75.

18. Rita Charon, *Narrative Medicine—Honoring the Stories of Illness* (New York: Oxford University Press, 2008).

19. Antoon A Braembussche, "Historical Explanation and Comparative Method: Towards a Theory of the History of Society," *History and Theory* 28 (1989), 1–24.

20. Miguel Suárez Bosa, ed., *Atlantic Ports and the First Globalisation c. 1850–1930* (Basingstoke: Palgrave Macmillan, 2004).

21. Nils Hansson, Friedrich Moll, Thorsten Halling, and Bengt Uvelius, "Scientific Language Trends among Swedish Urologists and Surgeons 1900–1955," *World Journal of Urology*, https://doi.org/10.1007/s00345-018-2451-z; Michael Prinz and Jarmo Korhonen, eds., *Deutsch als Wissenschaftssprache im Ostseeraum—Geschichte und Gegenwart: Akten zum Humboldt-Kolleg an der Universität Helsinki, 27. Bis 29. Mai 2010* (Frankfurt: Peter Lang, 2011); Roswitha Reinbothe, *Deutsch als internationale Wissenschaftssprache und der Boykott nach dem Ersten Weltkrieg* (Frankfurt: Peter Lang, 2006).

22. Max Engman, *Petersburgska vägar* (Esbo: Schildts, 1995).

23. Bernd Henningsen, *On Identity—No Identity: An Essay on the Constructions, Possibilities and Necessities for Understanding a European Macro Region; The Baltic Sea* (Copenhagen: Baltic Development Forum, 2011), 37.

24. Hendriette Kliemann, *Koordinaten des Nordens: Wissenschaftliche Konstruktionen einer europäischen Region 1770–1850* (Berlin: Berliner Wissenschafts-Verlag, 2005).

25. Bruno Latour, *Science in Action: How to Follow Scientists and Engineers through Society* (Cambridge, MA: Harvard University Press, 1987).

26. Anne Whitehead, "The Medical Humanities: A Literary Perspective," in *Medicine, Health, and the Arts: Approaches to the Medical Humanities*, ed. Victoria Bates et al. (New York: Routledge, 2014), 108.

27. Mike Bury, "Illness Narratives: Fact or Fiction?," *Sociology of Health and Illness* 23, no. 3 (2001): 264.

Part One

Transfers of Medical Knowledge across the Baltic Sea

Chapter One

Gym Machines and the Migration of Medical Knowledge in the Nineteenth Century

ANDERS OTTOSSON

Around 1970 Arthur Jones (1926–2007), son of an American physician, launched his training concept, Nautilus.[1] It was a new type of gym machine intended to improve exercise and strength training. Bodybuilding had at the time become popular, as epitomized by the movie *Pumping Iron*, starring a young Arnold Schwarzenegger. Nautilus machines spread globally and became big business. They were also copied by others, and most modern gyms have machinery using similar principles.

Since his early teens Jones had dedicated himself to weight lifting, but despite his good results he had always thought that something was missing. At the time there was no scientific literature on "exercise physiology" to guide him. For that reason, he had to design his machines in a scientific vacuum. The shortage of adequate research resulted from the lack of scientists interested in strength training. This in turn was caused by the fact that "it was then impossible to determine the results of exercise for the simple reason that the required tools for any such measurements did not exist."[2]

It is tempting to consider whether Jones drafted his innovative concept in splendid isolation. New inventions and ideas are seldom the fruits of a single individual's labor and genius, although posterity may easily get this impression. Scholars of the sociology of knowledge and history of science often point this out. Investigations show that successful scientific breakthroughs and innovations are frequently linked to several individuals and intellectual milieus, forming a kind of critical mass enabling new ideas to be born. This phenomenon is sometimes highlighted by the Nobel Prize ceremonies. Did the laureate(s) actually contribute the most?

Instead of critically examining Jones as an innovative maverick, this chapter will use a similar approach to a person he honored greatly. Jones claimed splendid isolation, but he has revealed that there was a man whose work might have helped him greatly, if he had only known of its existence. About a hundred years before Jones, the Swedish physician Gustaf Zander (1835–1920) had invented a series of machines with basically the same design as Nautilus or, in Jones's words, in accordance with "simple laws of physics" and a full understanding of "muscular functions." Like the Nautilus concept, Zander's machines met the need for resistance: "direct, rotary-form, variable and balanced resistance." Jones insisted though that his innovations did not involve plagiarism: "I did not copy Zander's work and learned nothing from him, was not even aware of his work until long after I had made the same discoveries that he had made."[3]

In Zander Jones recognized a soul mate who, like him, had experienced a situation where scientific ignorance about exercise was monumental: "His only problem was that he lived about a century ahead of his time, at a time when very few people cared about exercise and even fewer knew anything about it."[4] Zander was thus ahead of his contemporaries, which was why he did not get the recognition he deserved. Jones's conclusion is my point of departure here in framing the emergence of Zander's machines historically and sociologically. We shall ask ourselves whether Zander really was as ahead of his times as Jones believed? The simple answer is no. Zander seems rather to have been a product of his times. Zander is in fact the Swedish physician who may have succeeded best in leaving an international footprint, in Jones's own homeland, the United States. Zander became famous thanks to his gym machines.[5]

Altogether Zander designed seventy-six different devices. They were introduced in Sweden in the early 1860s and soon spread out in all directions. The first destination was probably Finland and thence around the Baltic Sea, further into Europe, and finally the whole world. Their success was fully comparable to that of Nautilus. The greatest impact came in Germany where Zander institutes grew up like mushrooms until World War I, and as with Nautilus others began to develop similar machines.[6] Zander's machines had a strong scientific aura, not least because they made it easier to measure the effect of training. He received many awards and honors. [7] In 1916 Zander was even nominated for the Nobel Prize in physiology or medicine. After World War I, however, his machines quickly lost their attraction and disappeared as a social phenomenon.[8]

This raises several key questions. How was it possible for a doctor from a sparsely populated backwater in northern Europe to make such an impression outside Sweden? Although his machines were initially not received uncritically, it is unlikely that Zander's triumph could have taken place in a scientific void. He must have been part of a larger context that made the machines possible. Thus, the ambition here is to unearth the scientific infrastructure that enabled Zander's machines to succeed and to "migrate" globally.

This chapter establishes that Zander was not the pioneer one might easily be led to believe. His type of machine had admittedly not been seen before, but he was actually not innovative regarding what they were supposed to achieve. A better way to describe them is as the "technified" offspring of an older but equally influential scientific tradition, which thus deserves to be included here. This tradition too had a strong scientific provenance in Sweden and was as mechanically oriented as Zander's machines. The difference was that what Zander managed with machines was in the older tradition performed manually, that is, by human hands. This manual tradition and its representatives are now even more forgotten than Zander, but, as will be argued, they cannot be disregarded if we want to understand his success more fully. How and why this older tradition was institutionalized, thus paving the way for Zander, will be illustrated with examples mainly from Sweden and countries around the Baltic Sea where Germany will hold center stage. At the end I will discuss tentatively why Zander and the factors making his great success possible have disappeared from our historical awareness.

The Origin of Gym Machines: Zander's Inspiration

Although Zander's contemporaries, in contrast to Jones's beliefs, showed great interest in weight lifting, aspiring "strong men" were unwilling to use Zander's machines. The reason for this is simple but important to bear in mind: they were not designed to meet healthy people's desire for bigger muscles but intended to treat diseases.[9] This focus on illness reduced the resistance in Zander's machines. Some were even completely passive, with steam engines and not the patients powering the machines.[10] Many machines also executed different types of massage. Chronic and internal diseases were treated as well as orthopedic ailments, with scoliosis as the main therapeutic focus.[11]

Zander developed the first prototypes at his sisters' pension for girls outside Bårp, in southwestern Sweden. In 1857 he was made responsible for the girls' gymnastic training. Additionally, he was enrolled at Uppsala University, where he laid the foundation for the medical degree he took in 1864 at the Karolinska Institute in Stockholm.[12] While at the university he began to take an interest in gymnastics and physical exercises. He learned Pehr Henrik Ling's (1776–1839) system of gymnastics. The Ling system's great influence on international physical education is well researched, also internationally.[13] Millions have been drilled in "Swedish gymnastics" in schools worldwide.

Zander's main interest was not the Ling system's potential in the educational field, however, but its medical possibilities. The system included not only physical education (pedagogical gymnastics) but also military gymnastics (mostly fencing) and physiotherapy (medical gymnastics). The latter had become very popular at this time, even internationally, and Zander saw the opportunity to develop this treatment further but not to change the biomedical principles behind it. No, the important thing was that the manual techniques were "mechanized." As indicated above, Zander was convinced that machines could offer more than the human hand. They made the treatments mathematically precise, which appealed to him and his contemporaries who were increasingly fascinated by technology and measurability.[14]

This interest in "technology" also affected the many health resorts and spas that flourished at the end of the century, making them fertile grounds for the machines. Sanatoriums and hospitals were also keen on using them. A more materialistic historical explanation for Zander's success is, however, economy. His machines were less labor intensive. The administration of regular manual physiotherapy demanded up to five persons. Machines made the treatments cheaper and thus were of greater benefit to the suffering. This economic potential helped Zander to gain momentum, as the development in Germany in particular shows. As early as 1884, mandatory accident insurance was imposed there, making employers responsible for loss of income in case of accidents in the workplace. This made industrial enterprise and rehabilitation more economically interconnected, which made the machines attractive. In the long run, a set of Zander machines was cheaper than a staff of physiotherapists. The increased accessibility of physiotherapy was also a factor highlighted by the Nobel Committee in its nomination of Zander in 1916, although the historical background was different: World War I had left behind an unprecedented number of maimed soldiers for whom Zander machines were thought to provide the most effective rehabilitation. The Swedish orthopedic surgeon Professor Patrik Haglund, who had nominated Zander for the prize, justified his proposal using German physicians' view that Zander's invention provided the best treatment available for the care of war disabled.[15]

The German successes in particular probably made the Nobel Committee look favorably on Zander. At the time Swedish research and education were heavily influenced by Germany, and the importance of the German recognition of Zander shines through in the positive appraisal of his nomination. The extent of Zander's scientific impact in Germany is proved by his almost mandatory presence in standard German works on the history of medicine.[16]

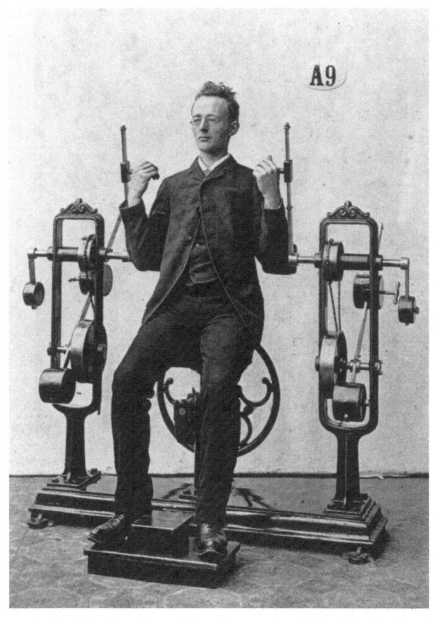

Figure 1.1. Zander machine used for flexion and extension of the arms.

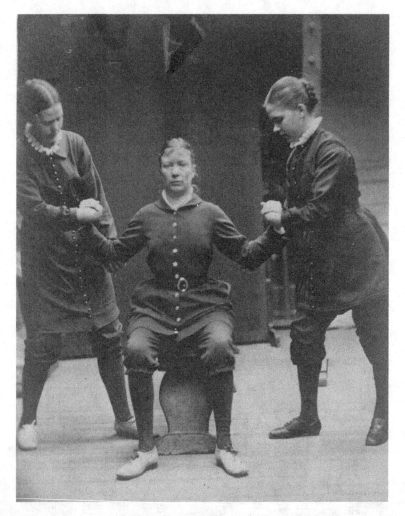

Figure 1.2. The manual "gym machine" for flexion and extension of the arms that Zander wanted to mimic in figure 1.1.

However, as has been implied, the launch of the machines was not completely smooth. And it took a few years before the resistance faded away. Objections came mostly from those who had invested their entire career in the older manual physiotherapy that Zander's weights and levelers were supposed to replace. Although Zander's skeptics soon became a minority, their criticism could be biting and an indication of how well embedded manual physiotherapy was in the therapeutic and scientific landscape of the second half of the 1800s. In Germany, physicians initially called the apparatus derisively "magnificent toys for big children," but the main bone of contention was the machines' potential. Could they really match the quality trained hands could offer?[17] In this respect, the criticism should also be weighed against a more cynical explanation: the objections had a streak of Luddism in them. The machines were unacceptable because they threatened to put many physicians and physiotherapists out of work. At a time when private practice was the dominant form of employment in the health-care sector, this explanation cannot be neglected.[18] Thus, some years of adjustment were needed before the old manual and the new mechanized methods could coexist. They never became mutually exclusive and could often complement each other.

The criticism of Zander is, however, most interesting because it can lead us further into the scientific and therapeutic infrastructure that he benefitted from on the one hand and on the other tried to develop, that is, scientifically sanctioned manual physiotherapy. In the above-mentioned German literature, regardless of whether it condemned or praised Zander's machines, its strong Swedish provenance is marked. Titles like H. Nebel's *Bewegungskuren mittelst schwedischer Heilgymnastik und Massage: Mit besonderer Berücksichtigung der mechanischen Behandlung des Dr. G. Zander* (1889) and J. Schreiber's *Beiträge zur mechanischen Behandlung: Mit besonderer Berücksichtigung der schwedischen Heilgymnastik speciell der mechanischen Gymnastik des Dr. Gust. Zander* (1888) speak thereof.[19] Zander's work was identified as a new branch of an established scientific Swedish physiotherapy tradition in Germany.

It will be argued below that just as German recognition helped Zander to be seen as worthy of a Nobel Prize, his Swedish origins made it easier for him to succeed not only in Germany but also in the rest of the world. To grasp why it was relatively easy to sell in the machines internationally, Zander's Swedishness must be analyzed. Why was Sweden such a scientific authority on the subject? The answers to that question can largely be related to the person already mentioned as Zander's greatest source of inspiration: Pehr Henrik Ling. One can gain an impression of how firmly rooted Ling was when Zander entered the stage by listening to Swedish criticism of him, here from the country's leading orthopedist at the time, Dr. Herman Sätherberg. The year is 1872: "It may seem that a cure [Ling's physiotherapy] which has officially been practiced in the nation's capital for a half a century should be so recognized and proven that it no longer need be defended . . . but because Mr. Zander has sought to substantiate his claim with an argument masquerading as scientific, it is not misplaced to show how misleading his reasoning in fact is."[20]

Understandably, Zander justified his "unscientific" venture and in doing so he emphasized specifically that he had not, as Sätherberg claimed, "[tried] to ruin our longstanding and so highly valued manual physiotherapy." Instead Zander underlined how well aligned his machines were with

Ling's heritage. He "informed Mr. S[ätherberg] that one of Ling's own disciples had assured [him] that Ling himself, on several occasions, had expressed the opinion that it was desirable for devices to be constructed for the execution of movements."[21]

Zander's rhetoric shows that Ling was without doubt an important scientific point of reference, and that he had been so for a long time. Historical research on Zander needs to be complimented with regard to this. That he was influenced by Ling's physiotherapy is of course nothing new, but how great Ling's influence actually was throughout most of the 1800s, even on many physicians, needs better attention. Today we do not remember this, but Ling left even bigger imprints on the medical world than Zander.[22] By adding Ling to the historical equation, it becomes possible to embrace the scientific discourse that precipitated the need for the mechanical treatment of diseases on which Zander could later capitalize. In this regard, Ling's gymnastic system is a key, not just because Zander professed to the same but also since it fused the sick and the healthy body into one organism that, in turn, led to the physical educator and the physiotherapist being the same person. They were amalgamated into a single professional unit. This meant that the mechanical treatment of diseases was intimately connected to physical education and the hardening of healthy bodies, ideologically and practically. In both these areas Ling was a giant. The reasons why will be dealt with in the following sections, starting with the healthy body.

The Arena of Physical Culture

Ling was a Swedish poet and fencing master who in 1813 founded and became director of the Royal Central Institute of Gymnastics (RCIG) in Stockholm, the world's first governmental institution in charge of an entire country's physical upbringing. The idea was for the RCIG to produce physical education teachers trained in Ling's gymnastic system to work in regiments and schools nationwide. It was hoped that physical educators could remedy the alarming weakness that seemed to have befallen the population. However, this condition was not confined to Sweden. Physical frailty was seen generally as a European phenomenon, and thus Ling was not alone in launching a gymnastic system. John C. Gutsmuth's *Gymnastik für die Jugend* (1793) has been identified as an influential pioneer work, but only after the turn of the century did loud advocates gain attention in the public debate.[23] Some of the most renowned system developers were the Spanish Francisco Amoros, the Swiss Heinrich Pestalozzi, and the German Friedrich Ludwig Jahn. With followers in tow they often competed intensely with each other as to whose system was best designed to strengthen the body.[24] Of the above, though, only Jahn's system—Turnen—could match Ling's international influence in the nineteenth century and well into the next.

Consequently, the climate for more gymnastics was optimal, a major reason being the Napoleonic Wars. They had given strong political muscle to pedagogical ideas encouraging improved physical education. The French emperor's continental ravages had abased the national pride of many countries, and the inhabitants' poor physical standard was seen to be one reason for their poor fortunes in war. The people had gone to seed and grown lazy, especially if compared with "before." National Romanticism flourished, and for Ling the Vikings became iconic, showing Swedes' earlier physique: ramrod straight with impressive torsos and prepared for combat. But it was in ancient Greece that the cure was to be found. The Greeks had realized the importance of being fit in both body and soul.[25] In their *gymnasions* the philosopher and the athlete were fused into one, enabling them to create the greatest of all civilizations.

Sweden had not been directly involved on the continental battlefields but had nevertheless been deeply humiliated. In a war with its archenemy, Russia, in 1809, the country had lost its eastern half—Finland. The need for restoration was acute. Thanks to the mighty spark of revanchism, Ling was able to win royal support for the RCIG and thus enjoy state protection. The RCIG was destined to make Sweden whole again, an outstanding and prestigious assignment. The RCIG's martial potential would also guarantee the institution a student body with a very high societal profile. The army began commanding its officers to attend the RCIG, and from 1830 few civilians entered the school, a trend lasting well into the 1900s. Physical education was institutionalized as a phenomenon and throughout the 1800s gymnastics found champions in all political camps. With its formidable formative capacity, gymnastics was viewed as an important weapon in fighting a range of complex problems faced throughout the century. Conservatives and liberals, and toward the end of the century also socialists, could see in gymnastics a tool to solve the societal problems identified by each respective political view.[26]

The RCIG's state protection is a major reason Ling's system could assert itself in the continental competition. It bestowed unique legitimacy upon the system, making it visible even to foreign governments. Invitations to give official demonstrations in other countries were received.[27] An associated factor that also contributed to the Ling system's competitiveness abroad was that it gained recognition as being scientifically grounded. No other system managed to capture as strong a reputation. Ling was convinced that his system, in contrast to the many other systems at the time, was the only one based on true scientific principles. He claimed it was founded on rigorous studies in natural science, anatomy, physiology, and

pathology, and hence these subjects became important parts in the education given at the RCIG. Every movement and exercise in the system was
said to have its physiological value confirmed by science. For that reason,
all other forms of gymnastics were forcefully rejected at the RCIG as being
inferior. Ling's followers were almost fanatical in their faith in the system's perfection and capacity for bringing up the young. Particularly badly
thought of was its toughest competitor in the arena of physical culture,
German Turnen. According to Ling followers, practicing Turnen inevitably
led to severe overstrain that would have prevented an all-around harmoni-
ous development of the body.[28]

Despite the Ling system's Swedish hallmark and nationalist sentiments, it
was perceived abroad as more politically neutral than other systems because
of its scientific affiliation. This could in turn drum up opportunities for
the dissemination of knowledge and culture but also cause turbulence.
This became evident in the system's charged relationship with the German
Turnen. The latter's father figure, Friedrich Ludwig Jahn, was an idealistic agitator, and with his Turnen he wanted to unite the German nation,
which at that time consisted of several city-states and electorates. Therefore,
Turnen became a threat to the prevailing political order of things and for
a time Jahn's gymnastics was even banned in Prussia. It was not until the
Turnen movement's unifying idealism began to harmonize with Prussia's
own goals that it became an accepted political tool. Before then, however,
Prussia's need for gymnastics had to be satisfied by other means. Prussia
turned to the RCIG for a substitute that was not subversive, which led to a
huge gymnastic conflict in Germany that broke out during the 1860s. It even
had its own name: "die Barrenstreit."[29] On the surface the showdown concerned whether parallel bars (and horizontal) should be used in German
gymnastics training. On one side were the many promoters of the native
Turnen, on the other, Ling proponents. The former group was in favor of
bars, the latter against.

The turmoil originated in Prussia's support of an RCIG replica.
Hugo Rothstein, an RCIG-trained German officer, had established Das
Centralinstitut für den gymnastischen Unterricht in der Armée in Berlin
in 1847, in the name of the Prussian state. The RCIG stood as a model.
From his center Rothstein propagated the advantages of Ling's system
over Jahn's.[30] In the nationalistically inflated era, Rothstein's craze for
Swedish gymnastics aggravated the *Vaterland.* It was an attack on an
authentic German cultural product. The issue was debated accordingly.
Feverish and infected as it was, it engaged both the Prussian parliament
and the scientific community. Among others, two of the history of medicine's scientific preeminent figures, Rudolf Virchow and Emil Dubois
Reymond, questioned the Ling system's scientific qualities as well as its
lack of bars.[31]

The Arena of Mechanical Medicine

What really helped Ling's system to reach wide distribution, however, was its usefulness not on healthy bodies but on sick ones. Its ability—via physiotherapy—to cure and relieve a variety of internal and chronic diseases, including orthopedic ailments, helped the system to root itself abroad. No other system placed such great importance on physiotherapy. Until recently, however, researchers on Ling have not grasped how fundamental physiotherapy was for his system's internationalization. One reason for this is that studies involving Ling have mainly been carried out by scholars interested in the history of physical education. The physiotherapy aspect has thus been seen as less interesting and less worth mentioning.[32] This is ironic since Ling believed that physiotherapy gave his system its scientific qualities, and his many followers agreed with him. Since physiotherapy bore the system's scientific credibility, it also became the professional spearhead for Ling's advocates. It was not until the closing decades of the nineteenth century that the RCIG's main scientific interest was directed toward the physical education segment of the system.[33]

Another reason why physiotherapy has not received much attention is the fact that research on the origins of the physiotherapy profession has not identified Ling and the RCIG as the source of physiotherapists' first formal training and professional identity. Instead, the cradle of the profession has been situated in England around the turn of the nineteenth century. This means that historical and sociological research on the physical therapy profession in different countries often takes for granted that the profession was originally gendered feminine, with women practitioners lacking both professional autonomy and a unique bulk of scientific knowledge.[34] Lost behind that perception, however, and this is important, is that the profession was originally a male-only occupation wearing the professional insignia of *autonomy* and *science*.[35] When the profession first appeared in Sweden during the first half of the nineteenth century, physiotherapists were either noblemen or members of the upper class. Because of the above-mentioned annual military commendations to the RCIG, they were also often men of the sword— officers in the Swedish army. Not until 1864 were women allowed to enter the profession. However, men remained in the majority in Sweden until the turn of the century.[36]

The epistemology that led to the RCIG's physical educators also becoming physiotherapists was a derivation of Ling's adamant conviction that the sick and the healthy body were scientifically inseparable. They were linked organically. The idea was that when diseases were handled mechanically, patients should be passed on to different levels of difficulty in pedagogical gymnastics. This dualism did not start to disappear until after the turn of the century.[37] Thus, a full RCIG training awarded the students a triple competence, permitting them to work outside their regiments, as physical educators and physiotherapists. Female students did not participate in military gymnastics, and hence their education took two years, not three. In 1887 the government took firm control of licensing physiotherapists. Male students entering the RCIG without officer's rank needed sufficient qualifications for admission to the university while only compulsory school was required for female applicants.[38] The right to open a licensed clinic and receive patients had no restrictions based on gender, however.

The breaches in historical and sociological research on physical education and the physiotherapy profession have obscured the fact that most of the first professionals to implement Ling's system abroad were primarily operating as physiotherapists, not physical educators.[39] For the same reasons the ideological force behind the RCIG alumni's eagerness to proselytize for Ling's system abroad has also been lost. Many of them acted like crusaders. They wanted to convert the medical sciences to a more mechanical way of understanding and curing disease, Ling physiotherapy's various movements and manipulations. In the eyes of Ling (and physiotherapists) mechanical cures were as potent as "chemistry" (pharmacology); it was a kind of *iatromechanics*. Ling claimed that "mechanical phenomena as well as chemical ones can underpin diagnosis . . . and one shall therefore not be surprised that mechanical means can affect illness in lungs, liver, viscera, brain, eyes, nose, etc."[40] Orthodox medicine was therefore seen as harmfully occupied with chemistry. Mechanical and chemical cures must be in balance, or medicine would be ineffective and even dangerous. Hence, medical science itself was one sided and unbalanced.[41] The faith in the cure's scientific qualities, potency, and importance to medicine was enormous. Physiotherapy's chief standard-bearer, Professor Gabriel Branting (1799–1881), Ling's successor as head of the RCIG, was confident that its "truths" would "force away a lot of what is now recognized as science," that is, pharmacology.[42]

In consequence, the RCIG did not just have a mission to ready Sweden for grand, new deeds, it also had to revolutionize the medical sciences across national borders. From the 1830s physiotherapists traveled to foreign cities and celebrated health resorts and spas to spread the word that their physiotherapy was a *new science*, indispensable to efforts at curing and preventing disease and ill health. The project of physical restoration was always present in their rhetoric, but doubtlessly it was the medical quest that made these missionaries leave Sweden. Though not spared from contemporary criticism, their "missionary work" was a success, and many laypeople, physicians, and patients from around the world went to the RCIG and other celebrated clinics to improve their knowledge and skills. The physiotherapists' status was so great that physicians sometimes even worked as their employees.[43] They have even been described as leading figures in a now forgotten but then prominent scientific discourse on how to cure and relieve disease mechanically.[44]

One main driving force placing physiotherapy in the scientific foreground was also economic. During much of the 1800s, the educational system in Sweden and elsewhere was scarcely developed. There were very few teaching positions in physical education. To make a living, especially as a missionary abroad, other sources of income were necessary. Physiotherapy could offer these, and patient fees were therefore the financial engine behind the spread of Ling's gymnastics for a long time. No wonder that early publications by Ling's followers had physiotherapy as their main theme![45] The pecuniary potential was also something that attracted physicians, providing further explanation as to why Ling's physiotherapy was embraced by the medical community.[46] As has already been mentioned, health care at this time was almost entirely a private market, and not being able to meet the therapeutic demand could be synonymous with social degradation.

Not surprisingly, the greatest impact was made in Sweden. Even though the RCIG was not linked to a faculty of medicine, it became officially responsible for the training of physicians in physiotherapy. The school's statutes from 1864 not only stated that it would educate "doctors of gymnastics" (ordinary "chemistry doctors" trained as physiotherapists), it also stated that without an RCIG diploma physicians were forbidden to open physiotherapy clinics.[47] In the second half of the 1800s, the medical Karolinska Institute also made several political attempts to include Ling's physiotherapy as a compulsory part of medical training, hence adding even more historical flavor to Zander's Nobel Prize nomination in 1916. Most passionate were orthopedists, and until circa 1900 Ling was their father figure, particularly in relation to curing chronic and internal diseases.[48]

As mentioned previously, though, Ling's influence on orthodox medicine was also very significant internationally, as is perhaps best illustrated by his name's accepted place in the plethora of literature on physical medicine (e.g., massage, electricity, hydropathy, physiotherapy) from the second half of the 1800s. Although his disciples rarely admitted any such thing, Ling was neither alone nor first to achieve scientific recognition in the field of mechanical medicine. There were others, also physicians, who tried to make a name for themselves as scientific authorities. A good example is the German orthopedist Daniel Gottlieb Schreber (1808–61), whose work was translated into Swedish.[49] However, not until the last decades of the century did physicians get a guru of their own to match Ling's patriarchal status as inventor of scientific mechanical cures. His name was Johann Mezger (1839–1909), a Dutch physician later known as "the father of scientific massage."[50] Interestingly enough, Mezger was a physical educator before taking his medical degree. The professional demarcation between the sick and the healthy body was still vague.

The Dynamics of Success

How then were Ling and his physiotherapists able to become so successful? How could a layperson's doctrines make such impression in the medical world and thus pave the way for Zander's machines? One important factor is that physiotherapists were indirectly able to benefit from the great interest in physical upbringing that characterized the period, something that naturally had also made physicians very interested in preventing bodies from becoming unhealthy. Consequently, the medical profession per se was very much part of the same "health discourse" as Ling's followers were. In that respect it has been noted that physicians often preferred Ling's gymnastics before other systems.[51] Another explanation lies even more within the medical community itself. Ling's main development took place during a time that is often described as a "crisis" for orthodox medicine. It was marked by therapeutic confusion and subjected frequently to criticism. Doctors and laypeople alike voiced strong concerns, often targeting the ineffectiveness and even danger of physicians' methods. Much slander was directed toward the pharmacopeia's "toxicity" and "unnaturalness." Ling's view that medicine was too "chemical" was therefore not atypical but, rather, contemporary. The intellectual milieu was thus receptive to "revolutionary systems." The ones to attain the greatest fame and most long-lasting reputations thanks to this were homeopathy and different types of mesmerism and hydropathy.[52]

Context-wise it must also be remembered that the professional muscles of the medical profession prior to 1850 were not particularly strong. The profession had not yet reached the strength that has since made it the subject of many volumes of sociological research on how professional monopoly is achieved through "occupational imperialism."[53] In other words, physicians' ability to control the medical field was relatively weak in the mid-1800s. Hence the professional status line between laymen and doctors was not clearly drawn, especially not in the area of "mechanical cures" since these methods had no formal platform in physicians' formal training. That the professional dividing line between physicians and laypeople could be miniscule is indicated by the title of the above-mentioned Dr. Schreber's work: *Kinesiatrik oder der gymnastische Heilmetode: Fur Ärtze und gebildete Nichtärtze nach eigenen Erfahrung dargestellt* (1852).[54] In the field of scientific mechanical cures, however, Ling had, through the RCIG, succeeded in creating a professional power structure with state protection, which physiotherapists rarely omitted to advertise. Since physiotherapists often came from a class background topping that of physicians, they had great leverage and could therefore influence doctors as well as patients.[55]

It is very important to include patients in the sociohistorical mix explaining transfer of medical knowledge. As already mentioned, being associated with rich patients was an advantage. Thanks to them, one could earn a good deal of money. Clients with high standing were also important for other reasons. For crusading entrepreneurs operating in the medical field, their political, social, and cultural capital were as desirable. The RCIG's principal teacher, Professor C. A. Georgii, also an army lieutenant, was well aware of this. In 1847 he was in Paris to convince the medical sciences, and he had come in contact with Frédéric Chopin among others, which he informed professor Branting in Stockholm about: "I'm negotiating with a couple of patients: one Russian family whose only daughter suffers from pulp. Cordis with hypertrophy; the other is the Composer Chopin suffering from asthma nervosum compliqia l'emphyseme et de bronchité chronique. *If my treatments are successful, the latter's great number of literary and high-born supporters might be of great importance, when it comes to getting the science or cure method adopted.*"[56]

Hence patients were more than money. They were also hothouses in terms of growing a reputation and carriers of medical knowledge.

Eastward Migration

One of Ling's "golden boys," Lieutenant Carl Frederick de Ron, is a good example of how successful RCIG alumni operating transnationally could be and how important patients were for the dispersion of knowledge. De Ron directed his mission eastward, and he was one of the few early alumni who also succeeded in physical education.[57] The majority of texts written about these early RCIG students are usually more than one hundred years old and authored by Ling's followers. As a result, they have an almost hagiographical aura, and the stories about de Ron are no exception. Readers are informed that de Ron, commissioned by Ling in 1835, first took service as a physical educator in Finland. Two years later he had moved to St. Petersburg of his own accord. He stayed there for more than twenty years. It has been claimed that he was encouraged by the czar to draw up the guidelines for an "imperial" RCIG whose size would have outshone the mother institution by far. His proposal is said to have flopped because of the enormous costs of such a large-scale project and "the Russian society's cultural backwardness, which would make the gymnastic programme seem like an anomaly in comparison with all the other neglected parts of the educational system."[58]

Nevertheless, it was as a physiotherapist de Ron reached his prime. Like many of his peers, he knew how to target the clients of high caliber, and if necessary he even remitted them to the RCIG for special treatment.[59] And it was also thanks to them that he was able to attract the Russian government's interest in his RCIG project. After having treated Empress Alexandra Feodorowna and then made her club-footed grandson, the Duke of Leuchtenberg, one of the capital's best waltz dancers, his fortune was made.

De Ron's physiotherapy clinic now became a nest for high society. It also grew very large. To meet the demand several physicians worked under his supervision, including the RCIG-trained physician Georg Berglind.[60] De Ron became a "physiotherapist by order of the Czar" and accompanied the court on several of its travels in Europe. His institute is said to have received a yearly subsidy of 10,000 rubles on the condition that de Ron annually treat sixty impecunious patients and trained thirty officers in gymnastics. There seems to be some validity in these stories. In a letter to the RCIG (1850) de Ron writes, "After 15 years of hard work Ling's system has been recognized as an independent science by the highest medical authorities, and the Czar has ordered that plans are to be made for a Central Institute and that governmental funds shall support my private establishment! I therefore dare to make notice of myself by sending [you] Collegii Medici's dictum issued, as can be seen, by request of the Czar."[61]

In 1858 de Ron returned to Sweden. He apparently made himself unpopular at the Russian court on account of his violent temper and lack of adaptability.[62] His institute was taken over by Dr. Berglind, who long kept clinics in St. Petersburg and in the fashionable Crimea. He also became a keen writer on physiotherapy.[63]

The Dynamics and Agency of Historical Forgetfulness

So far, I have unearthed the scientific and cultural infrastructure constructed jointly by physiotherapists and physicians that helped Zander and his machines on their way. However, why have this infrastructure and the ones building it been forgotten? In relation to the "father of homeopathy," Dr. Samuel Hahnemann, for example, Ling is a rather diminutive figure in scholarly work on the history of medicine. Yet Ling's footprints are probably both greater and deeper than Hahnemann's. For instance, physiotherapists, not homeopaths, have a mandatory presence in modern health care worldwide, but physiotherapists themselves are not even aware that Ling and the RCIG actually created their profession. And if Arthur Jones is to be believed, the world of gyms was equally oblivious about Zander. The simple answer is that Ling and Zander lost the symbolic relevance they had for physicians and physiotherapists. But why? I shall address this matter with a few words in conclusion. At the risk of simplifying and without the possibility of explaining adequately, Ling has become blurred out of the history.[64] Roughly speaking, the reason for this is that the professional dividing line between physicians and laypeople became increasingly evident during the second half of the nineteenth century. The strength and professional identity of the medical profession grew much stronger. The result was that one pyramid-like hierarchy developed the medical field, in which physicians' top positions became clearer, not least because they were effectively able to allocate professional power via the breakthrough of scientific biomedicine. They won the rights of scientific interpretation regarding these kinds of treatment, and other groups and interests were subordinated by them, a process full of professional conflicts.[65]

Although the biomedical breakthrough strongly favored the medical profession's professional power base, it was not until much later that the new scientific discoveries were translated into effective cures. Many physicians were therefore still dependent on therapies included in the previously mentioned generic term "physical medicine." That label covered a variety of methods like light therapy, electricity, hydropathy, massage, and physiotherapy. Like physiotherapy, these therapies were not explicitly included in orthodox medical training. They were usually *extracurricular*, with the consequence that laypeople also believed that they could stake scientific claims as therapists.

How then were doctors to distinguish themselves from laypeople in such an environment? The generic term "physical medicine" came into scientific fashion during the second half of the 1800s, perhaps as a direct consequence of physicians trying to distance themselves from competitive laymen. More research is needed, but conflicts evidently developed in these therapies regarding the scientific rights of interpretation. Physiotherapists constituted the strongest challenge to physicians in this arena. They had governmental sanction for their science and moreover they began supplementing their mechanical cures with other physical therapies. The last straw was the physiotherapists' "crusade mentality," itself a very offensive form of "occupational imperialism" aimed at the medical profession. It is thus clear that physicians and physiotherapists became increasingly antagonistic to each other. Strong tensions prevailed even though both groups were often in agreement about the scientific and curative potential of physiotherapy and other methods.[66] Thus, the primary problem was not about efficacy and scientific quality but about who would preside over whom: a matter of power.

With the growing strength of the medical profession, the notion gained ground that physiotherapists were too big for their boots. Why were they allowed to act without any supervision and, not infrequently, to speak in a derogatory tone about doctors and their science? Considering both groups' continued dependence on private patient fees, it is not hard to imagine the friction emerging.[67] A passage in a German textbook for physicians, *Lehrbuch der Schwedische Heilgymnastik unter Berücksichtung der Hertzkrankenheiten*, captures the problem. The author portrays physiotherapists as "prophets" using their titles "to dazzle" the public, not least "the higher ranks of the aristocracy." He also blames the "king of Sweden" for his "strange habit" of awarding professorial titles to army officers "notoriously unfamiliar with medical knowledge."[68]

When this was written, in 1896, physicians had attained a firmer collective advantage over physiotherapists. These harsh words should probably also be considered in relation to the rising scientific star of the massage specialist Dr. Mezger (and by then many other massage physicians).[69] Roughly put, physicians had long needed a scientific authority of their own over mechanical medicine. Ling as a laypeople undermined physicians' now much stronger claim to be the sole custodians of medical science. The common story since before 1850 was that Ling had put mechanical treatments on a scientific footing. As long as this story prevailed, criticism of physiotherapists threatened to hit back at physicians themselves. They often used the same historical authority (Ling). It was a kind of Catch-22. Consequently, and again simplified, this "history" had to be reformulated in physicians' own professional rhetoric to avoid giving physiotherapists scientific backing. Physicians needed an authority independent of Ling as a better weapon in the fight against physiotherapists' status, and Mezger rose to the occasion and gained many followers. A new history could be formulated that both separated Ling from science and made it easier to criticize him.[70] This eroded the scientific reputation of the RCIG, first abroad but later even in Sweden, despite the Ling tradition's stronger armor there. As physicians began monopolizing the scientific treatment of diseases, a further intertwined result was that the RCIG, a scientific institution authorizing non-physicians to deal with the sick body outside medical faculties and hospitals, slowly turned into a societal anachronism. This also helped to damage physiotherapists' professional power base.

What most helped to push Ling to the scientific fringes, however, was perhaps a shift of paradigm among the physicians most involved in the above-mentioned Catch-22. Around 1900 orthopedists stopped legitimizing their medical specialty with conservative methods. Developments in antiseptics, radiology, and anesthesia made orthopedic diagnoses more accessible to successful surgery. Orthopedists were therefore no longer in need of having their scientific status confirmed via orthotics, bandages, and spine-correcting beds. The scalpel sufficed. Their economic need to treat chronic and internal diseases mechanically declined equally, not least through employment at the emerging larger hospitals.[71] This did not, however, reduce orthopedists' interest in subjugating physiotherapists under their authority.

To cut a long story short, physiotherapists lost the power struggle with the orthopedic surgeons. The even power relation of the mid-1800s was very asymmetric by the start of the next century. The victors write history, and there was no room for independent, autonomous physiotherapists with a science of their own in the orthopedists' new history. Physiotherapists' old historical narrative was silenced by the orthopedists' new success story. Thus, the former played a small part in another profession's historical narrative, which stated that physiotherapists had always been dependent on the medical profession and that they had physicians to thank for their profession's existence as well as for their skills and knowledge.[72]

In summary, physiotherapists saw their previous professional status evaporate. There was still a demand for their skills, but they had to accept unconditionally the role of physicians' assistants. Here a key tactic was to dislocate physiotherapists from their old home turf: the hard-to-control private market. Put simply, physicians accomplished this in three intersecting ways. The first way was to stop working with the most disobedient physiotherapists, who often happened to be men. Gender warnings were even issued. In Sweden a governmental investigation, led by orthopedists, even recommended that the government prohibit men from becoming physiotherapists.[73] For that reason neither men nor the gospel of Ling were particularly welcome at the many physiotherapy schools founded by physicians around the turn of the century. Women were generally less of a problem because it was harder for them to work as autonomous professionals, not to mention to claim scientific status.[74]

The second way was to accept physiotherapists in the new big hospitals with their clear-cut medical hierarchies, where disobedient (autonomous) physiotherapists were not particularly welcome. These autonomous physiotherapists, often male, also tended to avoid hospitals. They found it unmanly to work under physicians. Female physiotherapists had less of a problem with this. Women even began preferring such employment. Unlike the male physiotherapists they started seeing benefits in medical patronage and did not mind as much losing the autonomy that came with private practice.[75]

The third way was to set new boundaries for physiotherapists' scope of practice. Their old regime favored *internal medicine* over *surgery*. In the new order, at the hospitals, physicians were to perform surgery while physiotherapists offered *rehabilitation*. When this came into full practice, a new but distinct order of rank was observed. Surgeons made diagnoses and prescribed suitable treatments, and physiotherapists then had to follow their instructions and incisions.[76] Physiotherapists' old fields of interests—chronic and internal diseases—were best dealt with by physicians, preferably those with special interests in physical medicine, a cadre whose numbers now had declined considerably.

This process can be found in most countries but, for obvious reasons, was most prolonged and charged in Sweden. The hierarchal problem was most deeply rooted there. The process also cut off physiotherapists' contact with the healthy body. The physiotherapist and physical educator went separate professional ways, a development that, of course, was also influenced by the development of medical science/practice away from "holism" toward specialization.[77] When physiotherapists gave in to the medical profession's authority, they also gave up Ling as a father figure, despite keeping "his" movements and manual techniques in their scope of practice. His revolutionary layperson status did not benefit them when they were working in the professional hierarchy of Hippocrates.

To finalize and return to where we started, to Zander, the tension-filled process described here probably affected his success story positively. Although Zander did not hide the fact that he regarded Ling highly, there are indications that he, like Dr. Mezger, became a tool in the ongoing efforts to mute physiotherapists' scientific rights of interpretation. His machines were used to create a unified order in the field of mechanical medicine. As a physician, albeit heavily affected by Ling's doctrines, Zander had scientifically refined what a layperson had invented but lacked the ability to perfect. That the scientific mind of a trained physician had surpassed that of Ling was a story that indirectly contributed to dethroning him. That impression is reinforced by contemplation of the fact that it was an orthopedic surgeon who recommended Zander for the Nobel Prize.[78]

One may also speculate whether the end result of the conflict, that hierarchical order was instated, had the opposite effect. Could it have helped to subdue scientific fascination with Zander? After World War I, his machines soon disappeared from the market. Of course, this may be explained first by the fact that physical medicine as such seemed obsolete by then to physicians in general and second by the postwar Depression that made investment in a set of Zander machines unrealistic.[79] However, what effect did the subjugation of physiotherapists to the medical profession's authority (except in Sweden possibly) have on physicians' decision to abandon Zander? Perhaps the Depression only made it apparent that his symbolic scientific value was no longer required. Further research will be needed to clarify this issue. Until then, anyone who wants to get acquainted with Ling and Zander can still do so by visiting a physiotherapist or a gym.

Notes

1. The company was founded 1971, but the concept's first prototype came as early as 1948.

2. Citations from "In Conversation with Arthur Jones," March 30, 2015, http://www.realfighting.com/exercise_science.php.

3. Ibid.

4. Ibid.

5. Sarah Bakewell, "Illustrations from the Wellcome Institute Library," *Medical History* 41 (1997): 487–95; H. C. Kreck, *Die Medico-mechanische Therapie Gustaf Zanders in Deutschland—Ein Beitrag zur Geschichte der Krankengymnastik* (Frankfurt am Main, 1987); Tomas Terlouw, "De Opkomst en Neergang van de Zander-insituten rond 1900 in Nederland," *Gewina* 27 (2004): 135–58.

6. In Germany it became close to self explanatory to say, "I will now go zandering" (Ger. *jetz gehe ich zandern*). A curiosa is that the large ocean liners often were

equipped with Zander machines. Zander machines can be found at the bottom of the sea, aboard the *Titanic*. For German physicians walking in Zander's footsteps, see M. Hertz and A. Bum, *Das Neue System der Maschinellen Gymnastik* (Berlin: Urban & Schwartzenberger, 1899).

7. E.g., Zander received awards at the World Exhibitions in Philadelphia 1876 and Paris 1878. The Swedish Society of Medicine honored Zander with its Gold Medal for his thesis *Om den habituela scoliosens behandling medels mekanisk gymnastik* (Stockholm, 1889).

8. Nils Hansson and Anders Ottosson, "A Nobel Prize for Physical Therapy? Rise, Fall, and Revival of Medico-mechanical Institutes," *Physical Therapy* no. 8 (2015): 1184–94.

9. David L. Chapman, *Sandow the Magnificent: Eugen Sandow and the Beginnings of Bodybuilding* (Chicago: University of Illinois Press, 1994); Jan Todd, "The Strength Builders: A History of Barbells, Dumbbells and Indian Clubs," *International Journal of the History of Sports* 20 (2003): 65–90. Here, the American physician Dudley Sargent became a leading figure. See Carloyn de la Penã, "Dudley Allen Sargent: Health Machines and the Energized Male Body," *Iron Game History* 8 (2003): 3–20.

10. Later, the machines could also be powered by electricity.

11. For this reason, Zander also designed antropometric devices.

12. Zander's first thesis came the same year and was titled "Om mekanisk gymnastik." See Anders Ottosson, Sjukgymnasten—vart tog han vägen? En undersökning av sjukgymnastyrkets maskuliniering och avmaskulinisering 1813–1934" (PhD diss.: Göteborgs Universitet, 2005), 266–61.

13. Sheila Fletcher, *Women First: The Female Tradition in English Physical Education 1880–1980* (London: Athlone Press, 1984), 17–55; David Kirk, *Defining Physical Education: The Social Construction of a School Subject in Postwar Britain* (London: Routledge, 1992).

14. See, e.g., Carolyn Thomas de la Penã, *Body Electric: How Strange Machines Built the Modern American* (New York: New York University Press, 2003); William F. Bynum and Roy Porter, *Medical Fringe and Medical Orthodoxy* (London: Croom Helm, 1987).

15. Hansson and Ottosson, "A Nobel Prize," 1190–91.

16. Max Neuburger and Julius Pagel, *Handbuch der Geschichte der Medizin*, vol. 3 (Jena: Fischer, 1905), 124, 339, 351–53.

17. Citation from Hünerfauth, *Handbuch der Massage*.

18. Hansson and Ottosson, "A Nobel Prize," 1190–94.

19. H. Nebel, *Bewegungskuren mittelst schwedischer Heilgymnastik und Massage: Mit besonderer Berücksichtigung der mechanischen Behandlung des Dr. G. Zander* (Wiesbaden: J. F. Bergmann, 1889); J. Schreiber, *Beiträge zur mechanischen Behandlung: Mit besonderer Berücksichtigung der schwedischen Heilgymnastik speciell der mechanischen Gymnastik des Dr. Gust. Zander* (Wiesbaden: J. F. Bergmann, 1888).

20. Citations from Herman Sätherberg, *Några ord till belysning af frågan om de tvenne olika gymnastikmetoderna, den manuella och den mekaniska* (Stockholm: n.p., 1872), 2–3. Sätherberg had first vocied his critisism in the newspaper *Nya Daglighanda* (January 15 and 16, 1872). Zander replied in the same paper. See also T. J. Hartelius, *Gymnastiska iakttagelser* (Stockholm: Zacharias Häggströms förlag, 1865), 51–60; Hartelius, *Den manuela metoden och maskinmetoden inom sjukgymnastiken* (Stockholm: Alb. Bonnier Boktryckeri, 1873).

21. Citations from Gustaf Zander, *Svar på "Några ord till belysning af frågan om de tvenne olika gymnastikmetoderna, den manuella och den mekaniska"* (Stockholm: Nya Dagl. Allehandas Aktiebolags Tryckeri, 1872), 4–5.

22. Anders Ottosson, "The Manipulated History of Manipulations of Spines and Joints: Rethinking Orthopaedic Medicine through a European 19th Century Discourse of Mechanical Medicine," *Medicine Studies* 3 (2011): 83–116; Anders Ottosson, "One History or Many Herstories? Gender Politics and the History of Physiotherapy's Origins in Nineteeth- and Early Twentieth-Century," *Women's History Review* (2015): 286–319; Anders Ottosson, "Androphopia, Demasculinization, and Professional Conflicts: The Herstories of the Physical Therapy Profession Deconstructed," *Social Science History* (2016): 433–61.

23. Jan Lindroth, *Idrottens väg till folkrörelse: Studier i svensk idrottsrörelse till 1915* (Uppsala, 1974), 23–25; Jens Ljunggren, *Kroppens bildning: Linggymnastikens man-lighetsprojekt 1790-1914* (Eslöv: Symposion, 1999), 41–42. Gutsmuths' work was translated into Swedish 1813. See J. C. F. Guthsmuts, *Gymnastik för swenska ungdomen eller kort anvisning till kroppsöfningar* (Lund: Berlingska, 1813).

24. Gertrud Pfister, "Cultural Confrontations: German Turnen, Swedish Gymnastics and English Sport—European Diversity in Physical Activities from a Historical Perspective," *Culture, Sport, Society* 6 (2003): 61–91; Pfister, "The Role of German Turners in American Physical Education," *International Journal of the History of Sport* 26 (2009): 1893–925.

25. Ljunggren, *Kroppens bildning.*

26. Jens Ljunggren, "The Masculine Road through Modernity: Ling Gymnastics and Male Socialisation in Ninetenth-Centrury Sweden," in *Making European Masculinities: Sport, Europe, Gender*, ed. J. A. Mangan (London: Routledge, 2000), 86–111; Ottosson, "Sjukgymnasten—Vart," 61–78.

27. The original invitation from Count Narcisse Achilles de Salvandy (Fr. Ministre de l'instruction publique) is not yet identified. However, it is mentioned in a letter from RCIG's principle teacher, professor Georgii, adressed to Salvady's sucessor: Carl August Georgii to the French minister [text loss], 12/3 1848, GCI:s enskilda arkiv, vol. 46, RA (National Archives). Ottosson, "The First Historical Movements," 1892–1919.

28. A quote from RCIG's principal teacher, Lieutenant Carl August Georgii, captures this view. The year is 1846: "In Berlin, Copenhagen, and Carlsruhe I have had the opportunity to study the German Turnkunst in all its guises, everywhere uncorrectable as to its principles, often being unnatural and one sided in practice. The advantages of Swedish gymnastics are astounding." Carl August Georgii to Lars Gabriel Branting, 21/9 1846, vol. 9, GCI:s enskilda arkiv, National Archives, Sweden. Author's translation.

29. Julia Shiöler, *Über die Anfänge der Schwedishen Heilgymnastik in Deutschland—ein Beitrag zur Geschichte der Krankengymnastik im 19. Jahrhundert* (Münster: Medizinische Fakultät der Westfälischen Wilhelms-Universität Münster, 2005), 70–74.

30. Rothstein also published a five-volume work on Ling's system: Hugo Rothstein, *Die Gymnastik nach dem schwedischen Gymnasiarchen P. H. Ling* (Berlin: E. H. Schröder, 1848–54).

31. Emil Dubois-Reymond, "Schwedische Gymnastik und deutsches Turnen," in *Das gesammte Turnwesen*, ed. Georg Hirth (Leipzig: Buch & Consult Ulrich Keip,

1865), 185–96; Rudolph Virchow, "Ueber das Barren turnen, vom ärtzlichen stand-punkte," in *Das gesammte Turnwesen,* ed. Georg Hirth (Leipzig: Buch & Consult Ulrich Keip, 1865), 196–206.

32. Ottosson, "Sjukgymnasten—Vart," 93–95; Ottosson, "One History," 296–319; Anders Ottosson, "Androphobia, Demasculinization, and Professional Conflicts: The Herstories of the Physical Therapy Profession Deconstructed," *Social Science History* 40, no. 3 (2016): 433–61; Anders Ottosson, "The Age of Scientific Gynecological Masseurs. 'Non-intrusive' Male Hands, Female Intimacy, and Women's Health around 1900," *Social History of Medicine* (2016): 802–28.

33. Jan Lindroth, *Ling—från storhet till upplösning: Studier i svenk gymnastikhistoria* (Stockholm: Symposion, 2004), 45–54; Ottosson, "Sjukgymnasten—Vart," 91–113.

34. Dale Larsen, "The Historical Development of Knowledge in Physiotherapeutic Spinal Manual Therapy" (PhD diss., University of Sydney, 2005), 78; Ruby Heap, "The Emergence of Physiotherapy as a New Profession for Canadian Women, 1914–1918," in *Framing Our Past: Canadian Women's History in the Twentieth Century,* ed. Sharon Anne Cook, Lorna R. McLean, and Kate O'Rourke (Montreal: McGill-Queen's University Press, 2001), 295–99; D. Nicholls and J. Cheek, "Physiotherapy and the Shadow of Prostitution," *Social Science Medicine* 61 (2006): 2336; Beth Linker, *War's Waste: Rehabilitation in World War 1. America* (Chicago: University Chicago Press, 2011); Rogers, *Polio Wars,* 16–18, 40–44.

35. Anne Witz, "Patriarchy and Profession: The Gendered Politics of Occupational Closure," *Sociology* 24 (1990): 675–90; J. Gilbert, "Science and Its 'Other': Looking Underneath 'Woman' and 'Science' for New Directions in Research on Gender and Science Education," *Gender and Education* (2001): 291–305.

36. Ottosson, "Sjukgymnasten—Vart," 300–13.

37. Jan Lindroth, *Ling—från storhet till upplösning. Studier i svenk gymnastikhisto-ria* (Stockholm: Symposion, 2004), 19–42; Anders Ottosson, "Svärdet, facklan och staven samt en ek på villovägar? Synen på sjuk och frisk vid GCI 1813 till cirka 1950," in *200 år av kroppsbildning: Gymnastiska Centralinstitutet/Gymnastik- och Idrottshögskolan 1813–2013,* ed. Hans Bolling and Leif Yttergren (Växjö, 2013), 51–76.

38. Svensk Författningssamling [Swedish Book of Statutes] (Stockholm: Svensk Författningssamling, 1864), 1864. See also Ottosson, "Sjukgymnasten—Vart," 61–72, 286–97.

39. Ottosson, "One History," 310–19.

40. P. H. Ling, *Samlade Arbeten* (Stockholm: Alb. Bonniers, 1866), 577. Author's translation.

41. The Italian physician and mathematician Giovanni A. Borelli is understood as the originator of iatromechanics (or iatromathematics). His theories had impact in the late seventeenth century, especially in London. M. Theodore Brown, "The College of Physicians and the Acceptance of Iatromechanics in England, 1665–1695," *Bulletin of the History of Medicine* 45 (197): 12–30. P. H. Ling believed that "iat-romathematics" had been suffocated by the hegemony of "chemiatrics." See Ling, *Samlade Arbeten,* 461.

42. Citations from Brantings tal 1840, GCI:s enskilda arkiv, vol. 6. National Archives, Sweden.

43. Physiotherapy was considered a scientific remedy, and physiotherapists were for that reason sometimes awarded the title of professor. See Ottosson,

"Sjukgymnasten—Vart," 72–78, 132–42; Ottosson, "First Historical," 1908–13; Lotta Holme, *Konsten att göra, barn raka: Ortopedi och vanförevård i Sverige till 1920* (Linköping: Carlsson, 1996), 39–52.

44. Ottosson, "The Manipulated," 83–116.

45. See, e.g., J. Govert In de Betou, *Therapeutic Manipulation, Or a Succeful Treatment of Varoius Disorders of the Human Body by Mechanical Applications* (London: J. Masters, 1842); E. E. Erenhoff, *Medicina Gymnastica or Therapeutic Manipulation: A Short Treatise on This Science as Practiced at the Royal Institution at Stockholm* (London: J. Masters, 1845); C. A. Georgii, *Kinésiethérapie ou traitements des maladies par le mouvement selon la méthod de Ling* (Paris: Germer Ballière, 1847); M. M. Eulenburg, *Die Schwedische Heil-Gymnastik Versuch einer wissenschaftlischen Begrundung derselben* (Berlin: August Hirschwald, 1853); J. Albert Neumann, *Die Heil-Gymnastik oder die Kunst der Leibesübungen, angewant zur Heilung von Krankheiten nach dem Systeme des Schweden Ling und seiner Schüler Branting, Georgii, de Ron, sowei nach eigenen Ansichten und Erfahrungen* (Berlin: P. Jeanrenaud, 1852).

46. Even the RCIG was for a long period dependent on patient fees. That source of income exceeded by far the institute's governmental funding. Ottosson, "Sjukgymnasten—Vart," 178–85.

47. Svensk Författningssamling, 5 § 1.

48. Ottosson, "The Manipulated," 101–12.

49. D. G. Moritz Schreber, *Kinesiatrik oder die gymnastische Heilmetod:. Für Ärtze und gebildete Nichtärtze nach eigenen Erfahrung dargstellt* (Leipzig: Friedrich Fleischer, 1852); Schreber, *Aerztliche Zimmer-Gymnastik*. See also: Schiöler, *Über die Anfänge*, 101–11. The French physician Joseph-Clément Tissot's work *Gymnastique Médicinale et Chirurgicale* (1780) is especially worth mentioning since it was translated into Swedish in 1797. Joseph-Clément Tissot, *Gymnastique Médicinale et Chirurgicale* (Paris: P. Bastien, 1780); Ottosson, "Sjukgymnasten—Vart," 63.

50. On Metzger, see N. Robert Calvert, *History of Massage* (Rochester, VT: Healing Art Press, 2002), 99–110. Many physicians would become "massage specialists" with international reputation, which perhaps is interesting given that massage of today is included in the "Big Five" among the therapies captured by the generic term "alternative medicine." See also: Motzi Eklöf, "Svensk Massage: En internationell historia," in *In på bara huden: Medicinhistoriska studier tillägnade Karin Johannisson*, ed. A. Berg et al. (Nora: Nya Doxa, 2010), 65–85.

51. W. Jack Berryman, "Exercise in Medicine: A Historical Perspective," *Current Sports Medicine Reports* 9 (2010): 195–201; Roberta Park, "Edward M. Hartwell and Physical Training at the John Hopkins University, 1879–1890," *Journal of Sport History* 14 (1986): 108–19; Park, "Sharing, Arguing," 519–48.

52. Bynum and Porter, *Medical Fringe*, N. D. Jewson, "The Disappearance of the Sick-Man from Medical Cosmology, 1770–1870," *Sociology* 10 (1976): 225–44.

53. G. Larkin, *Occupational Monopoly and Modern Medicine* (London: Tavistock, 1983).

54. D. G. M. Schreber, *Kinesiatrik oder der gymnastische Heilmetode: Fur Ärtze und gebildete Nichtärtze nach eigenen Erfahrung dargestellt* (Leipzig: Fleischer, 1852).

55. Ottosson, "The Manipulated," 93–105.

56. Carl August Georgii to Lars Gabriel Branting, 26/8 1847, Törngrens Arkiv, vol. 12: LVII, National Archives, Sweden. Translation and italics made by the author.

57. One of the first to try out Ling's physiotherapy outside Sweden was in fact Franz Berwald (1796–1868), probably Sweden's most famed composer internationally. Before Berwald's career in music took off, he ran an orthopedic and physiotherapy practice in Berlin and then actually made several machines. Having done this in the early 1830s, Berwald could thus be seen as an early precursor to Zander. His work as a physiotherapist seems to have had a marginal effect (if any) in terms of adding a Swedish "identity" to physiotherapy. How much of Berwald's treatments were "Ling" are not easy to determine either. Berwald was also up to date with contemporary developments in German orthopedics. Holme, *Konsten att,* 37; Ingvar Andersson, *Franz Berwald* (Stockholm: Nortedts, 1971), 68–69, 92–97; Adolf Hillman, *Franz Berwald: En biografisk studie med kompositionsförteckning* (Stockholm: Wahlström & Widstrand, 1920), 37–38; Robert Layton, *Frans Berwald, a Critical Study of the 19th Century Swedish Symphonist* (London: Anthony Blond, 1959), 63–66.

58. Citation from Gustaf Moberg, *Svenska Gymnastikens märkesmän* (Stockholm: Hj. Hanssons tryckeri, 1920), 64. Author's translation.

59. Carl Fredrik de Ron to Lars Gabriel Branting, 18/6 1838, Törngrens arkiv, vol 12: LV, National Archives, Sweden.

60. Dr. Berglind took his RCIG exam 1848. See A. Georg Berglind, *Gymnastiska Centralinstitutets historia, 1813–1913* (Stockholm: P. A. Norstedt & Söner, 1913), 347.

61. Carl Fredrik de Ron to Lars Gabriel Branting, 24/5 1850, Lars Mauritz Törngrens arkiv, vol. 12: LV, National Archives, Sweden. Collegii Medici's dictum can be found in EIa: 2, nr. 514 (1850), GCI:s arkiv, National Archives, Sweden.

62. De Ron apparently had to to leave Russia because he impudently rebuked a young Russian grand duke for not being devoted enough to his gymnastic training. The empress is then supposed to have said, "Fredrik Carlowitsch, what have you done, now I can no longer save you." Citation from Moberg, *Svenska Gymnastikens,* 64. See also Louise Wikström, *Carl Fredrik de Ron: Ett glömdt geni* (Stockholm: Bille, 1904).

63. A. Georg Berglind, *Ueber die Bedeutung der Gymnastik in medizinischer, hygienischer und pädagogischer Beziehung* (St. Petersburg: Buchdruckerei von Jul. Stauff, 1869).

64. Ottosson, "One History," 296–319.

65. The most influential work in this field is probably Magali Sarfatti-Larsson's *The Rise of Professionalism: A Sociological Analysis.*

66. Ottosson, "The Age."

67. The RCIG, for instance, had (until c. 1860) the polyclinic in Sweden that likely served the highest numbers of celebrities. Members of the royal court and Stockholm's economic, political, and cultural elite were patients there. Even famous scientists and physicians consulted the RCIG for their illness, like professor Anders Retzius and his brother Magnus, physician in order of the king. See Brantings receptböcker, vol 22, GCI:s enskilda arkiv, National Archives, Sweden. Magnus Retzius's physiotherapy prescription is dated January 14, 1841, and Anders Retzius's is dated August 31, 1842.

68. Citations from Henry Hughes, *Lehrbuch der Schwedische Heilgymnastik unter Berücksichtung der Hertzkrankenheiten* (Wiesbaden: J. F. Bergmann, 1896), 26–27. Author's translation.

69. For other famous "massage-physicians" see Alfons Cornelius, *Druckpunkte, ihre Entstehung, Bedeutung bei Neuralgien, Nervosität, Neurasthenie, Hysterie, Epilepsie,*

Geisteskrankheiten, sowie ihre Behandlung durch Nervenmassage (Berlin: Verlag Otto Enslin, 1902); Isidor Zabludowski, *Tecknik der Massage* (Berlin: Thieme, 1900); Douglas Graham, *A Treatise on Massage* (St. Louis: J. H. Vail, 1890); Albert Hoffa, *Der Technik der Massage* (Berlin: Enke, 1893); Just Lucas-Champonniére, *Precis du Traitement des Fractures par le massage et la mobilization* (Paris: Rueff et Cie, 1895).

70. Ottosson, "One History," 301–7; Ottosson, "The Age," 820–28.

71. Roger Cooter, *Surgery and Society in Peace and War: Orthopaedics and the Organization of Modern Medicine, 1880–1948* (London: MacMillan, 1993); D. Joel Howell. D. *Technology in the Hospital: Transforming Patient Care in the Early Twentieth Century* (Baltimore: Johns Hopkins University Press, 1995).

72. Ottosson, "The Manipulated," 83–87; Ottosson, "Androphobia," 451–60.

73. Hughes, *Lehrbuch der Schwedische*, 245; Betänkande med förslag angående ordnandet av sjukgymnastutbildningen i riket avgivet av sakkunniga inom Ecklesiastikdepartementet, *Ecklesiastikdepartementets konseljakter*, 19310220, no. 64 (3), National Archives, Sweden.

74. St. Thomas' Hospital's physiotherapy school in London did not allow men to enter; neither did Christiania Ortopedisk og Mekaniske Institutt in Norway. The first two Swedish schools reaching governmental sanction (in 1902 and 1909) after RCIG were also closed to male applicants. See, Rannvieg Dahle, *Arbeidsdelning—makt—identitetBetydningen av kjönn i fysioterapiyrket* (Trondheim, 1990), 80–82; Ottosson, "Sjukgymnasten—Vart," 313–27.

75. Lindroth, *Ling—från storhet*, 65–71; Ottosson, "One History," 296–319; Ottosson, "The Age," 802–28. Regarding the field of orthopedics in Germany, see Doris Schwarzmann-Schafhauser, *Orthopädie im Wandel: Die Herausbildung von disziplin und Berufsstand in Bund und Kaiserreich (1815–1914)* (Stuttgart: Franz Steiner Verlag, 2004).

76. Ottosson, "The Manipulated," 106–15.

77. During the 1920s specialists in "physical medicine" could sense that they were looked down upon by their colleagues. Gerry Larkin, "Orthodox and Osteopathic Medicine in the Inter-war Years," in *Alternative Medicine in Britain*, ed. Mike Saks (Oxford: Claredon Press, 1992), 112–23. See also Roger Cooter, "Bones of Connection? Orthodox Medicine and the Mystery of the Bone-Setter's Craft," in *Medical fringe and medical orthodoxy, 1750–1850*, ed. W. F. Bynum and R. Porter (London: Croom Helm, 1987), 158–73.

78. Hanson and Ottosson, *A Nobel Prize*, 1190–94.

79. Kreck, *Die Mediko-Mechanische*; Terlouw, *De Opkomst*, 148–58; Hansson and Ottosson, *A Nobel Prize*, 1191–93.

Chapter Two

Gynecological Massage

Gender, Conflict, and the Transfer of Knowledge in Medicine during the Fin de Siècle

MICHAELA MALMBERG

In the late nineteenth century, a new gynecological method arose that became hugely popular in Western medicine. Despite having been developed and used during the Victorian era—a period renowned for its rigid attitudes toward nudity, sexuality, and personal interaction—the treatment was indeed an intimate one. A brief description: the doctor or therapist inserted a finger in the vagina, anus, or both of the patient, holding the other hand on the stomach and massaging the uterus from the outside while the internal finger was held up toward the massaging hand. The massage also included different movements, such as bending, pressing, and stretching, as well as different exercises to strengthen the pelvic area. Sometimes the therapy was administered with the aid of an assistant.

Invented in Sweden, this method quickly spread around the Western world, and was used during the last part of the nineteenth century by a large number of gynecologists in Europe and North America. It also spread to South Africa and Australia. In English, it was mostly referred to as pelvic or uterine massage. The method was described as being almost a panacea for female diseases, for which there were, at the time, few if any treatments. In 1898, Chicago-based F. H. Westerschulte wrote: "The medical world to-day becomes more and more fully convinced of the fact that pelvic massage is to be classed among the most important therapeutic measures of gynecology."[1]

After only a short period of development and application, and despite its considerable success, the promising method suddenly disappeared from gynecology around the 1920s. Interestingly enough, it also virtually disappeared from the history of medicine. Records of its influence and practice among prestigious doctors nearly vanished.

Recently, however, this massage has reemerged in popular fiction as part of a historical discourse about sexuality. In 2011, it resurfaced in the British film *Hysteria*, a romantic period comedy that constructs a fanciful narrative around the development, practice, and replacement of this method. In the movie, the patients are portrayed as wealthy, bored, and sexually repressed Victorian women who pay frequent visits to the doctor, claiming to be ill in order to solicit treatment with an intimate massage that leads to orgasm. The doctor, unaware of the women's ruse, misdiagnoses the orgasms as "hysterical paroxysms." The version presented in this film is fairly typical of popular culture treatments of hysteria from recent years, which present the massage as a cultural metaphor signifying an emergence from sexual repression.[2]

It is not only in popular culture that such myths around female sexuality proliferate; in fact, this particular myth has its basis in the work of the historian Rachel Maines, particularly her 1999 book *The Technology of Orgasm*, which posits the sexual nature of the massage. Maines claims that because of an androgenic view of sexuality, women—since ancient times and continuing into the twentieth century—have been sexually under-stimulated in such a fashion as to produce illness. The cure was to be found in the hands of doctors or midwives, who unknowingly massaged them to orgasm. This view has been popularized in the media but also by scholars in academic studies.[3] It first met with criticism in 2010, when classicist Helen King, in "Galen and the Widow: Towards a History of Therapeutic Masturbation in Ancient Gynaecology," described how Maines misreads the ancient and medieval sources.[4]

In what follows, I will examine the discourses surrounding the massage in fin-de-siècle society and offer a contemporary interpretation of them. Two intertwined topics will be addressed: First, I ask why the method's original practitioners, who produced earnest descriptions written in technical and scientific language, went silent before the reappropriation of the topic in the popular, sexualized discourse we see today. Second, in addressing this question, I will ask why women of the Victorian era would consider undergoing such an intimate treatment, and why doctors would dare suggest it. In this regard, the analysis is also an attempt to better understand why the method was able to find its way out of Sweden and proliferate in medical discourse and practice. Here, I highlight an often overlooked factor in the spatial transfer of medical knowledge, that of patients as carriers and "pull factors" for the spread of new treatments.

Initially skeptical of the method because of the professional background of its creator, the Swedish Society of Medicine eventually, by and large, embraced pelvic massage as a legitimate treatment. As I will show, this can partly be explained by the connections through which the method was received around the Baltic Sea region.

Development

Although massage—even in intimate versions—has likely existed across history as a treatment for pain and as an aid in pregnancy and childbirth, its modern version is ascribed to one man: Major Thure Brandt (1819–95) of the Swedish army. While at first it seems odd that Brandt would interest himself in creating and practicing a gynecological massage, the explanation for how this came about is unexceptional.

In Sweden, physiotherapy (or medical gymnastics as it was then called) was organically linked to military and pedagogical gymnastics, a holistic gymnastic system created by Per Henrik Ling (1776–1839) and taught since 1813 at the Royal Central Institute of Gymnastics (RCIG). In the institution's early days, the majority of students were officers of the Swedish army. This meant that physiotherapists were men from the upper classes, and even nobility, and had the same or higher socioeconomic status as doctors. Physiotherapists did not lack professional confidence and believed their mechanical medicine was equal to the chemical and surgical medicine practiced by regular doctors. In short, the theory stated that, for the body to stay healthy, it required a balance among its mechanics (movement), chemistry (food and medications), and dynamics (intellectual stimulation). Each part of the body was seen as connected to, and affecting, every other part. A rivalry between equally strong participants—doctors and physiotherapists—for the top spot in the medical hierarchy took place in Sweden during the nineteenth century.[5]

One of the methods debated as this rivalry played out was Brandt's pelvic massage. Brandt matriculated at the RCIG in 1841 and began teaching there the following year. He also spent two summers at a spa, where he came into contact with sick female patients. According to Brandt's own publication, *Gymnastiken såsom botemedel mot qvinliga underlifssjukdomar: Jemte strödda anteckningar i allmän sjukgymnastik* (1884), he developed his method in steps; the first patient he cured was a soldier with a rectal prolapse, which Brandt was able to put back in place. Later, this led him to think that the same kind of massage could be used for prolapses of the uterus, and, in 1861, he treated his first female patient, a forty-seven-year-old woman who for twenty-seven years had supported her prolapsed uterus in a sort of "halter."[6] That Brandt did not think it strange to treat women in this fashion can be explained by the prevailing mode of self-perception among physiotherapists. Brandt (and his patients) saw him as being equal to a doctor and believed that physiotherapy could cure just as many diseases and complaints, including gynecological ailments. In other words, the doctor/physiotherapist hierarchy that would later emerge, and persists to the present day, had not yet crystallized. However well established his medical credentials were, Brandt's willingness to use this method on female patients must also be examined in the context of the perceptions and practices of femininity in this particular era.

Theoretical Considerations

That this was a period of rapid and momentous transformation is well known; industrialization, urbanization, the rise of the middle class, and the new struggle of workers and women for equality are all relevant contexts. One of the most fascinating changes of the period—and for this chapter one of the most important—was the well-documented rise of the natural sciences, which displaced the previously dominant role of the church in explaining the world and its "natural" order. The study of the biological body became an important tool for explaining all things human and included the notorious propositions that attempted to validate social hierarchies by referring to biology (especially heredity). The working class, people of color, and women were described as biologically and fundamentally different from the white middle-class man, a belief whose resonance echoed throughout the discourses of sex and gender.

The dominant view of sex in this era characterized it as static and dimorphic. This filled a gap left by the absence of the preindustrial and early modern theological explanations of gender roles and sexual difference, while continuing to function as a constraining force keeping women separated from positions of power in the emerging social reality. It prevented middle-class women from undertaking male-gendered work, instead confining them to the domestic sphere as the separation of the home and the workplace solidified. (Working women and women of color were seen as degenerate and could therefore still be exploited in factories, as servants, or in prostitution.) In some ways, the new system was even more rigid than the old. In the preindustrial era women were, under certain circumstances, permitted to perform the work typically ascribed to men—for instance, tending to all the tasks on a farm during times of war or governing the kingdom when there was no suitable male heir. She was the "little man," not as good as, but still of the same stock.[7] Under the rubric of dimorphism, the essentialized female subject was still viewed as weaker and inferior, though now immutably so; she could not do what the male could. Instead, she had other virtues—albeit ones that were not connected with power in the public sphere—such as caring for the young. She was also seen as the vessel of a higher morality: "She is priest, not king. The house, the chamber, the closet, are the centers of her social life and power, as surely as the sun is the centre of the solar system," as one physician put it.[8]

Part of this antagonistic binary relationship between male and female was the pathologization of female bodies as the abnormal Other to the male's supposedly superior biology. As medical studies of the female body rapidly became popular, the modern medical specialization of gynecology took shape. This was a male quest to decipher the mystery of the female and reveal knowledge about the Other. Throughout its inception this field was dominated by male practitioners who developed a culture of machismo, with doctors comparing themselves to explorers of Africa and the female body, following colonial rhetoric, termed by Freud a "dark continent."[9] One of the influential theories that meshed well with these views was the ancient notion that women's illnesses stemmed directly from the uterus, an organ seen as prone to sickness that could spread to all other parts of the body. The era's "reflexion theory" stated that the uterus was the hub of a network of nerves from which disease was disseminated throughout the body.[10]

The view that the uterus was able to infect other parts of the body resonated well with the holistic view of physiotherapy and thus attracted the attention of Brandt and other practitioners. Given that this holistic view was still prevalent in medical practice, it is unsurprising that the pelvic massage was used for various ailments beyond those of the uterus, such as fatigue, headaches, backaches, depression, drug addiction, although the primary focus was on gynecological problems. There is, however, seldom any mention of hysteria in relation to the treatment; the term "hysterical paroxysm" is seemingly unrelated to the practice. So, for what reasons, if not for hedonistic ones, did patients choose to undergo such a treatment?

Treatments of Gynecology

To begin with, in the nineteenth century, most women bore many children, and destitute patients were just as likely as those of the middle classes to be treated with the massage.[11] Women often lived in harsh, impoverished conditions, had very little protection against sexual abuse and sexually transmitted infections, and thus had very real needs for gynecological health care. To view women of this period as merely bored, hysterical, or sexually repressed is to trivialize and risk abstracting them as historical Others. The choices most women had when it came to treatments were nothing short of nightmarish. Chemical treatments were often toxic, with severe side effects and little promise of cure. Some treatments led to addiction, which was observed in some of Brandt's patients who had consulted physicians prior to being treated by him.[12] The other option was surgery. In an era in which particular body parts were read as feminine, and therefore seen as causing various types of illness, operations were frenetic, experimental, and overused. Patients lost ovaries and uteruses—often completely healthy—in treatments for sundry ailments. Operations often rendered them infertile and led to intense pain, inflammation, scarring, and, not infrequently, death. In one common treatment, the uterus, believed to lie in a pathological position (but today seen as within normal variation), would be sewn to the abdominal wall, which often led to severe inflammation and death. Another treatment was cauterization with a heated iron—without access to modern anesthesia—where, as Ann Wood Douglas writes, "in a successful case, the uterus was left 'raw and bleeding' and the patient in severe pain for several days; in an unsuccessful one, severe hemorrhage and terrible pain might result."[13] Another treatment was to apply leeches to the vagina, from where they sometimes moved into the cervical cavity of the uterus itself. One doctor comments, "I think I have scarcely ever seen more acute pain than that experienced by several of my patients under these circumstances."[14] The alternative to these invasive procedures—physiotherapy and massage—must have seemed a benign and inviting course of treatment by comparison. This might also explain why the method was adopted by numerous gynecologists, who did not want to take part in rendering females infertile given the contemporaneous view that a woman's priority was to bear and raise children.

When Brandt's method was introduced to the Swedish Society of Medicine, however, it was roundly rejected—partly because Brandt was a physiotherapist and not a doctor. As mentioned above, the competition between different medical practitioners of gynecology had at this time grown vicious in Sweden, and doctors did not want to give credit to a method developed by a physiotherapist. The method's use could very well have ended there, since other male physiotherapists were, for the most part, uninterested in such techniques. However, it was around this time that women became engaged in physical therapy, as well as becoming doctors—a point to which I will return.

Sexualization of Gynecological Massage

One of the early male proponents of the massage was Finland's Dr. Georg Asp. In his 1878 publication *Om Lifmodersmassage* (On uterus massage), Asp describes how in the summer of 1874 he felt compelled to visit Sweden to learn the massage from Brandt. This had become necessary because women were traveling from Finland to Stockholm for the treatment; physiotherapists, in turn, had to travel there to learn it.[15] These professional and therapeutic journeys demonstrate the role patients played in the transfer of medical knowledge and treatments. Patients—at least those wealthy enough to do so—traveled abroad to receive treatments they could not access at home, and medical practitioners followed in their footsteps, a point to which I soon will return.

But first, let us have a look at the claimed sexual function of the treatment. As with many other doctors writing about pelvic massage, Asp does broach the issue of sexual stimulation. Like many others, he accuses other practitioners, including Brandt himself, of massaging in a way that could possibly lead to sexual stimulation. This contention allows Asp to claim that his own method circumvents any sexual excitation, freeing himself from the suspicion that he might have covert motives for performing the practice, or that it might lead to unintended results. Much of the early literature on pelvic massage, including Asp's, does refer to things like the necessity of avoiding the clitoris—contradicting Maines's assertion that it was an ignorance of the sexual function of this body part that made the sexual function of the massage possible.

How the pelvic massage came to be seen by commentators like Maines as a sexual procedure is a long story that will not be addressed here; in any case, notes by Asp and other practitioners make it clear that the supposed sexual stimulation of the patient was an issue that was familiar to the them, and one they were extremely wary of.[16]

With the rising middle class came a new moral discourse, in which pleasure seeking was seen as an immoral behavior of the upper and lower classes, while the bourgeoisie defined themselves by their restraint. The knowledge that female orgasms during (heterosexual) intercourse were not necessary for pregnancy, combined with the existence of an organ (the clitoris) whose sole purpose seemed to be to give pleasure, inflected female sexuality as immoral and obscene—something to be hidden away and to not "awaken." Knowledge of the clitoris did not disappear, but the organ was to be avoided at all costs. It is within this discourse—in which women might have a sexuality hiding like a monster inside "the dark continent" of their bodies—that it became so utterly important not to evoke this monster at any costs and to keep (middle-class) women away from all possible stimulation. In contradiction to Maines, who claims that the clitoris could be stimulated without understanding its effect due to an androgenic focus on penetration, the clitoris was not stimulated in the pelvic massage but studiously avoided precisely because of this fear. Moreover, the digits of the masseur were used internally, thus (often painfully) penetrating the patient.[17] That some of the members of the Swedish Society of Medicine accused the method of possible sexual stimulation should instead be viewed in the light of interprofessional power struggles and a misogynist fear of female sexuality.[18] The popular-culture depiction of the massage as a folly of middle- and upper-class women is further contradicted by the fact that a great number of documented patients treated with the procedure belonged to less privileged socioeconomic groups who dealt with painful medical problems in harsh conditions, as mentioned above.[19]

The Spatial Transfer of Pelvic Massage

A breakthrough for Brandt's method came in 1886. That year, he met with Austrian physician Paul Profanter, who worked at the university hospital in Vienna and the spa resort of Franzensbad, in Bohemia (Czech Republic). Profanter apparently visited Brandt at his clinic in Sweden and was so impressed with the method that he later wrote about it in his monograph *Die Massage in der Gynäkologie: Mit einer Vorrede des Herrn Geheimrath Prof. Dr. BS Schultze in Jena* (1887), which led to the dissemination of the method in the Baltic Sea region and from there out into the world. Supposedly, Profanter also convinced the physician who wrote the preface, Bernhard Sigmund Schulze (1827–1919), to invite Brandt to visit him at the University of Jena in Germany. Brandt accepted the invitation, and traveled to Jena in 1887, in the company of Norwegian physician and politician Oscar Nissen and Brandt's assistant, Miss Johannsson. According to Dr. Richard Hogner (1852–1930), "The Germans were surprised with the capability of Brandt to perform such a thorough and painless examination."[20] Schulze, a professor of gynecology, was also the director of the lying-in-institution and the gynecological clinic in Jena, and he too published monographs in which he specifically mentions Thure Brandt and asserts that his method should be received as an important innovation.[21] In 1888, the monograph's translation, *The Pathology and Treatment of Displacement of the Uterus,* was distributed in both Europe and the United States and reviewed by medical journals such as the *Journal of the American Medical Association.*[22] Profanter's texts on the pelvic massage were also translated in 1888 into Ukrainian as *Rukovodstvo k massazhu: Dlia uchashchikhsia i vračeĭ.* During the 1880s and 1890s, hundreds of texts discussing the massage—from articles to theses, in many different languages—were produced and circulated in the gynecological medical communities of Europe and the United States. In 1891, Brandt published—in collaboration with Swedish physician and physiotherapist Frans Lindbom—*Behandlung weiblicher geschlechtskrankheiten,* which gave the method further recognition abroad.[23] It was well known among practitioners at the turn of that century that the recommendations by Profanter and Schulze served as icebreakers, after which Swedish doctors also began to embrace the massage, safe in the knowledge that it had been approved by internationally renowned doctors. But methods are not spread only through medical journals. As Motzi Eklöf has pointed out, the examination of patients as medical agents has often been neglected within the field of medical history. This is despite the fact that patients often played a crucial role in the transfer of medical information and practice by acting as intermediaries and by seeking and conveying information about novel treatments to patients, doctors, and the general public.[24]

As mentioned earlier, both Profanter and Brandt spent a lot of time working at spas, and these places—baths, spas, and sanatoriums—became melting pots for medical exchange at the turn of the century. The resorts in the Alps were particularly popular. Here, practitioners and patients from around the world met and tried out new cures for all sorts of ailments. At many of these resorts, the Brandt massage was practiced, including at the famous Kellogg Institute in the United States and Lebendige Kraft in Zürich, an institution founded by Swiss physician Maximilian Bircher-Benner (1867–1939). The Lebendige Kraft sanatorium was a big rendezvous point for health travelers from all over the world, who often wrote home about the treatments they received. A significant amount of the patients came from Sweden: during 1904–1939, as many as 16 percent were Swedish citizens. Another big group came from the Baltic states. (In the guestbook, notes can be found from patients from Buenos Aires to the Philippines, Tel Aviv to St. Petersburg, and so on.)[25] Sanatoriums were also meeting points for doctors and nutritionists seeking to learn new methods—the gynecological massage among them. At Lebendige Kraft, it seems to have lived on long after its heyday; patient journals shows that it was practiced well into the 1930s.[26]

One of many competing with the importance of Profanter in spreading the Brandt method was Swedish physician Emil Kleen, well known at the time for his knowledge and interest in massage treatments in general but also for propagating the gynecological massage. In his *Handbook of Massage* (1892), Brandt's method is discussed and recommended, albeit with the reservation that is should solely be used by doctors. (Kleen was deeply entrenched in the aforementioned battle between Swedish physicians and physiotherapists.) The book was translated from Swedish into English, with help from the German edition. In its foreword, US physician Weir Mitchell (1829–1914), states, "I read with care much of Dr. Kleen's book in its German dress, and was glad to find so calmly scientific a statement of the uses and effects of massage. . . . I know of no other book on this subject which is so good as this."[27] The German-Swedish connection seems to have been important when the method was being introduced into the United States. The translator specifically points out the advanced uses of massage in Sweden and Germany (compared with the United States), although the authors and methods mentioned by him are all Swedish.[28]

A Patient's Perspective on the
Transfer of Medical Knowledge

What really caused this breakthrough for the gynecological massage, however, is less well known. It is mentioned by German American doctor Sofie Nordhoff-Jung in a speech to the Medical Society of Washington, DC, in 1895: "Thirty-eight years passed from the date of [Brandt's] first work before he received the recognition from the profession he so well deserved. Having successfully treated the wife of a wealthy merchant, the husband succeeded in getting a physician in Vienna interested in the methods employed. Thus it came about that later Brandt was invited to Stockholm and in a short time the most skillful gynecologists were his pupils."[29] Nordhoff-Jung's is the one voice among many that describes how the method became a success through the influence of the wife of a wealthy merchant. The husband is mentioned by Brandt in an article in *Wood's Medical and Surgical Monographs* from 1891.[30] His name was Robert Nobel, and he was likely the brother of the famed Alfred Nobel. As such, the honor of popularizing the method should partly fall to Paulina Nobel (née Lenngren, 1840–1918), as *she* is the one who convinced Profanter of its benefits in the first place. But Nobel is, as a matter of course, omitted in Profanter's own description of how he came to learn about the method, which includes praise only for other male physicians (and, of course, Brandt himself). This could perhaps be attributed to his desire to create an aura of professionalism around the method and to not damage (by association) his own reputation. This was a preoccupation with many physicians of the era, who carefully guarded their reputations of professionalism, since they faced challenges from so many other practitioners in the health-care business, including physiotherapists. One has to keep in mind that, in spite of some breakthroughs in medical knowledge around the turn of the century, the ability to cure had not increased significantly (and would not do so until the 1930s). The heroic status doctors had risen to during the past hundred years was in danger of collapsing and had to be defended at all costs.

Emil Kleen, writing in the tradition of the male-physician success story, states:

> In 1870 the talented Dr. Sven Skoldberg, since dead, took full cognisance of the "Brandt-method." . . . This facilitated the introduction of the method to many Scandinavian physicians and gynaecologists. Netzel and Sahlin, in Stockholm, Asp, in Helsingfors, and Howitz, in Copenhagen, took up the massage, and in this connection I must also make recognition of Nissen, of Christiania. On the continent Mezger was also active in this field, but Bunge was the first to write anything serviceable about it. Bandl, Hegar, Martin, Schroder, and other gynaecologists of great authority, by their recognition of gynaecological massage, soon contributed greatly to its spread; and in addition a considerable

number of German physicians obtained from Brandt himself a knowledge of his method.[31]

Just as in the case of the mythologized meeting of Profanter, Brandt, and Schulze, there is another story hidden away in this Whiggish interpretation of history that Kleen neglects to mention. This could be seen as *textual silencing*—a very specific form of exerting power that functions by ensuring that some aspects of an event or phenomenon never so much as even enter the discussion or the discourse around a subject.[32] Here, I have tried to uncover just these types of silences in the history of pelvic massage, which shed light on the power relationships in this field, and also suggest reasons for the disappearance of the practice. With regard to the practice of this massage reaching Finland and Dr. Asp, as in Mrs. Nobel's case, it was women—in this instance female physiotherapists and patients—who were responsible for its spread between institutions and locations. Asp writes that since physiotherapists learned the technique in Sweden, he felt obliged to do the same. This was in 1878, when the method was still viewed as questionable. Asp safeguards his own reputation by emphasizing that he is in no way interested in defending Brandt from his adversaries, and that he was compelled to look into the method because of the interest from these physiotherapists—he is merely a critical investigator. But by 1892, in Kleens's retelling of events, after the method had become approved of and celebrated, the participation of female patients and practitioners as agents had been excised from the narrative. As we shall see, in 1878 Asp himself had begun to intentionally obscure the participation of women in the method's rise.

Female Practitioners to the Front

In 1864, women were admitted to the RCIG, providing an early and uncommon opportunity for women to undergo professional training. Women came from all over Europe to study in Sweden, among them the first female doctor in Scandinavia, Dr. Rosina Heikel (1842–1929), from Finland.

Heikel's story is representative of that of a significant number of women who set out to become doctors but were forbidden to do so; these women instead trained as physiotherapists first, then took up pelvic massage, and subsequently entered gynecology. As was the case with patients, women with the means to do so went abroad for the medical training that they often could not access at home, and thus medical knowledge was transferred through them and their experiences. This was especially the case with physiotherapy. At the RCIG, the belief, in accordance with Ling's teachings, was that medicine needed to incorporate mechanical techniques to balance what was—in the view of Ling's followers—the overuse of medications, and students were encouraged to go out into the world and "evangelize," which many of them did.[33] Else Trangbæk has described the training of female physiotherapists in this era as an important part of the emancipatory struggle:

> They went out in large numbers into the world with a good education from the RCIG under their belts, and a vision of taking part in what I have chosen to term the modern women's project, where gymnastics, health and hygiene went hand in hand. The Swedish gymnastics played an important role in the physical upbringing for women, for children, in school and for women's education over a big part of the world.[34]

Like Heikel, many of these female physiotherapists and physicians were also feminists, active in caring for the poor and for women in prostitution, and supporters of sexual education. Among them was one of Sweden's earliest and most famous doctors, Karolina Widerström (1856–1949), and German neuroanatomist Elisabeth Harmine Winterhalter (1856–1952), who was the first scientist to discover that human ovaries contain nerve cells.[35] In 1884, Winterhalter started her medical studies in Zürich and Bern, and, after graduating in 1889, she went to Paris, Münich, and Stockholm to study surgery and gynecology. It is likely that this is when she learned the pelvic massage.[36] Because of her sex, Winterhalter was not permitted a full medical degree but instead had to work as an assistant to two male physicians in Frankfurt. During this time, she also wrote up her research and findings, which unfortunately were not accepted for publication at the time. As a result, she never published any further research but became renowned for her work as a feminist and for founding a popular health clinic for women in Frankfurt. She obtained her full medical degree in 1904. Richard Tucker writes, "Not one to shy from controversy, Winterhalter lived openly in Frankfurt with her [female] life partner Ottilie Roederstein (1859–1937), a renowned painter whom she met while studying in Zürich. With Roederstein, she championed the cause of women's education and cofounded a high school for girls."[37]

Brandt was also visited by French physician Madame P. Peltier, who later wrote a 144-page monograph about pelvic massage in 1895.[38] Some of the physiotherapists who conveyed the method around the world include the Swede Anna Sieurin, who worked in Köningsberg, among many other places in Europe; Alma Häckner, who in her work at Ramlösa Spa in southern Sweden treated many international patients; and Agnes Slettengren, who practiced in Massachusetts, California, and Seattle.[39]

In this chapter, however, the focus will remain on Heikel, who knew early on that she wanted to become a doctor. Because that profession was closed to women, she applied to the RCIG and was accepted in 1865. Here she could study anatomy, which at the time was also viewed as unsuitable for women. Self-motivated in the face of adversity, Heikel apparently even bought corpses herself to practice autopsy in her spare time at the school. She also learned the pelvic massage from Brandt.[40]

In 1878, she finally found work as a doctor in Finland within gynecology and obstetrics, working without a full license, though she did pass the exam. She was a women's rights activist who was supported in her struggle to become a doctor by other women. Upon receiving her permit to begin work, Heikel's achievement was celebrated by a large number of women in Helsinki.[41]

Gender Issues in Gynecology

Female doctors—and especially gynecologists—were likely sought after by women who had suffered misogynistic and insensitive treatment at the hands of male doctors, as well as for reasons of privacy. At this time, when a woman could be ostracized as fallen for simply being out alone in a public space, a visit to a male gynecologist must surely have been a cause for insecurity and anxiety. The famous doctor Anna Fischer-Dückelman—who in the 1890s was one of the very first women to become a physician in Germany and was also a feminist and practitioner of the pelvic massage—had argued the case for more female physicians. This was partly because of the method of pelvic massage, which could "hurt the female senses" when practiced by a man, as Fischer-Dückelman wrote in the widely distributed *Die Frau als Hausärztin* (The wife as family doctor) in 1901.[42] Dückelman's work was translated into thirteen languages, and her publications sold more than 1,000,000 copies.[43]

Heikel was a close friend of Asp and is likely one of the physiotherapists who was anonymously described in Asp's article. Perhaps more interesting is the likelihood that another of them was Asp's own wife; Mathilda Wetterhof-Asp (1840–1920). Wetterhof studied at the RCIG at the same time as Heikel, and she too learned the massage from Brandt. Following her time at the RCIG, she studied in several other schools around Europe—just as Heikel did. Any mention of Wetterhof in relation to the medical history of pelvic massage or in her husband's publications is omitted, however, in spite of the fact that they founded and owned the institute where the pelvic massage was practiced together and she was its director. In his publication, Asp consistently refers to the institute as his own.

Close to the end of the article, however, Asp makes casual mention of a crucial point: all the treatment carried out at his institute was actually performed by a female practitioner.[44] This brief and anonymous mention is the sum total of recognition offered to the female practitioner and indeed reads more like a disclosure clause than an acknowledgment of credit. Instead, it is Georg Asp who is cited as an expert on the method in numerous publications around the world.[45] The mention of the female masseur is probably intended to safeguard Asp's purity and professionalism, a defense against any accusations of improper behavior. Whether the practitioner mentioned was Wetterhof, Heikel, or someone else, I have so far not been able to determine, but it is a perfect example of textual silencing, wherein women's participation in medical practice and exchange of knowledge is made invisible, written out of history. Throughout the literature of the period on the topic, there is a clear current of male practitioners seeking to withhold the method from women who seek to make use of it on their own and to diminish their role in making its practice possible.

Brandt and Asp's need of, and assistance from, female practitioners is typical of the wider application of the method. From the perspective of the medical establishment, female practitioners ensured professionalism and lent an aura of propriety for the benefit of both patient and doctor.

In spite of that—or perhaps because of it—many male doctors practicing this method stated that women could not practice it on their own in a manner that was adequately professional. These assistants are seldom mentioned by name, and, to ensure their subordination to male practitioners, they were accused of having fingers too short for the task or lacking the strength and stamina of the male physician to persevere through the strenuous massage. Brandt himself claims this, in spite of the fact that all his assistants and many of his students were women.[46] (As the reader may recall, an assistant, Miss Johannsson, also participated in the famous meeting in Jena, though nothing more is known about her.)

Another physician who makes a similar claim about the unfitness of female practitioners is the Swedish gynecologist Gustaf Norström, though he targeted midwives in particular, since they had taken an interest in the method. Norström left Sweden after a failed gynecological surgery that was harshly criticized by other doctors, alighting in France to lick his wounds; he worked there with famed French surgeon Jules-Émile Péan (1830–98).[47] The patient he had operated on in Sweden had died because of his mistakes and because he did not listen to the warnings of the midwife present, who also reported what had happened to the Swedish Society of Medicine. But abroad Norström's name was clear, and he could rebuild his reputation. Norström wrote many articles about pelvic massage during this time, which he now seems to have been practicing instead of surgery. His hostility toward midwives is remarkable in its virulence. In one passage, he issues the stern warning: "Many . . . believe themselves possessed of gynecological knowledge, and do not hesitate to practice pelvic massage. If by chance they ran across a favorable case, they might cure it and there would be no way to repair the evil."[48]

Norström's misogynist prediction became perhaps something of a self-fulfilling prophesy, since before the disappearance of the method, sources suggest that women had become its main practitioners. One reason for this is the aforementioned seeking out of female practitioners by female patients. Probably—and paradoxically—the new dimorphic view on gender—intended to keep women away from male institutions like parliament, higher office and science—was cleverly used by many feminists and other women. If women were completely different and opposite, they argued, then women must be needed to add the "feminine view." In health care, as we have seen, the relationship of male physician and female patient could become very problematic in the prevailing discourse of (hetero)sexuality, and a female practitioner could guarantee professionalism. This, and the fact that there were a lot of single, middle-class women who, for economic reasons, had to participate in the labor market, led to the professions of doctor and physiotherapist slowly opening up to women, since they did, after all involve the feminine trait of "caretaking." Since patients of female physicians had to be women (to challenge the discourse with a female doctor treating a male patient was still too disturbing a thought), many ended up in the previously highly masculinized area of gynecology.[49]

The Disappearance

That male physicians eventually gave up the fight and abandoned the treatment can partly be explained by some significant shifts in the discourse of femininity at the beginning of the twentieth century. One of the more influential actors in this process was Sigmund Freud. In an early case study, that of Mrs. Emmy in *Studien über Hysterie* (1895), Freud describes recommending pelvic massage with Dr. N. for Emmy's daughter—the N. perhaps standing for Norström—which suggests that Freud, at least at this point, did not perform gynecological massage himself (contrary to Maines's claims) but approved of it.[50] Unfortunately, Emmy's daughter's health improved only temporarily after visiting Dr. N., and following her return tensions arose between Freud and Emmy. An upset Emmy wished to end her own treatment under Freud, and despite the persuasive campaign launched by both Freud and Dr. Josef Breuer for Emmy to stay in treatment, she left for a sanatorium in northern Germany. Freud, however, arrogantly ascribing "hysterical residue" to Emmy's behavior, is not so easily shaken off. Instead, he contacts the doctor at the sanatorium and instructs him on how to treat Emmy. Within a year, she is back with Freud in Vienna. In this power struggle between patient and doctor, the latter, in collaboration with his colleagues, wins. However, the question remains whether, or to what extent, this episode led to Freud's decision to cease physical-dietetic treatments and referrals for pelvic massage, in favor of focusing on the talking cure and listening to the patient. What has been documented by other scholars is the importance of Freud's own patients in motivating his shift to analytic listening as a primary therapeutic practice.[51] Freud is also interesting in that he developed the androcentric model that powerfully affected Western discourse on sex and sexuality over the course of the twentieth century. As touched on above, this model puts penile penetration of the vagina at the center of human sexuality, championing this as the most desirable and normal sexual behavior. This idea has a much later genesis than Maines claims. Freud is the one who displaced the clitoral orgasm in favor of the vaginal orgasm, claiming that the former was identified with an early developmental stage, and that the latter was the proper form of orgasm for adult women and—unlike the masculine clitoral orgasm—indicated true womanhood.[52] Since the gynecological massage was penetrative, and it is after Freud that penetration starts to be described as the highest form of female sexuality, it is unsurprising that the reputation of the massage as a threat to chastity really takes hold as Freud's theories spread. Another Freudian notion, however, has an even bigger impact on the fate of the massage. Karin Johannisson has documented how under Freud's influence the locus of women's pathologization is relocated from the supposedly pathogenic uterus to the neurotic brain. Johannisson shows how the supposedly fragile female psyche served as justification for female marginalization, and "subjective bodily symptoms [were seen as] psychogenic, that is to say born in the soul of the woman."[53] In other words, women's medical problems were seated in the mind and were to be treated diagnostically as psychological rather than physiological phenomena. Johannisson includes a chart documenting how new diagnoses like neurasthenia skyrocketed in the early decades of the twentieth century and goes on to explain that, "around the turn of the century, pioneers like Josef Breuer, Sigmund Freud and Pierre Janet were on their way to put forward psychodynamic interpretations of an array of symptoms that earlier were believed to have somatic origins."[54] This new discourse has persisted into the twenty-first century, whereby women are more frequently diagnosed with psychological problems than are men.[55] It has also been pointed out how the psychological life of men has not undergone the same scrutiny as that of women, allowing male violence or pursuit of power to slip through the cracks of pathologization.[56]

In this new era in which the problem with women was shifted onto the female psyche, gynecology was no longer an exploration into the "dark continent" of women's bodies but became the rather less glamorous task of caring for women's physical ailments. This was not an attractive enough proposition for male doctors to stay engaged. Men moved on to the now safer—because of medical advances—and therefore more attractive area of surgery. In the new discourse of medicine, a method like massage, practiced mainly by women, was deprived all its medical prestige, leading male practitioners to shun the treatment. Men who had practiced it were now seen as highly suspect, resulting in a dearth of publications on the matter and a glossing over of this chapter in medical history.

A New Medical Hegemony

The phenomenon of pelvic massage has many threads. It includes questions of body, sex, sexuality, gender, medicine, professionalism, and competition. It was part of a power struggle between medical practitioners, doctor and patient, and the sexes. For a long time, men were able to exclude women from medical professions and maintain the heteronormative and androcentric status quo, as well as the hierarchical relationship between male doctor and female patient, in which the latter was objectified and subordinated. At the same time, men from different medical professions fought each other over the rights to scientific interpretation, explanation, methods, and dominance in the medical hierarchy.

Through societal change and demands from patients and women who sought a medical profession, the field gradually changed. One of the first steps was women entering the field of physiotherapy, and through this channel gaining access to gynecology, and a treatment—pelvic massage—that was far less invasive than surgery. At the same time, physiotherapists gradually lost the battle and became subordinate to doctors, who created a ruling professional field in the medical hierarchy—surgery—where they continue to enjoy a position of dominance over other medical practitioners. For a while, female practitioners succeeded in wresting a method from the hands of male doctors, making them feel threatened. In response, the medical establishment managed to make the method disappear from professional medical practice altogether, by dividing gynecology and massage into different spheres. But women could no longer be shut out from the medical professions. The achievements of women like Heikel, Wetterhof, Fischer-Dückelman, and their patients is in this context quite remarkable; in spite of their inferior social and professional positions, they were able to break into the male-dominated professions of doctors and physiotherapist and insert themselves into, and influence, the course of medical history. To do so, they often had to travel and network across national borders. One can only speculate as to whether the competition from these noninvasive cures also helped to motivate an increased focus on safety and accuracy in the surgical field. Today, we also see a revival of this kind of health-care perspective within medical institutions, where in Sweden, for example, one can get a prescription for exercise from the doctor.

A significant task for the feminist movement of the twentieth century has been to reclaim the right for women to describe, explore, and use their (own) bodies and sexuality, without adhering to androcentric preconceptions about them. This struggle is one reason for the popularity of the anachronistic and loosely historical narrative about a secret sexual massage in the doctor's office. Nevertheless, the historical record requires that we turn away from such anachronistic descriptions and explore the original contexts of this episode in the history of medicine. To combat misogyny requires a recognition of how patriarchal structures over time have been fortified by the suppression of women and by creating confining boundaries for sex, gender, and sexuality as well as an acknowledgment of how the shifting parameters of such boundaries modify the course of history. To ignore this is to reinforce an asymmetrical set of social relations and, as historians, to render our subjects—in this case women—as mere passive recipients of historical events, rather than participants in their own right.

Notes

1. F. H. Westerschulte, foreword to *Massage Treatment (Thure Brandt) in Diseases of Women: For Practitioners*, by Robert Ziegenspeck (Chicago: n.p., 1898), 3.

2. Another recent and sustained example is found in the TV series *American Horror Story*, which started in 2011. Similar treatments of the topic can be found on popular history blogs and other web pages. *Hysteria*, dir. Tanya Wexler (United Kingdom: Scanbox Vision, 2011), DVD; *American Horror Story*, season 1, created by Brad Falchuk and Ryan Murphy (US, 20th Century Fox, 2011), DVD; Maya Dusenbery, "Timeline: Female Hysteria and the Sex Toys Used to Treat It—Vibrators, Douches, and Pelvic Massage: Curing Crazy Ladies for Centuries—One 'Hysterical Paroxysm' at a Time," *Mother Jones*, June 1, 2012, http://www.motherjones.com/media/2012/05/hysteria-sex-toy-history-timeline.

3. Rachel P. Maines, *The Technology of Orgasm: "Hysteria," the Vibrator, and Women's Sexual Satisfaction* (Baltimore: Johns Hopkins University Press, 1999); Helen King, "Galen and the Widow: Towards a History of Therapeutic Masturbation in Ancient Gynaecology," *Eugesta* 1 (2011): 206, http://eugesta.recherche.univ-lille3.fr/revue/pdf/2011/King.pdf; Peter Englund, *Tystnadens historia och andra essäer* (Stockholm: Atlantis, 2003), 121–33.

4. King, "Galen and the Widow," 205–35.

5. Anders Ottosson, "Sjukgymnasten—vart tog han vägen? En undersökning av sjukgymnastyrkets maskulinisering och avmaskulinisering 1813–1934" (PhD diss., Göteborgs Universitet, 2005), 64–70.

6. Thure Brandt, *Gymnastiken såsom botemedel mot qvinliga underlifssjukdomar: Jemte strödda anteckningar i allmän sjukgymnastik* (Stockholm: Albert Bonnier, 1884), 2.

7. Yvonne Hirdman, *Genus: Om det stabilas föränderliga former* (Malmö: Liber, 2001), 28–31. Thomas Walter Laqueur, *Making Sex: Body and Gender from the Greeks to Freud* (Cambridge, MA: Harvard University Press, 1990), 6–10, 139, 127.

8. William H. Holcombe, *The Sexes Here and Hereafter* (Philadelphia: J. B. Lippincott, 1869), 201–2, quoted in Carroll Smith-Rosenberg and Charles Rosenberg, "The Female Animal: Medical and Biological Views of Woman and Her Role in Nineteenth-Century America," *Journal of American History* 60, no. 2 (1973): 336, https://doi.org/10.2307/2936779.

9. Sigmund Freud, "Die Frage der Laienanalyse," *Gesammelte Werke* (Fischer, Frankfurt, 1926), 14:241, quoted in Ranjana Khanna, *Dark Continents: Psychoanalysis and Colonialism* (Durham, NC: Duke University Press, 2003), 48.

10. Brandt, *Gymnastiken såsom botemedel*, 1; Ann Wood Douglas, "The Fashionable Diseases: Women's Complaints and Their Treatment in Nineteenth-Century America," *Journal of Interdisciplinary History* 4, no. 1 (1973) 29–30, http://www.jstor.org/stable/202356; Karin Johannisson, *Den mörka kontinenten: Kvinnan, medicinen och fin-de-siècle* (Stockholm: Norstedt, 1994), 34.

11. Michaela Malmberg, "Major Brandt och den Mjuka metoden: Livmodermassage som fenomen och botemedel under 1800-talet" (BA thesis, Department of Historical Studies, Gothenburg University, 2011).

12. Brandt, *Gymnastiken som botemedel*, 247.

13. Douglas, "The Fashionable Diseases," 31.

14. James Henry Bennet, *A Practical Treatise on Inflammation of the Uterus, Its Cervix and Appendages and on Its Connection with Other Uterine Diseases* (Philadelphia: Blanchard and Lea 1864), 237, quoted in Douglas, "The Fashionable Diseases," 30.

15. Ulrika Nilsson, "Kampen om kvinnan: Professionalisering och konstruktioner av kön i svensk gynekologi 1860–1925" (PhD diss., Uppsala Universitet, 2003), 179.

16. In this era, it was not only pelvic massage that was accused of having possible sexual effects. When the speculum came into use in the 1840s, the same discussions arose; and again with bicycles, sewing machines, and so on. These examples are suggestive of the culture of fear surrounding perceptions of female sexuality that serves as a basis for the caution around the use and effects of the massage. For a more in-depth discussion on the sexual issue, see Michaela Malmberg, "Livmodersmassagens försvinnande, en nedtystad historia om medicin, kön och makt" (MA thesis, Göteborgs Universitet, 2014). See also Maines, *The Technology of Orgasm*, 3–9, 67–68; Georg Asp, "Om Lifmodersmassage," *Nordiskt Medicinskt Arkiv* 10, no. 22 (1878): 1–33.

17. Malmberg, "Livmodersmassagens försvinnande," 47.

18. Nilsson, "Kampen om kvinnan," 187.

19. Asp, "Om Lifmodersmassage," 15.

20. Richard Hogner, "On the Value of Kinesiotherapy in Gynecologic Practice," *Journal of the American Medical Association* 24, no. 4 (1895): 115, https://archive.org/details/journalamericanm24ameruoft.

21. Bernhard Sigmund Schultze, *The Pathology and Treatment of Displacements of the Uterus* (New York: D. Appelton, 1888), vii.

22. "Book Notices; The Pathology and Treatment of Displacement of the Uterus," *Journal of the American Medical Association* 12, no. 6 (1889): 213–14, https://doi.org/10.1001/jama.1889.02400830033012.

23. Malmberg, "Livmodersmassagens försvinnande," appendix 1.

24. Motzi Eklöf, *Kurkulturer, Bircher-Benner, patienterna och naturläkekonsten 1900–1945*, (Stockholm: Carlsson Förlag, 2008), 23, 117–42.

25. Ibid., 119–20.

26. Ibid., 140–41.

27. Emil Kleen, *Handbook of Massage*, trans. Edward Mussey Hartwell (Philadelphia: Blakiston, 1892), 5. Weir Mitchell was a physician from the United States who invented a form of "rest cure" for sick women, whereby patients were forced to lie in bed for weeks or months on end while being fed and massaged. This treatment was harshly criticized by one of its recipients, Charlotte Perkins Gilman, in her famous story *The Yellow Wallpaper* in 1890. Douglas, "The Fashionable Diseases," 42–43.

28. Among the different aspects of this progress, Hartwell specifically mentions Brandt along with Ling and Swedish doctor Gustav Zander, who invented machines for use in physiotherapy—similar to modern-day exercise machines—that were exported to the United States, among other places. (Zander was actually nominated for a Nobel Prize in medicine in 1916.) This transatlantic connection testifies to the fame and reach of Brandt's method at the time. Kleen, *Handbook of Massage*, 5

29. Sofie Nordhoff-Jung, "Kinetic Therapeutics in Gynecology," *National Medical Review Washington, D.C.* 4, no. 3 (1895): 39–44, http://archive.org/details/nationalmedicalr3418unse.

30. Thure Brandt, "Treatment of the Diseases of Women," *Wood's Medical and Surgical Monographs* 12, no. 1 (1891), 11. Nobel is also pointed out as the merchant in *Svea Folkkalender* (Swedish calendar) from 1896, but only the husband is mentioned. *Svea Folkkalender* no. 52 (Stockholm: Albert Bonniers Förlag, 1896), 251–52, http://runeberg.org/svea/1896/0264.html.

31. Kleen, *Handbook of Massage*, 207.

32. Thomas Huckin, "Textual Silence and the Discourse of Homelessness," *Discourse and Society* 13 (2002): 347–72, http://das.sagepub.com/content/13/3/347.

33. Anders Ottosson, "The First Historical Movements of Kinesiology: Scientification into Borderland between Medicine and Physical Culture around 1850," *International Journal of the History of Sport* 27 (2010a): 1892–919

34. My translation. The original reads, "De svenske gymnastiklærerinder fik en afgørende betydning for systemets udbredelse især i pigeskolerne. De drog i stort omfang ud i verden med en god uddannelse fra KCI i bagagen, og en vision om, at medvirke til det, jeg her har valgt at kalde det moderne kvindeprojekt, hvor gymnastik, sundhed og hygiejne gik hånd i hånd. Den svenske gymnastik fik som nævnt stor betydning for den fysiske opdragelse for kvinder, for børn, i skolen og for kvinders uddannelse over det meste af verden." Else Trangbæk, "Sally Högström og det moderne kvindeprojekt: Svensk gymnastik og GCI's betydning i Danmark," in *200 år av kroppsbildning, Gymnastiska Centralinstitutet/Gymnastik—och Idrottshögskolan 1813–2013*, ed. Hans Bolling and Leif Yttergren (Växjö: Davidsons Tryckeri AB, 2013), 143–47, quote 134–35.

35. Richard P. Tucker, "Elisabeth H. Winterhalter (1856–1952): The Pioneer and Her Eponymous Ovarian Ganglion," *Journal of the History of the Neurosciences: Basic and Clinical Perspectives* 22, no. 2 (2013): 191–97, http://dx.doi.org/10.1080/15332845.2012.728422.

36. Alma Häckner, "Något om Major Thure Brandt och hans livsgärning," *Hälsovännen, Tidskrift för Allmän och Enskild Hälsovård* 42, no. 3 (April 15, 1927): 15.

37. Widerström also lived with a female partner and was active in different women's rights movements. Tucker, "Elisabeth H. Winterhalter," 195. Nilsson, "Kampen om kvinnan," 161, 280–95.

38. "Reviews: La Méthode de Thure Brandt, et son Application au Traitment des Maladies des Femme, Par Madame P. Peltier, Ancine Externe des Hôpitaux, Docteur en Médecine de la Faculté de Paris, Paris: L. Batallie et Cie, 1895," *British Medical Journal*, April 27, 1895, 931.

39. Malmberg, "Livmodersmassagens försvinnande," 75–76

40. Helena Westermarck, *Finlands första kvinnliga läkare, Rosina Heikel—Kvinnospår i finländskt kulturliv*, Helsingfors: Söderström & co Förlagsaktiebolag Östra Nylands

Tryckeri, 1930, 70. Alma Häckner, "Något om Major Thure Brandt och hans livsgärning," *Hälsovännen, Tidskrift för Allmän och Enskild Hälsovård*, Årg. 42, N: o 3, April 15, 1927, 15

41. Heikel also started funds for female students of medicine, and was active in the debate on prostitution, demanding that all people afflicted with syphilis should undergo the same treatment and surveillance (not just the prostitutes), and arguing that the focus in combating prostitution should be moved from seller to buyer. Westermarck, *Finlands första kvinnliga läkare*, 9–10, 46–47, 125–128, 148; *Nordisk Familjebok, Uggleupplagan* 11 (1909), 256, http://runeberg.org/nfbk/0144.html; *Historiskt bibliotek*, no 5, (1875–1880), 636, http://runeberg.org/histbib/5/0644.html.

42. The Swedish edition from 1905 is used here; Anna Fischer-Dückelman, *Kvinnan som hemmets läkare: En oumbärlig uppslagsbok för hvarje kvinna* (Stockholm, Aktiebolaget Litterära verk, 1905), 628. See also Michael Hau, *The Cult of Health and Beauty in Germany: A Social History, 1890–1930* (Chicago: University of Chicago Press, 2003), 72–73.

43. Paulette Meyer, "Physiatrie and German maternal feminism: Dr. Anna Fischer-Dückelmann critiques academic medicine," *Canadian Bulletin of Medical History* 23, no. 1 (2006): 145–82, http://www.ncbi.nlm.nih.gov/pubmed/17152243.

44. Asp, *Om Lifmodersmassage*, 33.

45. Malmberg, "Livmodersmassagens försvinnande," 71.

46. Brandt, *Gymnastiken som botemedel*, 78–79. Gustaf Mauritz Norström, *The Manual Treatment of Diseases of Women* (New York: n.p., 1903), 5, http://www.archive.org/details/manualtreatment00norsgoog; Axel Grafstrom, *A Textbook of Mechano–therapy (Massage and Medical Gymnastics), Especially Prepared for the Use of Medical Students, Trained Nurses and Medical Gymnastics*, 2nd ed. (Philadelphia: W. B. Saunders, 1904), 187, https://archive.org/details/textbookofmechan00graf.

47. Péan also introduced hysterectomy (removal of the uterus) during the 1870s and likewise had an unflattering reputation for being something of a "butcher." *British Medical Journal*, June 6, 1891, 1236–37; *British Medical Journal* June 4, 1892, 1198–99; Johannisson, *Den mörka kontinenten*, 197.

48. Norström, *The Manual Treatment*, 32.

49. Nilsson, *Kampen om kvinnan*, 7.

50. Maines claims that Freud engaged in the gynecological massage himself, and her interpretation of it is that it was a sexual procedure. Norström worked with Péan in Paris at about the same time as Freud with Charcot, who himself had been an inspiration to Péan. Nilsson, *Kampen om kvinnan*, 201–2. Sigmund Freud and Josef Breuer, *Studies in Hysteria*, repr., vol. 2 (New York: Basic Books, ca. 1908), 67–77, http://www.archive.org/details/studiesonhysteri037649mbp; Ilse Grubrich-Simitis, *Early Freud and Late Freud: Reading Anew Studies on Hysteria and Moses and Monotheism* (London: Routledge, 1997), 25; Rachel Maines, "Freud and the Steam-Powered Vibrator," *Longing: Psychoanalytic Musings on Desire* (London: H. Karnac, 2006), 122; Maines, *The Technology of Orgasm*, 44.

51. Grubrich-Simitis, *Early Freud and Late Freud*, 27–28; Patrick Miller, "How Emmy Silenced Freud into Analytic Listening," in *On Freud's "On Beginning the Treatment,"* ed. Christian Seulin and Gennaro Saragnano (London: Karnac Books, 2012), 116.

52. Laqueur, *Making Sex*, 265–76; Maines, *The Technology of Orgasm*, 9; Jane Gerhard, "Revisiting 'The Myth of the Vaginal Orgasm': The Female Orgasm in

American Sexual Thought and Second Wave Feminism," *Feminist Studies*, 26, no. 2, (2000): 450–52.

53. Johannisson, *Den mörka kontinenten*, 29–39.

54. Ibid., 146; Malmberg, "Livmodersmassagens försvinnande," 81–87; Hans Glimell, *Den Produktiva kroppen: En studie om arbetsvetenskap som idé, praktik och politik* (Brutus Östlings Förlag Symposium, Stockholm/Stenhag, 1997), 103.

55. Johannisson, *Den mörka kontinenten*, 29–39.

56. Catherine Kohler Riessman, "Women and Medicalization: A New Perspective," in *The Politics of Women's Bodies, Sexuality, Appearance, and Behavior*, 2nd ed., ed. Rose Weitz (New York: Oxford University Press, 2003), 57–58.

Chapter Three

Worlds Unexplored

Medicine in Stettin, 1800–1945

JOANNA NIEZNANOWSKA

When discussing the place and significance of Stettin/Szczecin in the medical history of the Baltic Sea region in 1850–2000, one must begin by pointing to a crucial difference between the German city of Stettin and the Polish city of Szczecin: there is a medical university in Szczecin, whereas no pregraduate training of physicians took place in Stettin. Since the establishment of the Akademia Lekarska (Medical Academy; now Pomorski Uniwersytet Medyczny, Pomeranian Medical University; hereafter PMU) in 1948, and especially since the fall of communism and the opening of the borders at the turn of the 1980s and 1990s, Szczecin has had both the means and opportunities to participate actively in an international and constantly growing exchange of people, thoughts, and ideas. The PMU's (and thus Szczecin's) participation in the transfer of medical knowledge in the Baltic Sea region is evident and significant on many levels. Students from Norway, Sweden, and Germany come to PMU to study medicine (the English program was established in 1996) and dentistry (established in 2002). Within the Erasmus+ program, PMU cooperates with, among others, the medical faculties at the universities of Greifswald, Leipzig, and Würzburg in Germany; Linköping in Sweden; and Trondheim in Norway. There are postgraduate medical education exchange programs, with PMU hosting trainees from countries in the Baltic Sea region, and Szczecin's medical professionals pursuing training in Germany, Sweden, or Norway. PMU's researchers have designed or participated in multiple international research projects in collaboration with colleagues from other academic centers in the Baltic Sea region.[1] Last but not least, PMU's scientists publish a great deal, with some of their writings read, discussed, and referred to worldwide. One of the most spectacular examples is the Very Small Embryonic-Like (VSEL) stem cell research by Prof. Mariusz Z. Ratajczak and his team, with VSELs alleged to be nonexistent by some scholars, and proven to be real by others.[2] Another example of Szczecin's significant contribution to the transfer of medical knowledge at an international level (including the Baltic Sea region), is the PMU's International Hereditary Cancer Center, directed by Prof. Jan Lubiński, and *Hereditary Cancer in Clinical Practice*, an internationally recognized journal that is frequently chosen by authors from Baltic Sea countries for publication of their work.[3]

So while Szczecin of today plays a vital role on the international stage of medicine, the existing literature sheds no particular light on Stettin's participation in the spread of medical knowledge, either on a national (German) or international level. Is this because Stettin never played any vital part in the development of medical knowledge or because its contribution has not thus far been acknowledged? In my opinion, the latter is more probable. This chapter is aimed at explaining why Stettin's medical history has been wiped from our collective memories and finding out what part the German city of Stettin actually took in the production and transfer of medical knowledge in the Baltic Sea region. The answer to the first of these questions is intimately connected to the city's fate during and after World War II.

Stettin/Szczecin: A Deracinated City in Search of Its Identity.

In 1998, when preparing for the Cambridge Certificate of Proficiency in English exams, I read an article written by an English journalist for a British weekly. The article was about my city, Szczecin, and the impression it made on the writer. I do not remember anything from it but one striking adjective the journalist used to describe the place I called my home: "deracinated." Indeed, "deracinated" epitomizes the fate World War II bestowed upon the city: Stettin was renamed Szczecin, its German population was expelled, and the city was repopulated with Polish citizens, the vast majority of whom had been forced to leave their homes in the eastern territories that no longer belonged to Poland. The thread of Stettin's history was broken. The creation of Szczecin began with the deliberate avoidance or erasure of any connections to the city's previous history and owners. For several decades, many of the city's new inhabitants felt neither safe nor at home in Szczecin, one of the many reasons for this being the unclear status of the postwar Polish-German border. Only in November 1990, after the border treaty between Poland and the newly united Germany was signed in Warsaw, did my parents, who moved to Szczecin in 1968, feel they could finally settle down there for good. It is only for the past twenty-five years that we, the Szczeciners, have felt secure enough to explore the nineteenth- and twentieth-century history of Stettin. In 1994, a monumental volume on the city's history during 1806–1945 was published.[4] It was the third part of an editorial series by Polish scholars[5] and the first new publication on that scale on the history of the city since Martin Wehrmann's 1911 work.[6] In 2004, a group of Stettin/Szczecin lovers launched www.sedina.pl, a portal dedicated to the city's history, which has gained enormous popularity. With more than two million registered visitors and thousands of articles, photographs, and threads posted,[7] it provides firm evidence of how many inhabitants of Szczecin have turned into true Szczeciners, fascinated by and identifying themselves with the city's complicated past. Within the past quarter-century much has been written, both in Polish and German, on the political, economic, industrial, architectural, social, and scientific history of Stettin and Szczecin.[8] Most important is Jan Musekamp's *Stettin and Szczecin: Metamorphoses of a City, 1945–2000*, published in both German and Polish and widely recognized as relevant and exemplary in the field of the historiography of cities exposed to massive population changes and deracination due to World War II and its aftermath.[9]

Stettin/Szczecin and the Historiography of Forced Migration and Deracinated Cities in Postwar Europe

The colossal population transfer that took place in Europe during and after World War II was neither the first nor the last such event in the history of humankind. Yet it seems that it was not until after it had happened that the phenomenon of forced migration was recognized as a valid field of research in political, economic, or social history.[10] The forced transfer of Europe's population, one of the many consequences of the continent's new geopolitical order determined at the conferences of Yalta and Potsdam, has been a subject of scientific interest since the end of the war. Which elements of this phenomenon were studied, however, and how they were evaluated or interpreted, depended strongly on the language of narration, the national background of the researchers, and the geopolitical situation in Europe at the time. Before the fall of communism in Europe, the so-called expulsion of Germans (*die Vertreibung*) was the most prominent element of the English-language narrative on the postwar forced migrations in Europe.[11] The same subject dominated (Western) German research in this field.[12] In both English and German historiography of the German expulsion at that time, *die Vertreibung* was usually presented from a one-sided perspective as a kind of ruthless vengeance ordered by Stalin and inflicted on innocent civilians, having no direct connection whatsoever with the way the Nazis carried out their policies and the war itself. During the three decades after 1945 in Poland, as in other European countries falling under the USSR's control, the only research on war-related population transfer allowed to be published was that providing arguments justifying Poland's rights to the so-called reclaimed territories. Officially, the deportation of Poles from what had become the Soviet republics of Ukraine, Belarus, and Lithuania, or other parts of the USSR, could only be presented as a return to the homeland: repatriation. The publication and distribution of unabridged narratives of the Polish experience of deportation and expulsion was only possible abroad[13] or, from the mid-1970s, as a part of the so-called Second Circulation (the term that we Poles prefer to the Russian samizdat).[14] Starting in the late 1970s, and especially after the rise of the Solidarity movement in 1980, the forced migration of Poles during and after World War II was researched and discussed in a somewhat more open way, although access to archival sources was still restricted and possibilities for unabridged publication of research results remained limited.[15] A major, global change in the historiographic approach to the postwar population transfer in Central and Eastern Europe took place after the fall of communism, with the declassification of archives in countries previously under Soviet rule or control. For the English-language historiography of the midcentury forced migrations in Europe, two books were seminal: 1990's *The Uprooted*, resulting from an international conference held at the University of Lund, and edited by Göran Rystad;[16] and, particularly, 2001's *Redrawing Nations*, the proceedings of an international conference organized in 1997 in Gliwice, Poland (prior to 1945, Gleiwitz, Germany), edited by Philipp Ther and Ana Siljak.[17] Both books presented a number of aspects of forced population transfer due to World War II that had previously been barely acknowledged or discussed in English. The first focused on the consequences of the forced transfer of large populations. The second contained a number of papers on forced transfers of Poles and Ukrainians due to World War II and its aftermath. What is more, the authors of *Redrawing Nations* proposed a new insight into the motivations behind the postwar forced migrations. They point to the drive of the decision-makers at the Yalta and Potsdam conferences (with an emphasis on Stalin) toward the creation of a Europe built of ethnically monolithic states, thus presenting the deportations and expulsions of Germans, Poles, Ukrainians, and others as elements of ethnic cleansing. For the past twenty-five years, hundreds of scholars all over the world have been working on the construction of an in-depth, multidimensional, and multilateral presentation and discussion of the causes and consequences of forced migration (the phenomena resulting from World War II and the aftermath in Europe being but one in a long list of research topics on forced migration and deracination worldwide).[18]

Stettin/Szczecin is not the only city that suffered from deracination due to forced population transfer during or after World War II. Other obvious examples include Breslau/Wrocław, Danzig/Gdańsk, Königsberg/ Kaliningrad (Germany–USSR–Russia), Wilno/Vilna/Vilnius (Poland– Lithuanian Soviet Republic–Lithuania) and Lwów/L'vov/L'viv (Poland– Ukrainian Soviet Republic–Ukraine). Of these, only Breslau/Wrocław has so far been given a comprehensive, multidimensional, objective portrait of its complicated twentieth-century history, with the process of deracination and reconstruction of the city's identity thoroughly discussed: "Microcosm," by Norman Davies and Roger Moorhouse.[19] As for Wilno/Vilna/Vilnius and Lwów/L'vov/L'viv, these cities were multiethnic prior to the war, with Poles/ Jews and Poles/Jews/Ukrainians, respectively, as their main inhabitants, and they remained multiethnic in the postwar period, with Lithuanian/Russian and Ukrainian/Russian populations. Here, any account of the city's identity proposed by a representative of one of the groups (usually Poles and Lithuanians or Poles and Ukrainians, respectively, with Jewish narration painfully underrepresented because of the Holocaust) is usually attacked by the other groups as one sided, or even nationalistic, and thus unreliable. Only recently have projects been announced that arouse hopes of objective, multidimensional accounts of the history of these cities, embracing the issues of ethnic cleansing, forced migration, and deracination. For example, Theodore R. Weeks is working on a history of 1795–2000 Vilnius as a multiethnic city;[20] Christine Kulke of the University of California, Berkley, is preparing a dissertation on the communities of 1939–53 L'viv/Lwów/ L'vov/Lemberg;[21] Edmund Kizik of the Polish Academy of Sciences, Jacek Froedrich of the University of Gdańsk, Alvydas Nikzentaitis of the Lithuanian Institute of History, and Peter Oliver Loew of the Deutsches Polen Institut, Darmstadt, are working on a joint project exploring the parallel histories of Gdańsk/Danzig and Vilnius/Wilno from the perspective of transformations of collective memories in central Europe, 1939–2013.[22]

Stettin: A City with No Medical History?

Regarding the processes of being uprooted and pursuing identity, the case of Stettin/Szczecin appears most similar to that of Breslau/Wrocław. Yet there is at least one specific aspect of the history of Stettin's transformation into Szczecin that seems to be unique: the fact that not only Stettin's German population but also the city's medical history disappeared. Unlike the cases of prewar Breslau, Danzig, Wilno, or Lwów, the history of medicine in Stettin still remains largely unexplored. The most important reasons for this are strictly associated with the city's history and fate before, during, and after World War II. As explained below, these reasons are accompanied by a list of common assumptions shared by both German and Polish historians of Stettin/Szczecin as to why medicine in Stettin was (is) not worthy of their time and effort. A closer look at these reasons and assumptions must be taken before I address the question of what part Stettin actually played in the production and maintenance of medical knowledge on a national or wider scale.

First and foremost, the German city of Stettin had neither a university (and thus no medical faculty) nor, later, a medical academy. This, in my opinion, is the most important reason for the absence of medicine in the city's historiography. In the case of the prewar cities of Breslau and Danzig (or Wilno and Lwów), the people affiliated with their medical schools (in the case of Danzig, the medical academy; in other cities, the medical faculties at their respective universities), after surviving the forced migration, preserved and carried on the legacies of their schools and the memories of their teachers and masters. In the case of Stettin's physicians (and nurses, for that matter), there was no such common "nest"; thus, the individual memories, unanchored, were dispersed and, eventually, lost. In addition, because there was no medical faculty/academy in Stettin, it is commonly assumed that nothing and no one of particular relevance to the development of modern German (or international) medicine has ever existed here: no game-changing discoveries, no groundbreaking research studies, no inspirational trailblazers or role models. The common assumption follows that if there was any transfer of medical knowledge worth mentioning in reference to Stettin in an international context, it was a one-way, import-only flow.

Second, Stettin suffered devastating and irreparable damage during the war. The tremendous destruction of the city's architectural tissue by bombings and fires is still evident, since the obliterated districts have never been reconstructed. For historians, however, the most disastrous loss was Stettin's entire municipal archives, accompanied by less massive, yet substantial, losses to other collections.[23] With the documents lost, there is little, if anything, left to explore—this mournful phrase is repeated in many texts about Stettin's past. What makes the loss particularly painful with reference to the later decades of Stettin's existence is the fact that these were times that were too recent for the prewar historians of the city to consider history and therefore to mention or discuss. And it was in these municipal archives that the vast majority of documents concerning medicine and medical practitioners in Stettin was collected. With the archival sources lost, even the existence and character of the supposed import-only transfer of medical knowledge in Stettin is difficult to examine, since we do not have any detailed knowledge about where (or what, or from whom) Stettin's physicians learned. This is not the case in other, less unfortunate cities without universities, where collections of doctoral theses from physicians applying to the municipal authorities for the right to open a practice are available for research.

Third, given how little was written on medicine and its practitioners in Stettin pre-1945, it is generally assumed that they did not play any pivotal role in the social, cultural, or scientific life of the city. The highly valued, two-volume *Geschichte der Stadt Stettin* by Heinrich Berghaus does not contain any explicit information on medicine in Stettin.[24] In Martin Wehrmann's work we find the names of thirteen doctors deceased between the years 1827 and 1910 who were considered worthy of grateful memories for their contributions to Stettin's sanitary safety and a mention of the establishment of a Scientific Society of Stettin's Physicians (Wissenschaftlicher Verein der Ärzte zu Stettin) in 1857.[25] Yet, when discussing the city's intellectual life, Wehrmann does not utter a single word about this organization, as though the physicians' society added nothing meaningful to Stettin's cultural and scientific atmosphere. Separate publications on medicine in Stettin, predominantly devoted to its health-care facilities, were mostly commemorative booklets, yearly reports, and more or less lengthy entries in lexicons and encyclopedias. They contained statistical and administrative data, and many of them apparently were lost in the wartime turmoil. What has survived sheds some light on the role these institutions played in the city's life but does not reveal much detailed information on their personnel. Of these remnants, several publications, preserved in the Pomeranian Library and containing data on the history of Stettin's medical facilities (especially those that continued to operate in Szczecin), were referred to and quoted in three concise works by Bronisław Seyda (1912–2008),[26] the first head of the PMU's Department of the History of Medicine. In the most lengthy of these three, numbering sixty-five pages (and, unfortunately, never published), Seyda wrote, "Whoever shows interest in the medical past of Pomerania in general, and of Szczecin in particular, must admit with much astonishment that the German literature contains but scarce and fragmentary information on this subject."[27] Out of approximately twenty pre-1945 sources listed by Seyda, only three were used in the 1994 Polish monograph on the nineteenth-century history of Stettin; of this book's 996 pages, fewer than five are devoted to what is broadly understood as medicine (public health, epidemics, hospitals, physicians).[28] No monograph on any aspect of medicine in Stettin during 1800–1945 has been written in Polish.[29] A recently published book on the history of the Pomeranian University's Clinical Hospital in Pomorzany, the former municipal hospital of Stettin, devotes only sixteen of its 112 pages to the period before 1945, even though, according to its title, it covers the hospital's history from the Middle Ages.[30] Polish authors have published a few journal articles discussing selected persons and institutions related to medicine in Stettin, such as the department of urology at the municipal hospital and its first head, Dr. Felix Hagen,[31] or the Tuberculosis Hospital in Stettin-Hohenkrug.[32] Finally, there are a number of more or less detailed entries related to some aspects of medicine in Stettin in online encyclopedias.[33] Post-1945 German publications on medicine in Stettin are somewhat more comprehensive. There is a monograph on Dr.

August Steffen, the physician in chief at Stettin's pediatric hospital and the cofounder and first president of the German Pediatric Society,[34] and a book on the Kückenmühler Anstalten, a long-term care and treatment facility for the mentally disabled and ill,[35] but neither explores the documents in the State Archives of Szczecin, clearly suggesting that there is nothing there to refer to. Apart from monographs, some information on medicine in Stettin is retrievable from German electronic and printed encyclopedias, lexicons, journals, and magazines, as well as popular publications on the city's history. However, most of the evidence used in these publications comes from the scarce sources listed in Seyda's publications.[36]

To summarize, according to popular opinion, medicine in Stettin in 1800–1945 remains an unexplored field because there is nothing interesting about it, and because scarcely any documents or sources exist, and those that do have already been used. What has been published on this topic post-1945 is dispersed and mostly not very detailed.

The eighteen months I spent searching through the collections of the State Archives in Szczecin, however, as well as through books, journals, and web resources, have produced enough material to prove that all three of these assumptions are untrue. The following is by no means a finished work. It is a preliminary report on the sources identified thus far covering Stettin's medical history in 1800–1945 and on the reasons why this history deserves to finally be discovered and made known. It also addresses some promising leads indicating that the medical representatives of Stettin actually did participate on both national and international levels, with an emphasis on the Baltic Sea region.

The Myth That There Is Nothing Left to Explore

Though Stettin's municipal archives seem to be irrevocably lost, some parts of other collections covering medical topics in relation to Stettin have survived. The collections belonging to the Prefect of Pomerania (Oberpäsidium von Pommern—Naczelne Prezydium Prowincji Pomorskiej), the Land Directorate / Provincial Association of Pomerania (Landes-Directorium/ Provinzialverband von Pommern—Zespół Samorządowy Prowincji Pomorskiej), the Government District of Stettin (Regierungspräsidium zu Stettin—Rejencja Szczecińska, Wydział Prezydialny), and the District Office of Randow (Landratsamt Randow—Starostwo Powiatowe Szczecin[37]) contain altogether no fewer than three hundred files related to medical matters in Stettin. There are documents concerning the city's public and nonpublic hospitals (e.g., five extensive files on the municipal hospital for 1835–1937,[38] administrative documentation from the Diakonissen-und-Krankenhaus "Bethanien," Stettin's first modern hospital,[39] and the

Kinderheil-und-Diakonissen-Anstalt, the pediatric hospital directed by the aforementioned Dr. Steffen[40]), documents from seventeen private clinics (approximately half of those mentioned in Stettin's address books[41]), as well as documentation from pharmacies (twenty-five volumes)[42] and on public health issues (e.g., child mortality statistics for 1905–22[43]). There is also documentation from the Provincial School for Midwives (Provinzial Hebammen-Lehr-Institut) that covers 1812–1934 and seems to be complete up to the late 1870s,[44] and a file documenting the preparations for the school's establishment in 1777–1800.[45] In addition, there is information on the members and the proceedings of the Provincial Medical and Sanitary Council of Stettin[46] and many other topics. Of course, not every page in these files discusses matters directly related to Stettin or necessarily contains relevant data, but the collection contains a great deal of fascinating, mostly unknown, information on medicine in Stettin. Apart from the State Archives of Szczecin, some material on medicine in Stettin might retrievable from German archives, especially the Geheimes Staatsarchiv Preußischer Kulturbesitz (Rep. 65a—Regierung Stettin) and the Landesarchiv Greifswald (Rep. 60—Oberpräsidium der Provinz Pommern, Rep. 61—Medizinalkollegium). It is possible that some data on Stettin's deaconesses could be found in the archives of Diakonie Deutschland (Archiv des Evangelischen Werkes für Diakonie und Entwicklung).

Other sources with information on medicine in Stettin, especially in relation to medical practice, are the city's address books, as well as books and papers authored by physicians and other medical practitioners from Stettin. Precious data on Stettin's public health can be found in the official journals (*Amtsblätter*). Interesting information on the city's most respected and popular doctors can be traced in local newspapers (mainly the obituaries).

The Myth That Nothing Interesting
Ever Happened Here

As to this assumption, the above information on sources that have yet to be explored should suffice to challenge it. In the history of Western medicine, the second half of the nineteenth century was an era of game-changing discoveries and innovations that had profound impacts on virtually every aspect of human life, both public and private. How were all these changes implemented in a city like Stettin, a provincial capital and a metropolis, yet without a university? The records in the address books give us basic insight into the scale of the transformations. In the early 1850s, Stettin had a population of 60,000 packed into a very tight space that was restricted by massive fortifications. There were forty to fifty doctors practicing general medicine as well as surgery and obstetrics, and several barber-surgeons. Medicine,

both noninvasive and invasive, was practiced predominantly in the homes
of patients. The municipal hospital was a mere hospice, devoted to the care
of the poorest. There was also a pediatric hospital (founded in 1851) and
a school for midwives (founded in 1803 but operating beginning in 1806).
In the 1920s, Stettin numbered 230,000 inhabitants, a demographic explo-
sion that was the result of the demolition of the fortifications in 1873 and
the rapid territorial expansion and industrial development of the city. There
were approximately 250 physicians: half of them general practitioners, the
other half specialists, with several women in each category. The medicine
practiced at this time in Stettin was hospital based. Apart from several public health-care facilities, funded by either the state (e.g., the new municipal
hospital, opened in 1879) or by charity (Kückenmühler Anstalten, founded
in 1863; Diakonissen-und-Krankenhaus "Bethanien," established in 1869),
there was a substantial number of private clinics. In 1943 (when the last
German address book was issued), Stettin's population numbered 350,000,
with the increase due mainly to the radical expansion of the city's administrative boundaries in 1939. The number of physicians had not changed
significantly since the 1920s, but the names had. Stettin did not have a large
Jewish population (around 2,500 people in 1925), but many of the city's doctors were of Jewish origin. By 1943, they were all gone: some had managed
to emigrate, some had been exterminated. Another striking change in the
medical landscape of Stettin that can be traced in the address books, which
was a result of the rise of the Third Reich, was the disappearance of the
medical associations in 1933. In 1932, there were six such organizations in
the city. A year later only one, the so-called Presentation Evenings (Referat-
Abende), survived. This is when the Wissenschaftlicher Verein der Ärzte zu
Stettin, mentioned so briefly in Wehrmann's monograph, allegedly came to
an end.

The disappearance of the Scientific Society of Stettin's Physicians preserved in the sources is one of the most painful wounds World War II
inflicted on my city. The only tangible body of evidence for the society's
thriving existence seems to consist of two items: a sixty-four-page commemorative fiftieth-anniversary book written in 1908 by Dr. Ludwig Freund[47] and a
printed eulogy for the society's cofounder and president for thirty-five years,
Carl Ludwig Schleich Sr., by the same author.[48] The former work is known to
the historians of both Stettin and its medicine (among others, the authors of
the 1994 history of Stettin and Seyda), yet it has never been used as a source
of knowledge about the society itself. The only content in the book that has
raised any interest so far is the comprehensive chronicle of Stettin's public
health-care facilities. Ironically, the reason Freund wrote this twenty-eight-
page chapter was that all of the physicians instrumental to the existence and
flourishing development of the institutions described in it were at the same
time the most active members of the society, as well as its most regular and

important scientific contributors. What we learn from the other thirty-six pages of Freund's commemorative work is the reason no documents from the society have survived, though it also gives hope that some information on its activities can be recovered.

The most important reason for the lack documents from the society in the archival collection is that its members never wanted to make the *Verein*'s proceedings available to the general public. Its documentation, therefore, was never transferred to the public archives, and the society never edited any journals. When the society was established, its most important task was not continuing education or the development of science (although these were mentioned) but the nurturing of collegial relationships in Stettin's medical community. In the mid-1850s, because of the dramatic paradigm shift in the medical sciences, a sharp and bitter conflict arose between the older and younger generations of physicians in Stettin. The latter, followers of the new medicine based on cellular pathology, experimental evidence, and the statistical evaluation of data, criticized the former for their attachment to ancient, disproved concepts and theories. In return, the former, many of them highly ranked, respected citizens and trusted physicians to the most influential people in the city, discredited the Young Turks in front of their patients. The antagonism between the two generations of Stettin's doctors was soon evident to the general public and threatened the entire community with a loss of professional credibility. Therefore, the most benevolent— or maybe the most farsighted—of both groups established the society as a place where physicians could discuss their issues, seek reconciliation, build community solidarity, and learn from each other in a private setting. The plan, Dr. Freund reported fifty years later, worked tremendously well, and the society played a pivotal role in both bringing the city's doctors together (approximately two of every three Stettin physicians were active members of the *Verein*) and stimulating their professional and scientific development. The meetings were held once a month, first at the Pomeranian Museum at Rosengarten 1, then, from 1877, at the Three Crowns Hotel at Breitestraße 29–30 (none of these buildings exists today). In 1884, the society moved its headquarters to the newly opened Concert and Club House (Konzert-und-Vereinhaus) at Augustastraße 48, where, according to the address books, it remained until its disbanding in 1933. The *Verein*'s book and journal collection was stored at its headquarters, together with correspondence and meeting protocols (excluding the documents from the first decade of the society's existence, which had long been lost when Freund prepared his anniversary book). Was this collection removed from the building in 1933? That remains unclear. A meeting protocol published in 1939 in *Münchener medizinische Wochenschrift*[49] shows that, despite the decision of the Nazi authorities, the society remained active, either disguised as an association of military physicians or perhaps using the Presentation Evenings as a cover.

In August 1944, the Konzerthaus was destroyed in a devastating night bombing, its interior completely burned out. It is probably then that the society's archives were annihilated and, with them, the memory of the society itself. Thus, the only easily accessible information on the society's history ends in 1908. Fortunately, there is a good chance of being able to at least partially reconstruct the *Verein's* scientific activity in later decades. From 1896 on, excerpts of the society's meeting protocols were published in the *Berliner klinische Wochenschrift.* From earlier times, all that exists is a list of the most relevant lectures and presentations, disclosed by Freund. However, thanks to Freund's book we have insight into the Verein's social life until 1908, while no information whatsoever on that matter is available after the time of the society's fiftieth anniversary. Nonetheless, the information we are able to gather, as fragmentary as it is, proves that the Scientific Society of Stettin's Physicians played a vital role in the city's transformation into a cleaner, healthier, modern metropolis[50] and allowed local doctors to become participants in, and not just receivers of, the major achievements in German medicine during the late nineteenth and early twentieth centuries.[51] For that, the society deserves a place in Stettin's history.

The Myth That Physicians Did Not Play Any Relevant Role in Stettin

To begin, let us confront the above assumption with some brief information on two physicians who played active and vital roles in Stettin's conversion into a modern metropolis.

In the topographic history of Stettin by Heinrich Berghaus—a book that is highly treasured by the city's historians, since it contains a significant amount of now-lost documents, quoted *in extenso*—we find information as to why Stettin's New Town was built in the early 1850s on the left bank of the Oder, and not at Lastadie on the river's right bank, as the royal authorities in Berlin had planned. In a memorandum dated November 16, 1835, Dr. Ernst Heinrich Carl Kölpin (1774–1846), head of the Medical and Sanitary Collegium of Stettin,[52] referred to studies by Dr. Wilhelm August Steffen, who held the office of physician to the poor and operated mainly at Lastadie (his son would later run the pediatric hospital). Dr. Kölpin had presented a long list of well-documented medical arguments opposing Stettin's expansion in the planned direction and advocating its spread south of the Old Town, on a higher, and therefore dryer and warmer plain, beyond the fortification lines. Dr. Kölpin's argument must have made a profound impression in Berlin, as the fortifications were moved to make space for a new district in the area suggested. Thus, the city's shape for generations to come was decided thanks to the opinions of a local—however prominent—physician.

Another physician who influenced the shape of Stettin, though less liter-
ally, was Gustav Bogislav Scharlau (1839–1914). He was a second-generation
physician educated in Göttingen and Berlin. Before he returned to Stettin
to open a successful practice, Dr. Scharlau spent four years as an assistant
to Professor Eduard Martin at the maternity hospital in Berlin, gathering
clinical experience, publishing, and participating in the work of the local
Society for Gynecology and Obstetrics. On returning to Stettin he was soon
elected to the city council, a post he held for thirty-seven years. For nearly
twenty-five years (March 1883–December 1907), he was the council's chairman. This was the time of the greatest prosperity in Stettin's history. In 1901,
Dr. Scharlau was honored with a street named after him. Scharlaustrasse
(today ulica Szczerbcowa) was, and still is, a beautiful avenue leading to the
most symbolic buildings of Stettin/Szczecin: what was then the Municipal
Museum and the seat of the district government, that is, *Regierung*, nowa-
days the National Museum and the Western Pomeranian Province Office.
Scharlau was also awarded honorary citizenship in Stettin. Interestingly, and
significantly, he is the only honorary citizen of Stettin with no individual
entry in the Digital Encyclopedia of Szczecin.[53]

In addition to shaping the city through political and administrative
actions, local physicians actively participated in the city's scientific life. The
preserved lists of members of scientific societies operating in Stettin reveal
that physicians constituted a considerable part of each of these groups.
Many of the numerous medical practitioners active in Stettin's scientific
societies seem to be quite well remembered, although not as physicians
(though they were all successful and renowned doctors). For example, Carl
Ludwig Schleich Sr. (1823–1907), one of the pillars of the Scientific Society
of Stettin's Physicians (and father to Carl Ludwig Schleich Jr., the inventor
of infiltration anesthesia)—was a longtime, active member of the renowned
Society for Entomology. He specialized in micromoths (*Microlepidoptera*),
identifying a few new species, and he was honored with a butterfly named
after him (*Nepticula schleichiella*, Frey 1870[54]). Many physicians contributed to the work of the Technical Society (Polytechnischer Verein); Dr.
August Wilhelm Schultze was elected to its board in 1897. Ludwig Eduard
Emil Behm (1800–80), who taught obstetrics at the Provincial School for
Midwives for nearly half a century (as second teacher from 1834, as first
teacher from 1840, and as the school's director from 1847 until his death)
and was the coleader of the first executive board of the Scientific Society
of Stettin's Physicians,[55] earned his greatest fame as a geologist. The initial sixty-one pages of Berghaus's book, a chapter on the formation of
the Lower Oder Valley in the Tertiary period, was entirely imported from
Behm's publications.[56] These[57] were, and still are, listed among the most
relevant scientific works on that topic.[58] Behm's predecessor at the School
of Midwives, Friedrich Wilhelm Gottlieb (Teophil) Rostkovius (1770–1842),

was the coauthor of monumental monographs on the flora of Stettin and Swinemünde (now Świnoujście),[59] as well as Germany's fungi,[60] and has *Wikipedia* entries in both German and English as a prominent botanist and mycologist. Dr. Ernst Bauer (1848–1930), Behm's successor, was the founder and longtime president of the local Society for Ornithology (Ornithologischer Verein zu Stettin) and the editor in chief of its bimonthly journal. Dr. Johann Carl Rudolph Lehmann (1812–71), born in Stettin to the family of a renowned physician, not only opened a successful medical practice in 1839 but conducted profound studies of local mollusks, published in Pfeiffer's *Malakozoologische Blätter*.[61] After his sudden death in 1871, his colleagues honored him with a posthumous edition of his major work, a monograph on Pomeranian snails and clams.[62] Georg Buschan (1863–1942), a neurologist and psychiatrist who settled in Stettin in 1892, was also a renowned ethnologist and anthropologist, and founder and president of the Gesellschaft für Völker- und Erdkunde (Society for Ethnology), as well as the founder and editor in chief of the *Centralblatt für Anthropologie, Ethnologie und Urgeschichte*.[63] Martin Bethe (1866–1956), a dedicated and successful pediatric surgeon and the head of the department of surgery and orthopedics at "Kinderheil-Anstalt" Stettin-Finkenwalde (1895–1945), was also the founder (1923) and president (1923–42) of the Pomeranian Union for Studies in Genealogy and Heraldry (Pommersche Vereinigung für Stamm-und Wappenkunde). His obituary in the 1959 issue of *Baltische Studien* praised Bethe as one of the most valuable and collaborative members of the Society for Pomeranian History and Archeology (Gesellschaft für pommersche Geschichte und Altertumskunde).[64] The same source reveals that the genealogical archive collected by Bethe on Pomerania's physicians, surgeons, and other medical practitioners had survived the war in Berlin and, after a few years in Warsaw, was transferred to Leipzig in 1959. It is still there, a part of the collection of State Archives, and offers reasonable hope for the retrieval of some precious, otherwise unavailable data on medicine in Stettin in the nineteenth and early twentieth centuries.[65]

Stettin's Physicians and Their International Contacts: Promising Leads

From the data shown above, it might seem that Stettin's doctors were so preoccupied with turning their hobbies into legitimate professions that they had little time or desire to contribute to the development of actual medicine. Indeed, as Freund wrote, up to the late 1870s there were hardly any genuine clinical scholars in Stettin, and the work of the Scientific Society of Physicians was more or less restricted to simple casuistry.[66] There were, however, exceptions to that rule. Stettin's pediatric hospital, under the leadership of Dr. August Steffen, soon became a genuine research center and a place to which German doctors interested in pediatrics traveled for education (especially during this era, when many German universities had no pediatric clinics). The list of publications by Steffen and other physicians affiliated with the Stettin pediatric hospital numbers 109,[67] most of them printed in the *Jahrbuch für Kinderheilkunde*, the journal where Dr. Steffen was editor in chief from 1868 to 1899. Most German universities, as well as many prominent clinical education and research centers worldwide, subscribed to the journal, and, under Steffen's direction, it was commonly viewed as one of the leading titles in the field of pediatrics. This is where, for example, Dr. Harald Hirschsprung of Copenhagen published his groundbreaking account on infantile megacolon, or Hirschsprung's disease.[68] Evaluation of the contents of the fifty volumes of the *Jahrbuch* edited by Dr. Steffen in relation to the affiliations of the authors may reveal interesting data on the journal's role in the transfer of medical knowledge in the Baltic Sea region.

Another physician participating in the export of medical knowledge from Stettin was Ernst Brand (1827–97). His work on the effectiveness of hydrotherapy in the treatment of typhoid fevers as compared to the gold standard therapies of the time, based mainly on extensive use of opium and emetics,[69] played a vital role in the rebuttal of old treatments based on humoral concepts. As such, it also contributed to the establishment of the new, evidence-based paradigm in the medical sciences, as well as to the transformation of hydrotherapy itself into a legitimate part of the new medicine, a starting point for the development of modern physical therapy. Brand's contributions were acknowledged and praised, both in Germany and abroad.[70] What was commonly stressed was the exquisite quality of the statistical evidence provided in his publications, as well as the fact that he was capable of conducting scientific research of such quality while being a mere "praktischer Arzt," a family doctor with no access to the means and measures of a clinical hospital.[71] It is possible that Brand's method was known and discussed internationally; this hypothesis, however, cannot be verified without access to local sources, which I lack.

Yet another example of a physician successfully exporting relevant medical knowledge from Stettin was Hermann Wasserfuhr (1823–97). Born in Stettin, he established a medical practice there in 1846. With epidemiology as his major field of scientific interest, he contributed to the establishment of the Section for Public Health at the annual Congresses of German Naturalists and Physicians and, in 1869, cofounded the influential journal *Deutsche Vierteljahrsschrift für öffentliche Gesundheitspflege*.[72] He left Stettin in 1870 and made a successful career as a public health officer in Alsace-Lorraine. His most important scientific works, devoted to the issue of child mortality, however, were written in Stettin.[73] It would be very interesting to investigate the status of his publications abroad, which, again, is impossible without access to local sources.

During my relatively short period of research, I came across a couple of clues pointing more or less directly to the involvement of Stettin's doctors in an international context with links across the Baltic Sea. One refers to Dr. Gustav Wilhelm Scharlau (1809–61), the father of the aforementioned long-term chairman of Stettin's City Council. Dr. Scharlau Sr. was both a pharmacist and a physician. He studied medicine in Greifswald and Leipzig, gathered clinical experience in hydrotherapy in France and England, and established a successful hydropathic facility, Schönsicht, in Frauendorf near Stettin (now Szczecin-Golęcino). Like Ernst Brand, his follower, Scharlau the Elder contributed significantly to the transformation of hydrotherapy into a branch of evidence-based medicine. He published a great deal: a two-volume pharmacy textbook,[74] several monographs on the hydrotherapeutic management of fevers (with an emphasis on typhoid fever),[75] a series of polemical writings on Schönlein's system of pathology,[76] and a book on nutrition and therapeutic diets,[77] among others. In the nutrition book, published in 1858, we find the intriguing information that the author was an honorary member of the Stockholm Society of Physicians and a knight of the Royal Order of Vasa. When, and in recognition of what merits, did he earn these honors? A search through the archives of the Stockholm Society might offer an answer to this question, possibly revealing a previously unrecognized scientific link between Stettin and Sweden.

Another example concerns Ernst Neisser (1863–1942). Educated at the universities of Berlin, Breslau, Freiburg, and Heidelberg, Neisser defended his PhD dissertation in 1888 in Berlin, with Prof. Paul Ehrlich as his advisor, and earned a habilitation degree in 1893 in Königsberg (now Kalliningrad, Russia). In 1895, he came to Stettin to take the post of physician in chief and head of the internal disorders department at the municipal hospital, a position he held until his retirement in 1931. Neisser was an innovative researcher and a prolific writer. Among several dozen relevant publications, his 1904 paper on a new, safer method of brain puncture for diagnostic purposes, developed in collaboration with Kurt Pollack,[78] attracted great interest worldwide. In a chapter on brain puncture published thirty years later for the monumental, seventeen-volume *Handbuch der Neurologie*, Neisser stated that the primary reason the overall results of brain surgery in Germany were significantly worse than in Sweden was that, in the latter country, in-depth preoperative diagnostics, including brain puncture, were performed more frequently, thus allowing a more reliable measurement of the pros and cons of surgical intervention.[79]

Does this statement mean that Neisser had personal, firsthand knowledge of the Swedish approach to his diagnostic method because he had visited Sweden, trained Swedish physicians, or was in contact with them? The sources available in Szczecin shed no light on the matter, but perhaps Swedish archives could. There is one hint in a later biography of Prof. Neisser that suggests that this might be the case. After 1933, Neisser, a German patriot of Jewish origins living in Berlin, suffered increasingly severe state harassment. In 1942, he obtained a visa to enter Sweden; the Nazi authorities, however, denied him a visa to exit Germany. On October 1, 1942, after he received a transportation order to Theresienstadt, Prof. Neisser took a lethal dose of morphine; he died a few days later, never regaining consciousness, in a Jewish hospital in Berlin.[80] Had Prof. Neisser obtained a Swedish visa because that was the only escape option open to him or because there were people waiting for him in Sweden? This is another question that Swedish sources might be able to answer.

Of course, medicine in Stettin in 1800–1945 had a dark side, too. This should be examined with as much effort as the brighter side and as far as the surviving sources allow. One of the "dark matters" I find most intriguing refers to the circumstances of the official dissolution of the Physicians' Society in 1933. In 1932, the president of the society was a Dr. Mühlmann, the head of the radiology department at the municipal hospital and the founder-president of the local Society for Radiology. In 1933, not only were both societies dissolved but Dr. Mühlmann lost his job. The latter event strongly suggests that he was of Jewish origin. At that time, the president of the Abend-Referate, the only doctors' society that officially existed in Stettin after 1933, was a Dr. Rudolf Lemke. He is mentioned as the head of the Scientific Society of Stettin's Physicians in the protocol published in *Münchener medizinische Wochenschrift* in 1939.[81] Does this mean that the society, though officially dissolved, was actually taken over by the supporters of the new power? Did the Jewish members of Stettin's medical community experience any displays of collegiality, that quality so highly treasured by the society's founders eighty years earlier, from the physicians of "pure German blood"? The chances that these questions—especially the last one—will ever be adequately answered are rather slim, but these answers should still be sought. There are also other questions more directly related to the question of Stettin's involvement in the transfer of knowledge in the Baltic Sea region. How many of Stettin's Jewish doctors who managed to escape from Germany settled in Sweden? Did they take an active role in the development of medical science there? It is possible that, with access to Swedish archival sources, some light will be shed on these matters, too.

Dark or bright, relevant on an international or merely local level, the medical portion of Stettin's history deserves to be made known. Without it, our understanding of the Baltic region's past will remain incomplete. Without it, the picture of Stettin that we, the Szczeciners, are trying to reconstruct in order to embrace our city's fate, both past and future, will be false and deformed. There are so many fascinating, inspiring (or even terrifying) people, places, and stories from the history of medicine in Stettin waiting to be restored to our common memory. Chances are that Stettin did contribute not only to a local but also a national and even international discussion about medicine as a science and practice. Stettin's role in the Baltic Sea region, when reassembled using the fragments found in the dispersed surviving sources, will prove to have been more relevant than previously expected. However difficult and time consuming this process of recovery may be, it must be done. This chapter represents the beginning of that journey.

Notes

1. An example of such cooperation is the German-Polish research program that aimed to improve the early diagnosis of rare genetic disorders in infants born in the Pomeranian region, launched in 2012. "Polish-German Newborn Screening in West Pomeranian Province" accessed October 10, 2018, http://naukawpolsce. pap.pl/aktualnosci/news%2C392942%2Cpolsko-niemieckie-badania-przesiewowe-noworodkow-w-zachodniopomorskim.html.

2. The literature on VSELs and the VSEL controversy is very rich, and easily accessible online. For the relatively latest developments in the debate on VSELs, consult the contents of the April 2014 issue of *Stem Cell and Development*, http://online.liebertpub. com/toc/scd/23/7#utm_source=PR&utm_medium=email&utm_campaign=SCD.

3. For example, in May and June 2015, two major research papers from Scandinavian countries were published there: one analyzing the tumor spectrum in non-BRCA hereditary breast cancer families in Sweden (Camilla Wendt, Annika Lindblom, Brita Arver, Anna von Wachenfeldt, and Sara Margolin, "Tumour Spectrum in Non-BRCA Hereditary Breast Cancer Families in Sweden," *Hereditary Cancer in Clinical Practice* 13, no. 15 [2015], http://www.hccpjournal. com/content/13/1/15), and the other validating the common modifiers of BRCA1 penetrance in BRCA1 mutation carriers in Norway (Cecilie Heramb, Per Olaf Ekstrøm, Kukatharmini Tharmaratnam, Eivind Hovig, Pål Møller, and Lovise Mæhle, "Ten Modifiers of BRCA1 Penetrance Validated in a Norwegian Series," *Hereditary Cancer in Clinical Practice* 13, no. 14 [2015], http://www.hccpjournal.com/ content/13/1/14).

4. Bogdan Wachowiak, ed., *Dzieje Szczecina*, vol. 3, *1806–1945* (Szczecin: 13 Muz, 1994).

5. These four volumes were published under the auspices of Prof. Gerard Labuda (1916–2010), one of the most renowned and respected Polish historians, who also coedited the two initial parts of the series. The first two volumes, covering from prehistory to the end of the 1700s, were released in 1983 and 1985, respectively; the last volume, covering 1945–90, was published in 1998. The gap between the second (1985) and third volumes (1994) clearly indicates that it was the Prussian/German past of the city that its citizens found difficult or dangerous to handle.

6. Martin Wehrmann, *Geschichte der Stadt Stettin* (Stettin: Saunier, 1911). This work was reprinted by Weltbild, Augsburg, in 1993.

7. "O nas," sedina.pl—Portal Miłośników Dawnego Szczecina, accessed February 25, 2015, http://sedina.pl/wordpress/index.php/sedina-pl/o-nas/.

8. The Bibliographical Database of Western Pomerania lists 179 books in the 1990–2015 period with "Szczecin" and "history" as keywords. Bibliografia Pomorza Zachodniego, accessed February 2, 2015, http://aleph.ksiaznica.szczecin.pl/F/MRAUXU5238LHFKEUX2Q9GDDNR94IYX66KS76BUB9D6SHCTF LJG-03043?func=short-0&set_number=013016.

9. Jan Musekamp, *Stettin und Szczecin: Metamorphosen einer Stadt von 1945 bis 2005* (Wiesbaden: Otto Harrassowitz, 2010). The Polish edition of this book was printed in 2013.

10. A brief overview of the history of the forced migrations historiography includes Jérôme Elie, "Histories of Refugee and Forced Migration Studies," in *The Oxford Handbook of Refugees & Forced Migration Studies*, ed. Elena Fiddian-Qasmiyeh, Gil Loeschner, Kaly Long and Nando Sigona (Oxford: Oxford University Press 2014), 23–36.

11. An interesting overview of the English language historiography of the German expulsions is Rebecca Strung, *From Expulsion to Ethnic Cleansing: The Historiography of the German Expulsion*, accessed July 1, 2015. http://www.academia.edu/474761/From_Expulsion_to_Ethnic_Cleansing_The_Historiography_of_the_German_Expulsion.

12. Much of this research was supported by the Western German Federal Ministry for Expellees, Refugees and War Victims. For example, Theodor Schieder, ed., *Dokumentation der Verteibung der Deutschen aus Ost-Mitteleuropa*, 6 vols. (Bonn: Bundesministerium für Vertriebene, 1953–63). Large parts of this collection were translated into English by Vivian Stranders (Bonn: Bundesministerium für Vertriebene, 1961).

13. For example: *Trzy pytania i trzy odpowiedzi: Prawda o deportacjach Polaków pod panowaniem sowieckim* [Three questions and three answers: The truth on the deportations of poles under the Soviet rule] (London: Egzekutywa Zjednoczenia Narodowego, 1964); *Documents of Polish-Soviet Relations*, vols. 1 and 2 (London: Instytut Historyczny im. gen. Sikorskiego, 1961 and 1968).

14. For example, Julian Siedlecki, *Losy Polaków w ZSRR w latach 1939–1986* (London: Gryf 1987); this book was reprinted in 1989 in Wrocław by the underground Agencja Wydawnicza Solidarności Walczącej (Publishing House of Fighting Solidarity).

15. The most important works published officially in Poland in that time (with the significant use of the word "repatriation" in reference to population transfer) were Krystyna Kersten, *Repatriacja ludności polskiej po II wojnie światowej (studium historyczne)* [Repatriation of Polish population after World War II (historical study)] (Wrocław: Zakład Narodowy im. Ossolińskich, 1974); Tadeusz Bugaj, *Dzieci polskie w ZSRR i ich repatriacja 1939–1952* [Polish children in the USSR and their repatriation, 1939–1952] (Jelenia Góra: Karkonoskie Towarzystwo Naukowe, 1986).

16. Göran Rystad, ed., *The Uprooted. Forced Migration as an International Problem in the Post-War Era* (Lund: Lund University Press; Bromley: Chartwell-Bratt, 1990).

17. Philipp Ther and Ana Siljak, eds., *Redrawing Nations: Ethnic Cleansing in East-Central Europe, 1944–1948* (Lanham, MD: Rowman & Littlefield, 2001). The final shape and scope of this seminal publication resulted from and was influenced by the

devastating ethnic conflicts in the former Yugoslavia, still ongoing at the time of the Gliwice conference.

18. Consult the table of contents in Fiddian-Qasmiyeh et al., *Refugees and Forced Migration*, xiii–xvii.

19. Norman Davies and Roger Moorhouse, *Microcosm: Portrait of a Central European City* (London: Jonathan Cape, 2002). Several editions of the book have been published in English; it has also been published in Polish, German, French, Italian, and Czech.

20. "Theodore R. Weeks," Southern Illinois University, accessed July 7, 2015, http://cola.siu.edu/history/faculty-and-staff/faculty/weeks.php. A list of selected works by Weeks is available on the website of the Center for Urban History of East Central Europe , http://www.lvivcenter.org/download.php?downloadid=341, accessed July 7, 2015.

21. Christine Kulke, dissertation prospectus, University of California at Berkeley, accessed July 7, 2015, http://www.sscnet.ucla.edu/soc/groups/scr/kulke.htm.

22. "Edmund Kizik," accessed October 10, 2018, https://ihpan.edu.pl/pracownicy/45-edmund-kizik/.

23. Radosław Gaziński, Paweł Gut, and Maciej Szukała, eds., *Staatsarchiv Stettin— Wegweiser durch die Bestände bis zum Jahr 1945* (Munich: R. Oldenburg, 2004), 69–71, 75–78, 344–46.

24. Heinrich Berghaus, *Geschichte der Stadt Stettin*, 2 vols. (Berlin: Verlag von J. Riemschneider, 1875–76).

25. Wehrmann, *Geschichte*, 486.

26. Bronisław Seyda, "Z dziejów dawnych aptek szczecińskich" [On the history of Stettin's drugstores], *Farmacja Polska*, no. 4 (1961): 79–83; Seyda, "Z dziejów szczecińskich szpitali" [On the history of Stettin's hospitals], *Przegląd Zachodniopomorski*, no. 5 (1966): 41–53; Seyda, "Szpitale, apteki i epidemie w dawnym Szczecinie" [Hospitals, pharmacies and epidemics in the old Stettin], unpublished manuscript, 1969.

27. Seyda, *Szpitale*, 2.

28. Wachowiak, *Dzieje Szczecina*, 225–27, 475–77.

29. According to my knowledge, there are two Polish monographs on medicine in Stettin in earlier times, both unpublished. Iwona Gosk, "Praktyka lekarska i problemy medyczne Pomorza u schyłku epoki napoleońskiej" [Medical practice and medical problems in Pomerania at the end of Napoleonic era] (PhD diss., Pomeranian Medical Academy, 2000); Dorota Gosk, "Walka z zarazami na Pomorzu na początku XVII wieku" [The fight against pestilences in Pomerania in the early 17th century] (PhD diss., Pomeranian Medical Academy, 2001). There is also a book on public care for the poor in the districts of Stettin and Köslin prior to 1872, published by the University of Szczecin Press. Agnieszka Chlebowska, *Między miłosierdziem a obowiązkiem: Publiczna opieka nad ubogimi na Pomorzu w latach 1815–1872 na przykładzie rejencji szczecińskiej i koszalińskiej* (Szczecin: Wydawnictwo Naukowe Uniwersytetu Szczecińskiego 2002).

30. Zbigniew Machoy, ed., *Od średniowiecznego przytułku do Samodzielnego Publicznego Szpitala Klinicznego Nr 2 Pomorskiej Akademii Medycznej w Szczecinie* [From a medieval hospice to the Public Clinical Hospital No. 2 of the Pomeranian Medical Academy of Szczecin] (Szczecin: Wydawnictwo Pomorskiego Uniwersytetu Medycznego 2014).

31. Tadeusz Zajączkowski and Elżbieta M. Wojewska-Zajączkowska, "The Beginnings of Urology in Szczecin: Felix Hagen (1880–1962), the First Head of the Department of Urology in Stettin," *Annales Academiae Medicae Stettinensis* 56 (2010): 137–44.

32. Tadeusz Zajączkowski, "The Beginnings of the Antituberculosis Service in Stettin: Hermann Braeuning—the First Director of the Tuberculosis Hospital in Stettin-Hohenkrug (Szczecin-Zdunowo)," *Annales Academiae Medicae Stettinensis* 57 (2011): 105–9.

33. For example, "Zakład opiekuńczy Bethanien," *Wikipedia.pl*, accessed February 26, 2015, https://pl.wikipedia.org/wiki/Zak%C5%82ad_opieku%C5%84czy_%E2%80%9EBethanien%E2%80%9D.

34. Hermann Manzke, *Sanitätsrat Dr. August Steffen (1825–1910): Nestor und Spiritus rector der Kinderheilkunde in Deutschland und Mitteleuropa* (Kiel: Ludwig, 2005).

35. Friedrich Bartels, *Kückenmühler Spuren: Die Geschichte der Kückenmühler Anstalten in Stettin, von ihrer Gründung im Jahr 1863, über ihre Aufslösung im Jahr 1940, bis zu dem lebendigen Erbe im Jahr 2013* (Greifswald: Griepommern Verlag, 2013).

36. For example, Ilse Gudden-Lüddeke, ed., *Chronik des Stadt Stettin* (Leer: Verlag G. Rautenberg, 1993).

37. The city of Stettin as such was excluded from the District of Randow, yet large parts of the city as of the late 1930s (the Bredow, Grabow, Frauendorf, Nemitz, Eckerberg, Podejuch, Finkenwalde Districts and others) were not within Stettin's borders in the nineteenth century; these are included in the Randow collections.

38. Archiwum Państwowe w Szczecinie, Rejencja Szczecińska, Wydział Prezydialny, signatures 8051 and 8108–11.

39. Archiwum Państwowe w Szczecinie, Rejencja Szczecińska, Wydział Prezydialny, signatures 8093–94, 8114–15; Naczelne Prezydium Prowincji Pomorskiej, signatures 1894 and 2378.

40. Archiwum Państwowe w Szczecinie, Naczelne Prezydium Prowincji Pomorskiej, signature 2374.

41. Archiwum Państwowe w Szczecinie, Rejencja Szczecińska, Wydział Prezydialny, signatures 8133–48 and 8222.

42. Archiwum Państwowe w Szczecinie, Naczelne Prezydium Prowincji Pomorskiej, signatures 2422, 2424, 2458, 2463, 2470, 2474, 2482, 2487, 2508, 2510–19, 2537, and 2541; Rejencja Szczecińska, Wydział Prezydialny, signatures 8171–73 and 8180.

43. Archiwum Państwowe w Szczecinie, Rejencja Szczecińska, Wydział Prezydialny, signatures 8037–38.

44. Archiwum Państwowe w Szczecinie, Rejencja Szczecińska, Wydział Prezydialny, signatures 8210–12; Zespół Samorządowy Prowincji Pomorskiej, signatures 207–21; Naczelne Prezydium Prowincji Pomorskiej, signatures 2338–53.

45. Archiwum Państwowe w Szczecinie, Starostwo Powiatowe Szczecin, signature 609.

46. Archiwum Państwowe w Szczecinie, Naczelne Prezydium Prowincji Pomorskiej, signatures 2266–75, 2281–82 and 2307–10.

47. [Ludwig] Freund, *Der wissenschaftliche Verein der Ärzte und die öffentlichen Heilanstalten zu Stettin: Zum fünfzigjährigen Jubiläum 1858–1908 im Auftrage des Vereins herausgegeben* (Stettin: H. Susenbeth, 1908).

48. [Ludwig] Freund, *Gedächtnisrede für dem Geheimen Sanitätsrat Dr. Carl Ludwig Schleich* (Stettin: H. Susenbeth, 1907).

49. Rudolf Lemke, "Wissenschaftlicher Verein der Aerzte zu Stettin und Umgebung und Militärärztliche Gesellschaft Stetin. Sitzung vom 12. April 1938," *Münchener medizinische Wochenschrift*, no. 31 (1939): 1213–14.

50. Freund, *Der wissenschaftliche Verein*, 41–42, 46–47. Among other contributions, Freund mentions the society's relevant role in the planning of the municipal sewage system, the close cooperation with the city council in the campaign against high infant mortality, and the establishment of the *Rettungsgesellschaft* (providing first-aid education and emergency care to the city's inhabitants).

51. Freund, *Der wissenschaftliche Verein*, 27. For example, the society's members, Dr. Hans Schmid of the Bethanien Hospital and Prof. Karl Schuchardt of the Municipal Hospital, were among the first researchers to examine the clinical effect of Koch's tuberculin in the autumn of 1890.

52. Berghaus, *Geschichte*, 1:220–28.

53. "Honorowy Obywatel Miasta Szczecina," *Internetowa Encyklopedia Szczecina*, accessed February 2, 2015, http://encyklopedia.szczecin.pl/wiki/Honorowy_Obywatel_Miasta_Szczecina.

54. Heinrich Frey, "Ein Beitrag zur Kenntniss der Microlepidopteren," *Entomologische Zeitung*, nos. 4–6 (1871): 121–22.

55. Freund did not know the names of the society's first executive committee members, but he assumed that Dr. Behm was a member (*Der wissenschaftliche Verein*, 8). Behm's presidency seems to be confirmed by the fact that he was the cohost of the Thirty-Eighth Congress of German Naturalists and Physicians in 1863 (the only one that ever took place in Stettin), and the coeditor of the congress proceedings, together with Carl August Dohrn, the founder and president of the famous Stettiner Entomologische Verein. Indeed, a brief entry in the 1858 address book (the only issue up till 1880 to contain that sort of information) clarifies that Dr. Behm was the Society's copresident, together with Dr. Friedrich Herman Glubrecht.

56. Berghaus, *Geschichte*, 1–61.

57. [Ludwig Eduard Emil] Behm, "Tertiär bei Stettin," *Zeitschrift der Deutschen geologischen Gesellschaft* (1854): 270–73; Behm, "Die Tertiärformation von Stettin," *Zeitschrift der Deutschen geologischen Gesellschaft* (1857): 323–53, (1863): 420–34; Behm, "Tertiärformation von Stettin," in *Amtliche Bericht des 38. Versammlung deutscher Naturforscher und Aerzte* (Stettin, 1864), 90–98.

58. Wilhelm Deecke, *Geologie von Pommern* (Berlin: Gebr. Borntaeger, 1907), 120, 143, 160. "Literatura," in *Księga Puszczy Bukowej*, ed. Grażyna Domian and Krzysztof Ziarnko, (Szczecin: Regionalna Dyrekcja Ochrony Środowiska w Szczecinie, 2010), 1:462.

59. Friedrich Wilhelm Gottlieb Rostkovius and Ewald Ludwig Wilhelm Schmidt, *Flora Sedinensis exhibens plantas phanerogamas spontaneas nec non plantas praecipuas agri Sinemundii* (Sedini: Formis Struckianis, 1824).

60. L. P. F. Dittmar et al., *Die Pilze Deutschlands: Nürnberg 1817–1862*, ed. Jacob Sturm (Nürnberg, 1817–62). Detailed bibliographical information on Rostkovius's contribution to this series, as accessed February 2, 2015: "Bibliothek Christian Volbracht," Mikolibri, http://www.mykolibri.de/bibliothek/index.html?f=b&b=33023/html.

61. For example, Rudolph Lehmann, "Ueber eine neue Heliceen-Gattung," *Malakozoologische Blätter* 9 (1862): 111–12; Lehmann, "Die Nacktschnecken aus der Umgebung Stettins und in Pommern," *Malakozoologische Blätter* 9 (1862): 156–93, tabl. 2–5; Lehmann, "Neue Nacktschnecke aus Australien," *Malakozoologische Blätter* 11 (1864): 145–49.

62. Rudolph Lehmann, *Die lebenden Schnecken und Muscheln der Umgegend Stettins und in Pommern, mit besonderer Berücksichtigung ihres anatomischen Baues* (Cassel: Theodor Fischer, 1873). The book contains an introduction by E. Martens highlighting the importance of Dr. Lehmann's contribution to German malacology.

63. Eckhard Wendt, "Buschan, Georg," in *Stettiner Lebensbilder: Veröffentlichungen der Historischen Kommission für Pommern*, series 5, vol. 40 (Cologne: Böhlau Verlag, 2004), 106–8.

64. Otto Kunkel, "Martin Bethe (1866–1956)," *Baltische Studien*, n.s., 46 (1959): 10–11.

65· Bestand 21836, Genealogischer Nachlass Martin Bethe, 1 linear meter of material.

66. Freund, *Der wissenschaftliche Verein*, 8–9.

67. Out of these 109 publications (not counting book reviews, obituaries, etc.), August Steffen authored 74, including eight monographs. Manzke, *Sanitätsrat Dr. August Steffen*, 207–13.

68. Harald Hirschprung, "Stuhltragheit Neugeborener in Folge von Dilatation und Hypertrophie des Colons," *Jahrbuch für Kinderheilkunde*, n.s., no. 27 (1888): 1–7.

69. His most important publications on that matter: Ernst Brand, *Hydrotherapie des Typhus* (Stettin, 1863); Brand, *Zur Hydrotherapie des Typhus: Bericht über in St. Petersburg, Stettin und Luxemburg hydriatisch behandlte Fälle* (Stettin: Verlag von Th. von der Nahmer, 1863); Brand, *Die Heilung des Typhus* (Berlin, 1868); Brand, *Die Wasserbehandlung der typhösen Fieber* (Tübingen, 1877).

70. Brand's hydrotherapeutic management of typhoid fever, for example, became a subject of intense interest in Canada after his statistics were published in the *Union médicale du Canada* in 1874. John MacFarlane, "Les miasmes, les microbes et les médecines: La diffusion des idées anciennes et nouveles dans l'*Union médicale du Canada*; le cas de la fièvre typhoid (1872–1900)," *Scientia Canadensis*, no. 26 (2002): 68, https://www.doi.org/ 10.7202/800443ar.

71. "Ernst Brand, MD," *British Medical Journal* 1, no. 1889 (March 13, 1897): 692.

72. *Deutsche Vierteljahrsschrift für öffentliche Gesundheitspflege, herasugegeben von Dr. Göttisheim in Basel, Stadtbaurath Hobrecht in Stettin, Prof. Dr. C. Reclam in Leipzig, Dr. G. Varrentrapp in Frankfurt a. M., Dr. Wassefuhr in Stettin. Erste Ausgabe* (Braunschweig, 1869). There are three lengthy papers by Wasserfuhr in this volume: two strictly scientific publications and a polemical essay on the most desirable ways of implementing public health regulations in German lands.

73. Hermann Wasserfuhr, *Untersuchungen über die Kindersterblichkeit in Stettin, vom Standpunkte der öffentlichen Medicin* (Stettin: Leon Saunier, 1867); Wasserfuhr, "Die Sterblichkeit der Neugeborenen in Deutschland," *Deutsche Vierteljahrsschrift für öffentliche Gesundheitspflege* 1 (1868): 533–53.

74. G. W. Scharlau, *Lehrbuch der Pharmazie und ihrer Hülfswissenschaften zum Gebrauch für Aerzte, Apotheker und Studirende der Medizin* (Leipzig: Johann Ambrosius

Barth, 1837). The textbook was reprinted as a part of the series Literaturdenkmäler der Medizin- und Pharmaziegeschichte (Osnabrück: Kuballe, 1981).

75. For example, G. W. Scharlau, *Theoretisch-praktische Abhandlung über den Typhus, die Cholera, die Chlorosis u. die Harnröhren-Verengungen* (Stettin: Friedrich Nagel, 1853), http://www.mdz-nbn-resolving.de/urn/resolver.pl?urn=urn:nbn:de:bvb:12-bsb10479661-3; G. W. Scharlau, *Klinische Mittheilungen aus dem Gebiete der Wasser-Heilkunde* (Berlin: August Hirschwald, 1857), http://www.mdz-nbn-resolving.de/urn/resolver.pl?urn=urn:nbn:de:bvb:12-bsb10479662-9.

76. The publication that sparked the debate was [Ernst Siegfried] Lehrs and [Gustav Wilhelm] Scharlau, *Dr. Schönlein als Arzt und klinischer Lehrer aus der Schilderung des Dr. Güterbock einer unabweisbaren Kritik unterworfen* (Berlin: Enslin, 1842), http://www.mdz-nbn-resolving.de/urn/resolver.pl?urn=urn:nbn:de:bvb:12-bsb10473181-0.

77. G. W. Scharlau, *Die Nahrungsmittel und die Ernährung* (Leipzig: Ernst Keil, 1858), http://www.mdz-nbn-resolving.de/urn/resolver.pl?urn=urn:nbn:de:bvb:12-bsb10477745-1.

78. Ernst Neisser and Kurt Pollack, "Die Hirnpunktion: Probepunktion und Punktion des Gehirnes und seiner Häute durch den intakten Schädel," *Mitteilungen aus Grenzgebiete der Medizin und Chirurgie* 13 (1904): 807–96.

79. Ernst Neisser and Edmund Forster, "Die Hirnpunktion," in *Allgemeine Neurologie VII/2*, ed. Oswald Bumke and Otfrid Foerster (Berlin: Springer-Verlag 1936), 135.

80. Suse Vogel, "Die letzten Lebensjahre meines Vaters Prof. Ernst Neisser, 1939–1942" (unpublished manuscript, Kassel, 1947). Leo Baeck Institute Memoire Collection, accessed July 8, 2015, http://access.cjh.org/home.php?type=extid&term=1052600#1.

81. Rudolf Lemke, "Wissenschaftlicher Verein der Aerzte zu Stettin und Umgebung und Militärärztliche Gesellschaft Stetin: Sitzung vom 12. April 1938," *Münchener medizinische Wochenschrift*, no. 31 (1939): 1213–14.

Chapter Four

Smallpox in Malmö, Sweden, 1932

Disputed Knowledge of Infection, Contagion, and Vaccination in the Baltic Sea Region

Motzi Eklöf

In the beginning of 1932 a small epidemic of smallpox broke out in the coastal city of Malmö in southern Sweden. Ten people were afflicted, and one died. After the first cases of smallpox appeared, the first mass vaccination of an entire Swedish city took place. Both the decision to carry out mass vaccination and its implementation became the subjects of animated discussions and mutual accusations. The vaccine from the National Bacteriological Laboratory that was used also became the focus of a deep conflict among different medical experts. They were not in agreement as to how the vaccine should be manufactured, what contents were permissible, how the contents should be tested, and what the best methods of vaccination were. After vaccination a relatively large share of the population became ill, and four died after demonstrating symptoms of problems with the central nervous system. Experts disagreed as to what significance high virulence and varying contents of the vaccine had for people's health and what could be regarded as the normal reactions to vaccination versus unexpected and undesirable complications and side effects. On one side of this disagreement stood the highest medical authority in the country and, on the other, the general public that was affected in terms of both health and economics and that wanted to know what had gone wrong. It turned out to be difficult for the medical authorities to investigate the events, as the persons bearing the responsibility were reluctant to cooperate. The events during and after the Malmö epidemic form the basis for ethical and political judgments that remain relevant to today's public health policies.

Since the turn of the nineteenth century, the question of vaccination has been characterized by a rhetoric within which medical science and rationality have been placed in opposition to what has been said to be religious superstition, irrational skepticism, and myths of vaccination critics. At the same time, knowledge about infectious diseases, vaccines, and vaccination has always been characterized by uncertainty and changeability even within the framework of medicine. Doctors and scholars from various specialties, veterinarians, and health-care administrators, as well as individual and collective representatives for the general public, have maintained rival claims to the right to interpret current knowledge on smallpox, vaccination, and public health. Furthermore, there has been a lack of consensus concerning what should be considered legitimate grounds for knowledge: explanatory theoretical models, empirical experiments, epidemiologic statistics, or personal experience. There has been a flexible boundary between experimental and established measures concerned with vaccination and actually combating epidemics, where the need for a new order has as a rule appeared first when looking in the rearview mirror. In addition, there have been discussions as to whether vaccination should be compulsory or voluntary, and as to whether mass vaccination or selective measures directed toward persons at risk should be set in motion in times of threatening epidemics. The decisions made concerning safety and risks associated with vaccinations have been debated. All these questions were discussed in relation to smallpox vaccination and most recently in conjunction with the 2009 vaccination against swine influenza and its consequences.

On the basis of a combination of scientific and political reasons, various countries have developed differing strategies with regard to laws, regulations, and other measures dealing with contagious diseases. The strategies vary over time in accordance with new knowledge in bacteriology, hygiene, and disease treatment and in light of new estimations of the danger and risk of spreading diseases. These repeated changes have also been true for smallpox vaccination.

How can a threat to public health and uncertain knowledge be dealt with and communicated in a way that reassures and builds trust among the people who are going to allow themselves to be vaccinated and thus contribute to the operation of a preventive public health policy?

Smallpox in Sweden

Smallpox was and is a feared disease that is extremely contagious and has high mortality in its most virulent form, *Variola major*. In Sweden smallpox claimed many victims in the eighteenth century, particularly children. During the nineteenth century the disease occurred more seldom. The last great epidemic took place in the Stockholm area 1873–74.[1] The smaller outbreaks in the country during the twentieth century began with persons who had recently entered the country, both foreign citizens and Swedes returning home; the last cases occurred in 1963 in Stockholm.

Sweden early on tried the vaccine introduced by Jenner in 1796 and was among the first countries to pass national legislation making smallpox vaccination compulsory for children.[2] The Swedish law was in force from 1816 until 1976 and was revised and complemented during those years by demands for the revaccination of certain groups such as military recruits; foreign workers and prisoners; certain professions, for example, customs officers or general health-care practitioners; and, to the extent that it was deemed necessary, in case of an epidemic. During the nineteenth century it became clear that vaccination in childhood provided protection for a limited time, if at all, but vaccination was motivated with the argument that, in case of infection, those who were vaccinated would receive a milder form of the disease than those who were not. The age at which children should be vaccinated varied from two to six years; in the period after World War II, they were often vaccinated as infants.

The historian Peter Sköld has studied how smallpox was dealt with during the eighteenth and nineteenth centuries in Sweden with focus on vaccination's success factors.[3] He states that more than 90 percent of the population allowed their children to be vaccinated before the age of two years, and the remaining 10 percent in the years that followed. Summarily, he concludes that the number of cases of smallpox was reduced primarily as a result of compulsory vaccination, of general acceptance of vaccination, of vaccination coverage being very good, and of low opposition to the compulsory law. The obedience of the Swedish people to the vaccination law was attributed to belief in authority, pragmatism, and the will to appease the state. Peter Baldwin compares vaccination practices in Germany, England, France, and Sweden 1830–1930. He ends his historical description of Sweden in 1916 with the revision of the vaccination law that was supposed to make possible certain exceptions to the obligation to vaccinate.[4] Baldwin draws the conclusion that compulsion was modified in the same direction as in England, where the so-called conscience clause in the corresponding British legislation from 1907 made it simple to apply for exception from the obligation to be vaccinated, a right that some hundred thousand people were soon granted.[5]

During the twentieth century, the history of smallpox in Sweden, however, was characterized neither by lesser degree of compulsion in the beginning of the century nor a general acceptance of and obedience to the law. At a time when the disease was no longer endemic in the country, compulsory vaccination was questioned by the general public and in the parliament.[6] The arguments in favor of abolishing the requirement were reports that both children and adults who had not been recently vaccinated could become ill or die as a result of vaccination, as well as the view that in a democracy no more compulsion than was necessary should be used. During times when society was free of smallpox, many people reached the conclusion that the risks from vaccination were greater than the risk of being afflicted with smallpox. When smallpox entered the country, the tendency to vaccinate oneself and one's children increased.

Smallpox Comes to Town

On December 10, 1931, a Swedish bricklayer returned to Malmö after working for a week in the Urals in Russia.[7] After arriving home he had a slight illness for a time, but his daughter, who was only a few months old, became even sicker. On January 14 the mother took the child to the Flensburg Children's Hospital, where the head doctor, Greta Muhl, immediately suspected smallpox and saw to it that the child was transferred to the Epidemic Hospital, which was under the direction of Ebbe Petrén. The main responsibility for following the course of infectious diseases and leading the reaction to epidemics lay by law with the first city physician, J. Axel Höjer. Those persons who had been in the waiting room at the Flensburg hospital were vaccinated, as was the personnel in both places. The rooms at the hospital were disinfected, and so too were the homes of exposed persons. Contacts who might potentially have been infected were traced and vaccinated. The existing supply of vaccine was depleted, and new vaccine arrived from Stockholm on January 15.

Starting from January 16, there were initially small notices in the newspapers about a case of a milder form of smallpox, *alastrim*, and the situation was said to be under control: "No danger! Precautionary measures have been taken."[8] Two weeks later the danger of smallpox was generally spoken about with significantly bolder headlines. By that time it was obvious that it was a matter of *Variola major*. The disinfection had not been sufficiently thorough; all the people who had casually passed through the hospital rooms where the child had stayed had not been traced. The vaccine used the first days was deemed "weak" and "did not take," that is, no immunological reaction had taken place in a number of vaccinations. It had not been considered feasible to isolate all the staff members who had been in contact with the child, and these people could move around freely.[9] A nurse's aide from the Epidemic Hospital fell ill when she was in town. New cases of smallpox made their appearance.

The Vaccination Campaign

There were thus several paths of infection that had not been secured. At that point Axel Höjer convinced his Public Health Board, the County Administrative Board, and the Royal Medical Board to offer the entire population of Malmö and visitors general vaccination on January 30.

Fifty-five young doctors and medical students were assigned the task of vaccinating the general population in public locations. In addition, private doctors carried out vaccinations. Vaccination was voluntary, but, according to Höjer in his daily radio bulletins on the situation, those who did not get a vaccination could blame only themselves.

The vaccine was requisitioned from the National Bacteriological Laboratory (NBL) in Stockholm, which sent both small vials and bottles with vaccine for fifty persons.[10] A gap in access to vaccine appeared on the morning of January 31, when NBL had not read the train's timetable carefully and put the package with the vaccine on what was thought to be the night train to Malmö, but which stopped halfway. Höjer then appealed to Denmark for help. The head of the Danish serum institute, Thorvald Madsen, personally flew over the sound immediately with vaccine sufficient for several thousand people. From midday on January 31, Swedish vaccine was again available.

After a couple of weeks more than 112,000 residents of Malmö had been vaccinated, about 87 percent of the city's population; many of the remaining had been vaccinated recently, such as children and practitioners in professions where vaccination was required. The epidemic was prevented from spreading, and Höjer received credit for acting so resolutely. Besides the primary case with the bricklayer and the secondary case with his daughter, there were eight tertiary cases, seven of whom were infected at the Flensburg Children's Hospital, including the head doctor, Muhl, and the nurse's aide, both of whom had been vaccinated several times. One of the infected who had been vaccinated at a late stage succumbed.

In an early phase of the epidemic, Höjer had been criticized by a fellow physician on Malmö's Public Health Board for negligence in fighting the epidemic. If the contact cases from the Flensburg hospital had been carefully monitored, general vaccination could have been avoided.[11] A "weak" vaccine was only part of the problem.

Animal Vaccine

In comparison Sweden used human lymph longer than many other countries characterized by transfer of the smallpox infection from one individual to another. Animal vaccine had been manufactured on a small scale in Stockholm since 1884, but not until 1916 was it required by law as the first alternative. At the same time, primarily doctors or, eventually, medical students were designated as vaccinators. Previously, this had been a task mainly for the parish sextons, organists, midwives, and other specially commissioned persons, such as teachers.

According to the instructions issued by the Royal Medical Board in 1917, the vaccine, or lymph, should be produced in a calf's stomach.[12] The substance was to be taken from natural cowpox or real smallpox; in the latter case five passages through the calf were necessary. So-called retrovaccination could be performed; temporary passage through a human or a rabbit was then used to increase the weakened virulence of the vaccine. The calves were slaughtered after the vaccine was harvested, and their health was checked at the autopsy.[13] The vaccine, with assigned numbers that referred to a specific calf, was produced by lymph being mixed with glycerin for storage and to reduce the bacterial content from the hide of the calf. It was then ground and filtered through sterile gas. The occurrence of disease-causing bacteria was then checked using flat-bottomed culture plates, both after the harvest and after storage for at least a month.[14] The vaccine was to be checked by an inspector appointed by the Royal Medical Board.[15]

The conversion to animal vaccine was used as an argument for retention of the compulsory law when the law was challenged and revised in 1916. It was said that the risks of spreading diseases, such as syphilis and tuberculosis from person to person that accompanied human lymph were now totally ruled out.

Side Effects, Reactions, or Complications

Criticism soon arose not only concerning the use of "weak" vaccine during the first weeks of the vaccination campaign but also concerning vaccine that was too "strong." According to the newspapers, 10–15 percent of the vaccinated acquired the "vaccination disease."[16] They had swollen arms, fever, and were, in general, unable to work. But some also had deep and extensive necrotic, weeping pox that took weeks and months to heal; lymph glands were attacked, and on some patients extra pox appeared and spread over the entire body.

Most serious from the point of view of health were the ten or so cases of encephalitis (brain inflammation) following vaccination, four of whom died, including a woman whose death was attributed to smallpox.

This possible consequence of smallpox vaccination was well known; such cases had appeared in the European countries since the mid-1920s. This had caused the Royal Medical Board to issue new directives to the vaccinators to examine those who were to be vaccinated thoroughly and to make exceptions for persons with certain diseases or a predisposition to such diseases, such as the children and siblings of persons who had previously suffered from diseases of the central nervous system.[17] When several cases of encephalitis occurred almost simultaneously after the comprehensive vaccination campaign, the Royal Medical Board chose to cancel the campaign on February 15.[18] By then, the risk of further contagion was considered negligible.

A Veterinarian Starts a Debate

On February 17, the veterinarian Hilding Magnusson from the Agricultural Society in Malmö wrote a letter to the city physician, in which he encouraged Höjer to contact the director of the National Bacteriological Laboratory, Professor Carl Kling, and discretely ask him to withdraw the vaccine. Magnusson had also noted strong reactions to vaccination. He had examined vaccines of certain batch numbers and had found them to contain bacteria, especially streptococci and yellow staphylococci, in large quantities. He had tested the vaccines on animals—horses, cattle, rabbits, hamsters, and dogs— and, with the exception of the hamsters, they had experienced strong local reactions and developed necrosis. The rabbits died with puss-filled abscesses in their kidneys that were filled with the same bacteria. Magnusson argued that it was a question of lymph that was altogether too "fresh." He demanded a comparative study of different vaccines in relation to "vaccination injuries."[19]

Höjer forwarded Magnusson's request to Kling at NBL.[20] Höjer's and Kling's replies, however, were that that the bacteria in the vaccine, which they referred to as "associated bacteria," occurred normally and had no pathogenic effect on humans. According to NBL, vaccine that had a significantly higher bacteria content had earlier been dispensed without special complications; vaccine with more than five million bacteria per cubic centimeter had caused very weak reactions or none at all.[21] They made a clear distinction between reactions and complications. As an alternative explanation, the bacteria could also have been induced by the vaccinators. Some individuals had perhaps not been well at the time they were vaccinated, or they were old or possessed individual characteristics that reacted with the vaccine. The vaccine was simply strong with high virulence, which was desirable in this critical situation, and the reactions to vaccinations were just what one normally could expect.[22] Kling and Höjer did not think that any further investigation was necessary.[23]

Höjer and the NBL, as well as Magnusson, referred to different foreign scholars to support their side in the conflict about the possible effect of associated bacteria on health. Magnusson referred to the bacteriologist Landmann and to the regulations in other countries that established a far lower maximum limit for the number of bacteria in vaccine at levels than those found in the Swedish vaccine. In some countries the limit was zero. Höjer referred to, among others, a German committee that in 1896 found that the reactions that occurred in association with vaccination were not unusual, and that it was not probable that they were caused by staphylococci.

In Denmark there was an uproar over the fact that even a shadow of doubt could be cast on the vaccine that the country had contributed on January 31. At the request of the Danes, Höjer certified in writing that among those who lodged complaints with the Board of Health in Malmö concerning vaccination side effects, none had been treated with the Danish vaccine. Of course, not all who suffered side effects turned to that bureau, but the statement softened the criticism. However, it meant that the Swedish vaccine stood all the more in the limelight.[24]

Höjer gave professor of pathology John Forssman in Lund vaccine for a bacteriological study. Forssman also found bacteria, even though the level was lower than that found by Magnusson; some time had passed, and the bacterial content declines with time. His test rabbits also died with abscesses in their kidneys.[25]

At the request of the general director of the Royal Medical Board, Nils Hellström, Höjer wrote a report on the epidemic and the struggle against it. The report exists in several unpublished versions, the first dated February 25, the last May 2.[26] The report was immediately criticized by Magnusson and others because it did not seriously address the vaccination "injuries."[27] In the press it was found remarkable that the person who had been in charge of handling the epidemic was also called upon to evaluate himself without an impartial investigation.[28] On June 30 an increasingly pressed and irritated Höjer made a handwritten notation that he was leaving on vacation and had uttered his last word in the matter.[29]

The Scandinavian Pathological Congress in Lund 1932

Instead, the question received even more attention only a week later in conjunction with a conference in Lund held by the Nordic Pathology Association. One of the scheduled speakers was Hilding Magnusson, whose lecture was entitled "On Staphylococci in Vaccine as the Cause of Vaccination Injuries during the Mass Vaccination in Malmö in 1932." The title caused one of the arrangers, the Association for General Healthcare, to withdraw. The organization considered the matter far from substantiated and did not want to play into the hands of the anti-vaccination movement. Twelve scientists chose to stay at home, including Carl Kling.[30] Agitated voices were heard in the press about "the state vaccine" containing large amounts of yellow staphylococci, and, they argued, if this matter was not debated openly, it would *really* give the anti-vaccination movement support for their arguments.[31]

Magnusson delivered his lecture. He concluded that the *Stafylokokkus pyogenes aureus* must have been especially resistant to glycerin and to storage with "disastrous results." In his view the vaccine had probably retained its primary virulence, so that it was similar to a fresh vaccine or a so-called green virus.[32]

The senior physician from the Epidemic Hospital, Ebbe Petrén, had earlier seen strong reactions that could have been caused by staphylococci. He argued that "nervous" and older persons should not be vaccinated, as they could more easily develop complications.[33] The surgeon Gustaf Petrén reported that he had seen ten cases of extensive gangrenous processes in the wake of the Malmö vaccination and regarded them as effects of staphylococci.[34] Thorvald Madsen guaranteed the purity of the Danish vaccine; in Denmark they had been "alarmed" at the results in Malmö.[35] During the proceedings John Forssman demanded cleaner vaccine. He found it "dreadful that large quantities of virulent bacteria are inoculated into human beings on the assumption that the bacteria in question, being associated bacteria, are of no consequence, which of course is absolutely untrue if they are injected in sufficiently large numbers. Such an inoculation cannot but be condemned and it is astonishing that attempts are being made to defend it."[36] Forssman had captured the agitated mood in the working-class city of Malmö. Because of the long-term cases of illness, there had been demonstrations, meetings, and petitions submitted to the authorities.[37] The workers believed they had made great sacrifices. If they did not receive compensation for losses in income or for unemployment support, it would be difficult for the authorities to carry out vaccination and quarantine measures in similar epidemics. Forssman also stated later that the matter needed to be clarified for the general public. If the damage that had been caused was regarded as normal, people would think twice before allowing themselves to be vaccinated again.[38]

The disagreements were now made public. They concerned not only the obvious differences between the experiences of laymen and the (missing) actions of the authorities, but also among the experts. The Danish and Norwegian vaccine producers certified that they had very low maximum cut-offs regarding microbes in the vaccine, and complications after vaccination were very rare.[39]

The Royal Medical Board was forced to deal with the crisis that had arisen. General Director Hellström tried to get both parties mainly responsible to compile and deliver material for an investigation.

Axel Höjer and the Vaccination Administration

On August 18, Höjer sent a message to Hellström that it was "irresponsible" to arrange an investigation, and he did not under any circumstances wish to participate.[40] When he was called to attend the discussions at the

Royal Medical Board anyway, he pointed out that if one could not arrive at information that was useful for vaccination or for public health, then there should be no investigation. Furthermore, it was not possible to conduct the kind of comparative study that Magnusson called for. Höjer did have a point there.

The number of those vaccinated was recorded in the vaccination journals but not always exactly which vaccine had been used.[41] Sometimes the name and date of birth of the vaccinated person were recorded but not the address, nor was this information required on the form. There was no inspection made of all those who were vaccinated to check for any reactions. According to Höjer the vaccination lists that had been made hour by hour had been destroyed after the summation of the number of vaccinations per vaccinator, which was done to calculate the proper remuneration. The information that remained concerned only approximately six thousand children and ten thousand revaccinated persons. Certain companies had kept more detailed records of their employees, but Höjer argued that it would be hard to get in touch with these people because they had to be called in from their places of work throughout the town. The hospitals' surgical clinics had taken care of seventy cases of deep necrosis, but all those with serious reactions had not sought medical help. When Höjer sent out a questionnaire to all vaccinating physicians during the spring, the questions were not precise: for example, he did not ask for the vaccine numbers or the time of the vaccination. The replies were thus altogether too vague to serve as the basis for a study. His reporting of the results was also very selective both quantitatively and qualitatively.

Höjer reported that all vaccinators had submitted reports, and that ten or so doctors described revaccination with strong reactions and "ugly cases" that surpassed anything they had seen before.[42] Of the fifty-three doctors' reports preserved in the archives, about twenty described strong reactions or complications not earlier experienced.[43]

A Doctor Waller said that he had seen a number of patients vaccinated by others who had "especially large and ugly gangrenous changes."[44] He reported that vaccination had been carried out clumsily, carelessly, and with too many scratches, and that in a large numbers of cases unnecessarily large amounts of vaccine had been used. He questioned whether it was suitable and wise for the vaccinating doctors to allow their wives or others who were completely ignorant of health care to vaccinate. In several cases the doctors had not taken any hygienic precautions. Waller associated the complications after vaccination with these unsatisfactory conditions, and he said that he had nothing against being cited. Höjer reported two cases to the Royal Medical Board where the current regulations concerning vaccination had not been followed. "Considering the very small numbers vaccinated in this way, they could not have played a quantitatively large role." Höjer summarized by saying that "vaccination in comparable age groups has probably struck somewhat harder, but not essentially differently than in earlier vaccinations, which have previously been carried out by active vaccinators, just as the descriptions of this vaccination do not essentially differ from what we know from the literature as strong effects of vaccine."[45]

Vaccine Manufacturing at the
National Bacteriological Laboratory

Professor Carl Kling's first report from April 21 addressed the effects of vaccination, but mainly from other parts of the country and not just Malmö. Kling argued that the same vaccine had been used throughout the country without unusual reactions. The Royal Medical Board could counter, however, with reports that described severe reactions, including deaths of encephalitis involving not only older revaccinated persons but also children.[46]

At the NBL it was a nurse who produced all vaccine, from the calf to the consumer package, under the supervision of a veterinarian.[47] The lymph with which the cows were inoculated at the NBL came from rabbits in the second generation, she told the Royal Medical Board.[48] It was now said that experiments with sterile, so-called neurovaccine, cultured on the testicles or brain substance of rabbits, had shown drawbacks, so its use was not advised. No such neurolapin (passed through rabbits) had been added to the vaccine. In a newspaper interview in February, right in the middle of the vaccination campaign, however, Kling had promised quick delivery to the entire country of vaccine cultured on the brain substance of rabbits, "thanks to Levaditi's method."[49] It had been stated that such vaccine had been used in Spain with outstanding results. It did not need to be stored prior to use, and it could be produced in unlimited quantities.

For several years the laboratory had, without formal permission from the Royal Medical Board, used its own modified variation of animal trials on both rabbits and mice according to the Calmette-Guèrin method.[50] When the experiments had shown high virulence, the vaccine was sent out. According to the regulations, the vaccine should be tested on children—not to test for any eventual injurious qualities but for its virulence. For this purpose children from the Stockholm Public Orphanage or children called to the regular vaccination sessions were used. The tests on children were to be conducted by the inspector appointed by the Royal Medical Board. At the end of January, however, there was a rush to send out the vaccine, and it was not possible to obtain the number of children needed for testing on such short notice. Nor did the NBL consider the tests on children necessary. According to Kling, it was still only Sweden, Denmark, Tunisia, and Egypt that had regulations requiring testing on children. In countries such as Germany and England, animal trials were mandatory before tests could be made on humans. He regarded it also as wrong in principle to vaccinate people with a vaccine whose strength was unknown.[51]

In the middle of February, a check of the vaccine used in Malmö before that date showed that it caused very strong reactions. In his records the inspector questioned whether the vaccine should not be kept longer in storage before usage. Kling said that, even if he had received that report in time, he would have dispatched the vaccine anyway. According to the NBL, vaccines with high virulence that would clearly supply immunity should be used in the epidemic that threatened; it was the interest of the state that was prioritized.[52] The NBL chose not to send out a weaker vaccine that gave normal reactions.[53] Even though, according to Kling, the bacteria did not have any significance, he could consider trying to reduce their amount, as he put it, "for opportunistic reasons," as a concession to the vaccination critics.

After several reminders from Hellström, in December 1932 Kling submitted a more detailed report on the effect of the vaccine.[54] This report did not include Malmö in January to February 1932 but rather the rest of the country from March to June 1932. As far as the vaccinations in Malmö were concerned, Kling referred to Höjer's report. According to the NBL, there were no methods for determining whether the staphylococci and streptococci were human pathogens. Nor were there any connections between the bacteria count in the vaccine and the reactions and complications. Kling presented tables showing that selectively chosen vaccine batches with low bacteria count had caused strong reactions, and that vaccines with high bacteria count had produced weak or normal reactions. A vaccine that had contained sixteen million bacteria per cubic centimeter had produced normal pox in children.[55] There had been comparisons made between sterile neurovaccine and dermovaccine that were rich in bacteria, with the result that there was a tendency toward a milder course of events with vaccination with the latter.[56]

Vaccine number 38, which was used for vaccinations in Malmö on January 31, was not mentioned in Kling's December report. However, it is found in basic data that shows that, when it was inspected at the NBL on January 26, it contained 530,000 bacteria per cubic centimeter, and it belonged to the vaccines that were later reported by the inspector to cause "very strong reactions" in children. Furthermore, three of the cases of postvaccinal encephalitis, including one lethal case, were vaccinated with this number 38.[57]

In his report to the Royal Medical Board, Kling's conclusion was that all the vaccines used, including the vaccines that had been left over in Malmö and were later sent throughout the country, had been free from virulent bacteria. The reactions that had occurred did not depend upon "infected lymph" (his quotation marks) but rather on the reactions of certain individuals to the specific smallpox virus.[58]

Problems for the Royal Medical Board

General Director Hellström was early aware that the facts and standpoints presented would not satisfy the concerned and agitated public. During the discussions in October 1932, when both Kling and Höjer were present, on the initiative of the latter an agreement was reached concerning a short official declaration. The existing data could not serve as the foundation for an investigation, and, because such an investigation would not be able to illuminate the reasons for the reactions to the vaccine, it should not be carried out.

To try to have an independent external investigation when the country's leading bacteriologists disagreed, Hellström turned the issue over to the International Office of Public Hygiene in Paris (l'Office International d'Hygiene Publique) in the fall.[59] This was a situation where we might suspect partiality: Kling had been a member for several years and had already been in Paris and gained support for his views on the bacteria question.[60] Hellström tried to deal with the question of objectivity by also sending Forssman as an informant and observer. But, as the data were insufficient and uncertain concerning the vaccinations in Malmö, this organization was unable to reach conclusive results about what had caused the reactions or complications after vaccination. Similar effects had been observed in other countries, and it was not considered probable that there was a connection with the bacteria in the vaccine.[61]

Different Agendas and Priorities—but Still the Same

The different central figures in the wake of the smallpox epidemic in Malmö each had his own agenda. The city physician Axel Höjer wanted to defend his decision for mass vaccination, as well as the way in which it had been administrated. It would undeniably look bad if the local Public Health Board had encouraged vaccination with dangerous "state vaccine." Hilding Magnusson was a supporter of vaccination and regarded himself as the public's representative in the attempts to bring clarity into the reasons for the injuries and to prevent more cases. The NBL's director, Carl Kling, insisted that the laboratory's vaccine was "excellent" and that the Royal Medical Board's statement should not display any glimpse of criticism directed against the vaccine.[62] Professor John Forssman was sympathetic toward the public's wariness of the vaccine and was concerned about patients' trust in their doctors. Had they been alerted earlier that there was danger afoot and that it was not possible to take all precautions, then tolerance among people would have been greater.[63]

The Royal Medical Board also bore some responsibility. It had granted permission for mass vaccination. There was poor insight into the NBL's activities, and inadequate regulations concerning manufacturing of animal vaccine. No regulations existed concerning the desirable range of virulence or maximum bacteria counts. Authority over the NBL was apparently insufficient. The vaccination forms also made tracing and later control of the vaccinated impossible. General Director Nils Hellström expressly defended compulsory vaccination, which was constantly being questioned, particularly at that time. He stressed the importance of making vaccination as safe as possible, both from a medical and a psychological perspective. The matter was followed by "not just the opponents of vaccination, but also by an objective public that sought as best possible to judge the risks and advantages, which are associated with the process of vaccination."[64] All of those involved wanted to preserve public trust in medicine, authorities, and the principle of vaccination.

Relations across the Baltic Sea

But why were the contagion and later the vaccination risks initially toned down? Besides the fact that the contact cases were not properly traced and isolated, why did this quick and not entirely well-organized mass vaccination take place? Why were all the later attempts made to normalize the complications, regardless of the causes?

Smallpox and vaccination have a history that is several hundred years old, of being used both as a weapon and as defense. In 1932 the newspapers published daily reports on the uneasy political, economic, and military situation in Europe and the world. When it became apparent that smallpox had broken out in Malmö, important ships chose to bypass the harbor without docking. Orders to industry declined, as did exports; unemployment, though already high, grew. Höjer himself named the economy and trade as reasons why the city needed to be declared free of smallpox as soon as possible.[65]

There was also an incident fresh in people's minds that was called "an accident" or "experimental rage," depending on their perspective.[66] In 1930 two doctors in Lübeck had convinced the authorities to allow a whole age band of infants to be vaccinated with Calmette's new BCG-vaccine against tuberculosis. At least 250 children were vaccinated; 77 died of tuberculosis, and an additional 131 became seriously ill. In spite of early alarms about sick children, there was a delay in stopping the vaccinations, and the cases of illness were not directly examined.[67] In this case the bacterial experts were also in disagreement on what had happened. The hypothesis that this could have been a planned medical experiment was rejected. Nor was it possible for bacteriology in 1930 to prove that a spontaneous modification in the bacteria had not occurred, thus causing the catastrophe. The experts soon agreed that it was an accident caused by human error and poor scientific practice. The court drew the conclusion that the vaccine from the Pasteur Institute had been contaminated with live tuberculosis bacteria during its preparation at the laboratory in Lübeck. Both doctors were found responsible for this and for not having tested the vaccine on animals before it was used on children. According to later analyses, the verdict of the court was only a probable hypothesis; conclusive evidence had disappeared before the trial.[68] In Germany all vaccination with BCG-vaccine was prohibited until 1949.

The National Context and Personal Relations

In Sweden experiments with vaccination of children with BCG-vaccine were initiated in 1926. These campaigns continued without interruption, for example, in Sweden's northernmost county under the direction of bacteriologist Carl Naeslund, a project that he himself characterized as "in certain respects a successful scientific experiment."[69] Criticism of the requirement to vaccinate one's children against smallpox was already great in many parts of the country. Only about 60 percent of the children in Sweden were vaccinated, and in certain places in the country not more than a few percent.[70] The experts and authorities drew no parallels between the situation in Lübeck in 1930 and Malmö in 1932. According to the annual reports of the provincial doctors to the Royal Medical Board, however, the declining frequency of smallpox vaccination in the country was partly a result of the events in Lübeck that had received attention in the press.[71] One of the members of the three-man committee of experts that was supposed to present a proposal for the revision of the existing laws in this area that same year—the only physician on the committee—was present when it was decided not to more closely investigate the events in Malmö. The committee report proposed that smallpox vaccination should still be compulsory. Not much attention was paid to the effects of the Malmö vaccination in regard to Magnusson's vaccination injuries. Focus was instead directed to postvaccinal encephalitis, which was thought to be dependent upon individual factors, vaccination being only the trigger. However, this motivated precautionary measures.[72]

The mass vaccination in Malmö brought to light shortcomings in the education of medical students and doctors in vaccination. It had not been long since doctors in Sweden—partly under protest—had taken over the main responsibility for this procedure. Not much time elapsed before the responsibility for vaccination was transferred to the newly established Mother and Child Care Centers in 1940. The problematic compulsory vaccination with its roots in the turn of the nineteenth century was not the best precedent for winning public trust for the scientific endeavor, the authority of physicians, and the modernization of health care. Just as in Germany, England, France, and many other countries, doctors in Sweden were involved in the interwar debates on the "crisis" of medicine and the medical corps, and there was reason not to sabotage the trust of the general public even further.[73] The voluntary vaccination programs under development, furthermore, received more support among people than compulsory vaccination against smallpox.

From its establishment in 1909, the National Bacteriological Laboratory had a history of problems in the production of serum, which led to years of disagreements with the Royal Medical Board. One event made public in 1916 concerned five children who were infected with tetanus after injection with serum against diphtheria, one of whom died.[74] The Royal Medical Board called the director of the laboratory before the court and wanted to move manufacturing of the serum against tetanus to the National Veterinary Bacteriological Laboratory. The events left their mark on the relations between the NBL and the medical authorities.

Personal rivalries also played a role in the difficulties that the central figures had in cooperating to clarify in what had happened. At the beginning of the 1920s, Axel Höjer had competed with Greta Muhl for a doctor's post in Stockholm and in 1925 for the position of head doctor at the Flensburg Children's Hospital in Malmö and had lost both contests.[75] Höjer and Kling had earlier had a disagreement with Hilding Magnusson over the ways foot-and-mouth disease spread. Höjer was not named professor of hygiene in Lund, and in 1932, when he aspired to a professor's chair in public health at Karolinska Institutet, things did not go his way either. In his expert written opinion, John Forssman had ranked Höjer below his main competitor; Höjer's knowledge in bacteriology was not considered sufficient for a post in health care and hygiene. Höjer countered with the argument that bacteriology was part of general pathology and not hygiene. "Even when it comes to hygienic points of view concerning infectious diseases, bacteriology does not receive exclusive attention. The infected person stands in the foreground. Constitution, nutrition, climate and other influences from the environment receive increasing attention."[76] The chair was awarded to Carl Naeslund, who considered bacteriology still fundamental to scientific work in hygienics.[77] Höjer's opinion of bacteriology's subordinate position may be one of the explanations for his actions (or lack thereof) during the smallpox epidemic.

The Aftermath

The problems that arose during the sudden mass vaccination were used as arguments to retain compulsory smallpox vaccination in childhood, which was assumed to alleviate the effects of later revaccinations. The cases of postvaccinal encephalitis contributed to an adjustment of the law. Between the years 1924 and 1932, at least fifty-two cases of brain inflammation after vaccination had been diagnosed in Sweden alone, ten of which resulted in death.[78] During the same period, one out of the ten cases of smallpox had resulted in death—the revaccinated woman in Malmö for whom the cause of death was also listed as encephalitis. People who had a disposition toward neurological problems or fever cramps, and so on, could now also, according to the law, be excused from vaccination with the help of a doctor's certificate. The vaccine itself was not questioned.

An inspection of the NBL resulted in the suggestion that the scientific work there should be discontinued. The Royal Medical Board instead revised the regulations for the NBL concerning the manufacture and inspection of vaccine and the laboratory's scientific activities. The testing of vaccine on children continued, but from 1935 the child's name and age were to be given; previously, only the number of vaccinated "arms" was noted.[79] Everyone agreed that NBL's facilities—five small rented rooms in a building in central Stockholm—were not suitable for its tasks. "Certain important work which should be completely isolated, still must be carried out in spaces that are shared with others, which places great demands on the exactitude and alertness of the personnel," according to Kling in 1932.[80] Denmark and Norway were significantly better equipped. Five years later larger, newly constructed facilities for the NBL were dedicated in Solna, north of Stockholm.

Dealing with Uncertain Knowledge

The way smallpox was dealt with in Malmö in 1932 illustrates the uncertainty and changing character of medical knowledge. There was no consensus over the pathogenic role of various bacteria for infections and the margins of safety for vaccines and vaccination. Bacteriology's breakthrough during the latter part of the nineteenth century was just the start of a constant development of new discoveries and theories that often slowly, and sometimes under opposition, revised earlier conceptions. Into the twentieth century, bacteriology in Sweden was characterized by "theoretical confusion."[81] There were rival scientific collectives that called upon both older and newer theories of the role of different microbes and how infections were spread. With changeable bacteriological theories, the thought collective and society are responsible for validating what should be considered scientific fact, as described by the scientific theorist Ludwik Fleck.[82] In the case of Malmö an attempt was made to delegate these decisions to German bacteriologists and the International Office of Public Hygiene in Paris.

Fleck wrote his book about how scientific facts are created immediately after the events in Lübeck. During the 1920s and the 1930s, he was employed as a microbiologist in the German-speaking sphere, including working in the manufacture of vaccine.[83] Historian Christian Bonah describes the atmosphere in microbiology there in the 1930s as a crisis in scientific knowledge. Fleck saw the growing crisis in trust between medicine and the public as a sound opposition to the power of the medical elite. When the elite gains a strong position, the distance to the people increases, and dogmatism and secrecy dominate the thought collective, a development that can also be traced in the Malmö epidemic.

If an external and independent inspection committee for vaccine manufacture in Sweden had been quickly appointed to compare the various vaccines from the NBL and Denmark in relation to their effects on people and the possible complications, it could have provided further explanation to the authorities as well as to the general public. The question of what caused the vaccination injuries remains. Was the vaccine too "fresh"? Were the "associated bacteria" or the criticized vaccination techniques to blame? Were the reactions normal (in the terms of the experts and authorities) and to be expected with effective smallpox vaccinations? Or had neurovaccine from rabbit brains, known from other countries to cause necrosis, been sent out from the NBL because it was available, or had it become accidently mixed into the shipments in the primitive laboratory facilities? Could such vaccine also cause encephalitis? What actually took place at the National Bacteriological Laboratory during the period in question is difficult to trace afterward. The material concerning the manufacture and inspection of animal vaccine, especially from the end of the 1920s up until late 1940s, is to a large extent missing from the archives.

In his 1975 autobiography, J. Axel Höjer gives a description of the mass vaccination in Malmö that to a considerable extent deviates from available facts. Some older patients, he writes, who had not been vaccinated for thirty years, suffered from inflammations at the vaccination site, which "for several days caused pain and discomfort and which left them unable to work for three to five days."[84] Before "the conclusion based on facts was reached"—meaning that Magnusson's statement was unfounded—Höjer had had to take responsibility for a great deal of suffering, "especially among older people, nervous people, opponents of vaccination—or anti-socialist!"[85] The only thing that he could regret afterward was that he did not point out that retirees should have stayed home, so as to have avoided vaccination.

In 1935 J. Axel Höjer succeeded Nils Hellström as the general director of the Royal Medical Board, a position that he held for seventeen years.[86] He has been described by many researchers as one of the most important architects of Swedish health policy. In a double biography of Axel Höjer and his wife Signe Höjer, historian Annika Berg describes the former as one of the central figures in the building of the welfare state. His position as city physician in Malmö, starting in 1930, gave Höjer the opportunity to realize some of his ideas concerning public health in a more clearly political project. In spite of this statement, the smallpox epidemic in Malmö is mentioned in only one sentence, and Höjer's memoires are listed as the source.[87] Sköld and Baldwin concluded their respective studies of smallpox in Sweden around the year 1915.[88] In his study of polio epidemics in Sweden in the twentieth century, Per Axelsson describes the central role that Carl Kling had in polio research and the ways in which ideas concerning paths of infection and disease prevention differed from those in the United States; for natural reasons the roles of Kling and the NBL concerning smallpox are not treated here.[89]

Controversial Practices and Public Health Policy

There is reason to study in more depth Höjer's role as a civil servant and as the one who helped form the relationship of the state and the medical-bacteriological-hygienic experts to the people during times when epidemics were being fought, including the handling of smallpox in Malmö in 1932 and thereafter. A study of the development of the French-German-Swedish bacteriological scientific thought collectives during the 1920s and 1930s can also shed some light on the production of knowledge on which Swedish national health policies were based at that time. The Royal Medical Board required vaccines to be tested on children before they could be used on the general public, but authorities never raised any questions about whether any form of consent should be required from parents or legal guardians. Such views were advanced by the anti-vivisection movement. Thus, the Swedish conditions differed from the ethical discussions that were carried on in Germany with renewed vigor after the incident in Lübeck in 1930.[90]

The historical background concerning the differing nature and style of policies in the fight against epidemics of infectious diseases, as well as people's reactions to these policies, needs to be brought to light. Regardless of past or current epidemiological, hygienic, or bacteriological conclusions concerning the way with which smallpox and the mass vaccination in Malmö were handled, the ethical and political conclusions remain. As Bonah emphasizes, the ethical questions of our times also require an understanding of how science works and of how claims of knowledge and expertise gain legitimacy. The boundary between experimental and established vaccination practice has been flexible, as has been the border between voluntarism and compulsion. The oft-claimed dividing line in the vaccination debate—rational scientific and medical knowledge versus myths and irrational thinking— is not always easy to draw. Different experiences, knowledge, and agendas have generated different rationalities.

The events during and after the Malmö epidemic of 1932 show how difficult it is for the medical authorities to communicate evaluations of scientific knowledge and to tally the balance sheet of risk and safety to a general public that obviously has different experiences on which to base its considerations. Regardless of whether the choice is an in-depth comparative study resulting in informing the public of the results or—as was done here—not to report and analyze all the information possible to obtain, the events could not be expected to increase the public's confidence in vaccination and the medical authorities. But when the options are available, the question can still be asked whether citizens deserve this insight. It could generate more understanding of the production of scientific knowledge and of the actions of authorities, but it could also help them to better make their own decisions in matters of health. The ethical and practical aspects of public health policy still need to be discussed openly.

Notes

This article presented at the conference "Bridging the Baltic," Lund University, October 9, 2014. Elaborated in Motzi Eklöf, *Variola & Vaccinia: Om massvaccination och folkhälospolitik, vaccinforskning och läkaretik* (Malmköping: Exempla förlag, 2016).

I am indebted to Professor Emerita Marie C. Nelson for translation and helpful comments and to Ragnhild Blomquist Foundation (Uppsala University) and Maj and Lennart Lindgren's Foundation for Research in Medical History (Karolinska Institutet) for financial support.

1. Marie C. Nelson, and John Rogers, "The Right to Die? Anti-vaccination Activity and the 1874 Smallpox Epidemic in Stockholm," *Social History of Medicine* 5, no. 3 (1992): 369–88.

2. Neighboring Denmark and Norway required vaccination for entering school from the year 1810. See M. Tryland, "Kopper og koppe-virus—200 år sedan første vaksinasjon I Norge," *Tidskrift for Den norske legeforening* 121, no. 30 (2001): 3546–50. Bavaria required compulsory vaccination in 1807, but it was not until 1874, after the unification, that all of Germany was encompassed by this requirement. Finland passed a law on vaccination of children in 1883; the Soviet Union acted first in 1919 and made it compulsory for all in 1924. K. J. Pitkänen, J. H. Mielke, and L. B. Jorde, "Smallpox and Its Eradication in Finland: Implications for Disease Control," *Population Studies* 43 (1989): 95–111.

3. Peter Sköld, "The Two Faces of Smallpox: A Disease and Its Prevention in Eighteenth- and Nineteenth-Century Sweden" (Diss. Report No 12 from the Demographic Data Base, Umeå, Umeå University, 1996).

4. Peter Baldwin, *Contagion and the State in Europe, 1830–1930* (Cambridge: Cambridge University Press, 1999/2005).

5. Nadja Durbach, *Bodily Matters: The Anti-vaccination Movement in England, 1853–1907* (Durham, NC: Duke University Press, 2005).

6. Motzi Eklöf, "Conscientious Objections against Smallpox Vaccination in Sweden, 1900–1940" (conference paper, "Healthcare: Supply and Demand in Prehistory and History" in Gothenburg, May 6–8, 2015); also published as "Preventionens vapenvägrare: Samvete, vetenskap eller personlig erfarenhet—om (il)legitima skäl till undantag från obligatorisk smittkoppsvaccination," *Socialmedicinsk tidskrift* 62 no. 6 (2015): 662–73; also published as "Den obligatoriska smittkoppsvaccinationen ifrågasatt: Kättaren Israel Holmgren om kaninpassager, kårinstinkter och känsloskäl," *Svensk Medicinhistorisk Tidskrift* 19 no. 1 (2015): 157–80.

7. If not otherwise given, the story is based on several joint sources such as archival sources, newspaper articles, and publications.

8. "Smittkoppor i Malmö," *Sydsvenska dagbladet,* January 16, 1932.

9. According to the head physician, Ebbe Petrén, in "Smittoförhållandena vid smittkoppor," *Svenska dagbladet,* February 7, 1932. "Smittkopporna i Malmö 1931–1932 och deras bekämpande: En redogörelse av J. Axel Höjer. Förste stadsläkare," May 2, 1932, unpublished manuscipt.

10. P. Frédéric, "Smittkoppsvaccin för 50.000 personer i ett glasrör: Ansträngande dygn på bakteriologiska laboratoriet," *Sydsvenska dagbladet,* February 7, 1932.

11. Hugo Engleson, No 100, 1932, in the Archives of Malmö Public Health Board, Malmö City Archives, hereafter: AMHB.

12. Instructions from the Royal Medical Board concerning the production of animal vaccine: "Medicinalstyrelsens kungörelse den 29 januari 1917 om framställning vid Statsmedicinska anstalten av animal ympämne" SMA (1909–1918) was the forerunner to NBL, instituted in 1918.

13. When a contemporary textbook on vaccine describes "classic" production of vaccine from calves, it is described as a procedure that may have been used in the 1940s and the 1950s, but not in Sweden in the 1910s, 1920s, or 1930s. Richard B. Kennedy, Michael J. Lane, Donald A. Henderson, and Gregory A. Poland, "Smallpox and Vaccinia," in *Vaccines,* ed. Stanley A. Plotkin, Walter A. Orenstein, and Paul A. Offit, 6ht ed. (Philadelphia: Elsevier Saunders 2013), 718–45, esp. 729.

14. In 1906 the Royal Medical Board pointed out that vaccine was most powerful immediately after it was harvested; in 1914 it was stated that it should be stored for six to seven weeks before use and that vaccine older than four months should not be used. Instructions from the Medical Board to vaccinators concerning animal vaccine: Medicinalstyrelsens cirkulär den 14 november 1906 och 7 januari 1914 till vaccinatörer om animal vaccin. (Opinions on these matters changed later.)

15. Instructions from the Royal Medical Board to the inspector of animal vaccine: Medicinalstyrelsens instruktion från den 24 maj 1917 för kontrollant av animalt ympämne för skyddskoppympning.

16. E.g., "Epidemien svårast när den är över! Stor sjukprocent för vissa dagars vaccinering" (The epidemic is at its worst when it is over! Large percentage ill from vaccination on certain days), *Sydsvenska dagbladet,* February 12, 1932.

17. The circular from the Royal Medical Board January 9, 1928, addressed to doctors concerning animal vaccine and vaccination, was replaced on July 21, 1930, with one that more strongly emphasized for whom exemptions from vaccination should be made as well as information on disinfection of the instruments used in vaccination.

18. Höjer notified the appointed vaccinators from the public campaign in Malmö under the heading "Confidential," No 54/1932, Förste stadsläkarens konceptbok, AMHB.

19. Hilding Magnusson, "Om Ympskador: Granskning av viss del av stadsläkare J. A. Höjers rapport över smittkoppsepidemien i Malmö 1932," *Meddelande från Hushållningssällskapets Laboratorium* (Malmö, 1932), 13–14.

20. Letter from Höjer to Kling, exp. February 18, nr 56/1932, Förste stadsläkarens konceptbok 1932, AMHB. In translation: "Herewith is Mister Magnusson's *opus herostraticus* forwarded with no further comments. The simplicity with which he solves the difficult problems is priceless. Such a clever man harbors no doubts. How would it be to send him a tube of those vaccines that we got the first days, on Friday and Saturday, for a count. Perhaps he would have found as many there. Actually it should begin to fade away, but nothing of that has been noticed yet."

21. Hans Davide at NBL in a letter to H. Magnusson, April 20, 1932. Archives of the Health Bureau of The Royal Medical Board, State Archives in Stockholm, hereafter ARMB.

22. E.g., Höjer, "Anmärkningar till veterinär H. Magnussons granskning av vissa delar av undertecknads rapport över smittkoppsepidemin i Malmö 1932," June 14, 20, and 21, 1932 (different versions), AMHB.

23. At the end of February an epizootic outbreak of cowpox occurred. Revaccinated people spread the pox to the cows' udders, from which it spread to other animals and humans. The same thing had happened earlier in association with the annual vaccinations of children. "Kokopporna grassera allt mer i Skåne," *Sydsvenska dagbladet*, February 28, 1932.

24. Letter from Höjer to Madsen, exp. February 13, nr 51, 1932, Förste stadsläkarens konceptbok 1932, AMHB. "Vaccinen for stærk til Malmø. Læreranstalten og Realskolen lukket. Mange Skolebørn ligger med høj Feber. Det er Vaccinen fra København, det erg alt med," *Ekstrabladet*, February 10, 1932. Soon afterward the newspaper stated that the vaccine from Copenhagen and Stockholm had shared guilt. Later the Danish vaccine was completely without guilt. According to Höjer, "Inget tvivel om var orsaken är att finna" (No doubt about where to find the cause). See also the meeting at the Medical Board on October 11, 1932, Medicinalstyrelsen 11 oktober 1932, ARMB.

25. John Forssman's report to Höjer, dated April 20, 1932, in copy as attachment no 5 in Höjer, "Smittkopporna i Malmö," 1932.

26. Höjer, "Smittkopporna i Malmö," 1932.

27. Hugo Engleson, 6 februari § 41; June 22, 1932, letter dnr 100, bilaga § 447d. AMHB; Magnusson," Om ympskador," 1932.

28. "Orimliga anspråk," editorial, *Svenska Morgonbladet*, June 21, 1932.

29. Handwritten on a copy of a document that criticizes "D:r E." [meaning Hugo Engleson] June 30, 1932, AMHB.

30. "Föredragstitel vållar schism bland medicinera. Tolv vetenskapsmän strejka från kongress i Lund. Man fruktade vaccinationsmotståndarna," *Göteborgs handels- och sjöfartstidning*, July 5, 1932; "Vaccinfienderna har fått vatten på sin kvarn," *Sydsvenska dagbladet* July 7, 1932; "Utländska experter få döma i vaccinfrågan: Professor Kling svarar i stor utredning i stället för på patologkongressen," *Sydsvenska dagbladet*, July 8, 1932; "Intet fel på det svenska vaccinet: Professor Kling bemöter angreppen," *Nya Dagligt Allehanda*, July 8, 1932.

31. See, for example, "Föreläsarstrejken anses skandalös bland patologerna: 'Föreningen för allmän hälsovård' ger vaccinfienderna vatten på kvarn," *Göteborgs Handels- och sjöfartstidning*, July 6, 1932.

32. Hilding Magnusson, "Injuries Caused by Staphylococci in Smallpox Vaccine at the Mass Vaccination in Malmö 1932," *Transactions of the Fifth Scandinavian Pathological Congress*, held in Lund, July 3–6, 1932, ed. Arvid Lindau, *Acta Pathologica et microbiologica Scandinavica supplementum* 11, 1932, 204–16.

33. Ibid., 223–34.

34. Ibid., 227.

35. Ibid., 224–25.

36. Ibid., 220.

37. "Det arbetande folket skall ej bära följderna av skyddsåtgärder mot de epidemiska sjukdomarna," *Sydsvenska Kuriren* [paper of the Swedish Communist Party], March 12, 1932.

38. Forssman in discussions at the Royal Medical Board, October 11, 1932, p. no 44. ARMB.

39. A written copy of the message from Dr. Voss, Norway. The quotation is from O. Thomsen, Copenhagen, Archive of the National Bacteriological Laboratory, Professor Kling's Archive; the National Archives in Stockholm, ANBLK.

40. He used the word *lättsinnigt*. Letter from Höjer to Hellström, August 18, 1932, AHBRMB. Hellström noted on the letter, "Not an official document. No reply." In the letter Höjer also wrote that Magnusson surely wanted to humiliate Kling, against whom he certainly held repressed complexes. Höjer sent a copy of his letter to Kling, who was advised not to reveal that he knew about it.

41. The information is taken from Höjer's report of May 2, his letter to Hellström August 18, and the discussions at the Royal Medical Board, October 11, 1932.

42. Höjer to Madsen, 34.

43. The reports are preserved in AMHB.

44. W. Waller's report, March 17, 1932, AMHB.

45. Höjer's report, May 2, 1932, 34.

46. Wranne at The Royal Medical Board: "Rapporter över vissa skyddskoppympningar i Sverige under år 1932. 1) under februari och 2) under försommaren (maj-juni), vilka inkommit till Medicinalstyrelsen före den 5 oktober 1932." Unpublished. ARMB.

47. She had done this job since 1926, but no records had been kept of the vaccine production. Discussed at a meeting at the Medical Board September 15, 1932. ARMB.

48. According to NBL they had used the same method of production for more than twenty years. Hans Davide at NBL in a letter to Dr. Voss in Oslo, September 7, 1932, which was a reply to a request of August 30, NBL.

49. "Vaccin för hela Sverige ur 50 kaninhjärnor: Bakteriologiska laboratoriet redo leverera vaccin till hela landet," *Sydsvenska dagbladet*, February 2, 1932.

50. Kling and his associates had very close contacts with scholars at the Pasteur Institute in Paris, and he had presented much of his research in French fora.

51. Furthermore, NBL was always supposed to have a certain number of doses of vaccine on stock that had been completely checked and was ready for delivery. The Medical Board understood this to be vaccine that had been tried by its own inspector; Kling regarded it to be sufficient with the controls conducted in the laboratory.

52. Handwritten notes from a meeting at the Royal Medical Board in July 18, 1932. Davide's letter to Dr. Voss, September 1932. All documents ARMB.

53. Shortly before the outbreak of the epidemic, vaccine from 1929 was destroyed because of a lack of space, according to NBL.

54. Report from Carl Kling to the Royal Medical Board, December 21, 1932. ARMB.

55. Vaccine no. 22/1921.

56. Discussions with the Royal Medical Board, ARMB; Hans Davide, "Nya rön beträffande vaccinlymfans bacteriologi," offprint from *Svenska läkaresällskapets förhandlingar*, 1932, Stockholm 1933.

57. Eklöf, *Variola & Vaccinia*, 206.

58. An analysis by M. Kaiser at the Austrian Institute for the Production of Vaccine in Vienna pointed out that during the most recent fifteen years the effect of the lymph had increased in strength as a result of repeated passages and modified storage of the lymph to retain its virulence. No method for determining the titer (a way of expressing concentration) yet existed. Kaiser also noted a certain antagonism between the vaccine's virus and the staphylococci. His conclusion was that strong reactions during mass vaccinations depended upon high titer or a less suitable vaccination technique. M. Kaiser, "Ein Beitrag zur Beurteilung der vaccinalen Reaktionen nach den Massenimpfungen im Malmö" (January 1932) *Acta Pediatrica*, offprint 14, 1933, 430–48.

59. OIHP (1907–46) was the forerunner to WHO.

60. Höjer also had written to the office and complained that Magnusson had converted a detail in the Malmö vaccination to the main question. Copy in AMBH.

61. The French experts at Office International d'Hygiène Publique delivered two reports—*Rapport de la Commission de la Variole et de la Vaccination Antivariolique au sujet des accidents post-baccinaux de Malmö*—one arriving November 9, 1932, and a later, more extensive report from May 9, 1933, ARMB.

62. Kling in the meeting with the Royal Medical Board October 11, 1932. For the quotation, see clause 73, ARMB.

63. Meeting of the Royal Medical Board, October 11, 1932, 44, ARMB.

64. Hellström in the Swedish Medical Society, November 8, 1932, *Svenska läkaresällskapets förhandlingar*, 1932.

65. J. Axel Höjer, "Smittkopporna i Malmö 1931–1932 och deras bekämpande," *Hygienisk Revy*, 1932, 44–46. The article was listed as part 1, but no part 2 appeared because of the criticism concerning Höjer's presentation. Instead, the journal later published the conclusions from the French institute, "Ännu en gång smittkoppsepidemien i Malmö 1931–1932," *Hygiensk revy* 9 (1933): 99–102.

66. For "experimental rage," see Julius Moses, *Der Totentanz von Lübeck* (Radebeul: Madaus 1930).

67. Susanne Hahn, "'Der Lübecker Totentanz': Zur rechtlichen und ethischen Problematik der Katastrophe bei der Erprobung der Tuberkuloseimpfung 1930 in Deutschland," *Medizinhistorisches Journal* 30, no. 1 (1995): 61–79. The children were then treated with tuberculosis serum or an irritation therapy intended to cause fever. This implied vaccination with a combination of staphylococci and streptococci. In all thirty-one children received between one and nineteen injections at intervals of two to five days.

68. Christian Bonah, "'Experimental Rage': The Development of Medical Ethics and the Genesis of Scientific Facts," *Social History of Medicine* 15, no. 2 (2002): 187–202; Hahn, "'Der Lübecker Totentanz.'" One of the doctors had destroyed most of the remaining vaccine. In Sweden it was stated that the investigation had provided "full evidence" that the bacteria cultures were mixed up, and that the personnel had mistakenly vaccinated the infants with a culture of normally virulent tuberculosis bacteria and not with the Calmette vaccine. See Torsten Thunberg, "Annus Medicus 1932," *Svenska Dagbladets Årsbok*, ed. H. E. Kjellberg, vol. 10 (Stockholm: Svenska Dagbladet, 1932).

69. Carl Naeslund, *Till medlemmarna av Karolinska Institutets lärarekollegium: Svar å docent Axel Höjers skrivelse* (Uppsala: Almqvist & Wiksell, 1932). He was of the opinion that vaccinated children in general demonstrated a lower mortality than those who were not. This was assumed to depend on an unspecified immunization effect, a hypothesis that is still cited by scholars.

70. Statens Offentliga Utredningar (SOU) 1932:37, *Betänkande angående skyddskoppympningen,* Avgivet av inom socialdepartementet den 4 oktober 1930 tillkallade sakkunniga, Stockholm, 1932.

71. Sveriges Officiella Statistik, *Allmän hälso- och sjukvård år 1930, av Kungl. Medicinalstyrelsen* (Stockholm, 1932), 19–20.

72. SOU 1932:37.

73. Motzi Eklöf, "Läkarens ethos: Studier i den svenska läkarkårens identiteter, intressen och ideal 1890-1960" (Linköping Studies in Arts and Science No 216, Linköping, Linköping University, 2000; Linköping University Electronic Press, 2006).

74. Motzi Eklöf, *Fallet Blända: Statens serumtillverkning, en skandal och vetenskaplig krishantering* (Malmköping: Exempla förlag, 2018).

75. Annika Berg, "Den gränslösa hälsan: Signe och Axel Höjer, folkhälsan och expertisen" (Uppsala Studies in History of Ideas 39, Uppsala, Uppsala University, 2009), 182–84.

76. J. Axel Höjer, "Professor Forssmans sakkunnigutlåtande beträffande de sökande till den vid Karolinska Institutet ledigförklarade professuren i allmän hälsovårdslära," Lund 1932, citation p. 23.

77. Naeslund, *Till medlemmarna av Karolinska Institutets lärarekollegium.*

78. The figures differ slightly in different sources. Furthermore, the suspected encephalitis cases reported by doctors were forwarded by the Royal Medical Board to Carl Kling for his opinion on whether the encephalitis could be associated with vaccination. A glance at the material stored in the archives shows that his opinion was based to a large extent on the time that had elapsed between vaccination and the onset of symptoms. Today it is known that cases may also occur during the time span in which Kling judged that symptoms in the brain could not have to do with vaccination. The statistics should thus probably be revised.

79. Copies of the protocols in ANBL, Serological Dept.

80. Kling's annual report to the Royal Medical Board for the year 1931, dated March 31, 1932, ARMB.

81. "Teoretisk vilsenhet," according to Ulrika Graninger, "Osynligt blir synligt: Bakteriologins etablering i sekelskiftets svenska medicin" (diss., Linköping Studies in Arts and Science no 163, Stockholm: Carlssons, 1997).

82. Ludwik Fleck, *Genesis and Development of a Scientific Fact* (Chicago: University of Chicago Press, 1935).

83. Bonah, "'Experimental Rage.'"

84. J. Axel Höjer, *En läkares väg: Från Visby till Vietnam* (Stockholm: Bonnier, 1975), 130–32.

85. Höjer was a Social Democrat.

86. He got the position after five other candidates had declined, according to Berg, "Den gränslösa hälsan," 203.

87. Berg, "Den gränslösa hälsan," 201: "Axel Höjer höll en hög profil som stadsläkare. Bland annat gjorde han sig rikskänd genom att stoppa en hotande smittkoppsepidemi i Malmö med hjälp av massvaccinering och radiopropaganda."

88. Peter Sköld, "Smittkoppor—den nya tidens stora farsot," in *Svenska folkets hälsa i historiskt perspektiv*, ed. Jan Sundin et al. (Stockholm: Statens folkhälsoinstitut, 2005), 134–75; Sköld, "The Key to Success: The Role of Local Government in the Organization of Smallpox Vaccination in Sweden," *Medical History* 45 (2000): 201–26; Sköld, "Smittkoppor," 171.

89. Per Axelsson, *Höstens spöke: De svenska polioepidemiernas historia* (Stockholm: Carlssons, 2004).

90. Barbara Elkeles, "The German Debate on Human Experimentation between 1880 and 1914," in *Twentieth Century Ethics of Human Subjects Research: Historical Perspectives on Values, Practices, and Regulations*, ed. Volker Roelcke and Giovanni Maio (Stuttgart: Franz Steiner Verlag, 2004), 19–33; Christian Bonah and Philippe Menut, "BCG Vaccination around 1930: Dangerous Experiment or Established Prevention? Debates in France and Germany," in Roelcke and Maio, *Twentieth Century Ethics of Human Subjects Research*, 111–35.

Chapter Five

The Politicization of the Temperance Movement in Pre-independence Estonia

KEN KALLING AND ERKI TAMMIKSAAR

The early phase of the temperance movement, which was dominated by religious concerns, aimed to limit the abuse of hard alcohol. The pioneering countries in this fight during the first half of the nineteenth century were the United States, Great Britain, and Sweden. In the 1840s Germany also tried to limit the usage and abuse of hard alcohol.

In most countries wine and beer were not considered alcoholic beverages and as such were not targeted by abolitionists.[1] A change in attitude can be witnessed from 1832 onward, when the Preston Temperance Society, or the "Seven Men of Preston," established the first temperance society in England opposed to any alcohol. At approximately the same time a similar initiative emerged in Sweden.[2] The new movements aiming for teetotalism were initially rather modest in numbers and influence, until a new outburst in the temperance movement took place in the last quarter of the nineteenth century. From then on the rhetoric of the movement was increasingly influenced by natural sciences and medicine, the increasingly popular sources of arguments for political ideologies.

The biologizing of national discourse reached the Baltic shores relatively early, mostly due to the German intellectual domination in the region. The main gateway for German influence in Scandinavia was Sweden. Swedes after all constituted one-sixth of the membership of the Internationale Gesellschaft für Rassenhygienie established in Germany in 1905.[3]

For Russia the gateway for the introduction of German-related ideologies was the Russian Baltic provinces with their German-speaking elites. Yet the acceptance of new ideologies in the Baltic realm must not be oversimplified.

The Baltic community was complex: besides the German-speaking upper and middle classes there were the indigenous Estonians and Latvians, who belonged to the peasant layer of society at the time and whose national emancipation ideas and ideologies were steadily growing. This process created tension within the society, which took an ethnic character, to the extent that the 1905 Russian revolution there was even characterized as an anti-German pogrom.[4] In addition to the local players, the Russian central authorities increased tension in the region with their Russification initiative. A complex situation was emerging at the edge of one of the old European empires, where one group, the Baltic Germans, were trying to retain their traditional privileges; another group, the Estonians and Latvians, were challenging them; and the third, Russian state, was running the policy of divide et impera, aiming to bind the Western parts of the empire more tightly with the rest of it.

Because of this situation, the biologizing of national discourse in the Baltic realm must be viewed as a typical case from the turn of the nineteenth century, where emancipating ethnic groups in old European multiethnic empires were reacting to the attempts of the rulers to foster cultural homogeneity by additionally stressing the biological criteria in the ethnic singularity.[5] In this context the fight against alcohol became a factor uniting nationalism with natural sciences and public health concerns.

Gustav Piers von Bunge—a Baltic Temperance Activist

It is at this point that Gustav Piers von Bunge (1844–1920) comes into play. Bunge was the professor of physiology at the University of Basel. He was of Baltic German origin, a graduate and until 1885 an assistant professor of the University of Tartu (known then as the University of Dorpat). The latter was among the leading universities of the Russian Empire in the nineteenth century. The rather broad autonomy the Baltic provinces possessed at the time was reflected in the university—teaching was done in accordance with the German academic tradition. It was the alma mater for the ruling class of the then Russian Baltic provinces (Estland, Livland, and Kurland), modern-day Estonia and Latvia, the so-called Baltic Germans. In the period discussed in this chapter, they were still preserving their traditional economic and cultural domination over ethnic Estonians and Latvians. This social division paralleled by an ethnic (linguistic) one was established in the thirteenth century as a result of the so-called Baltic Crusades and lasted until the emergence of the independent Baltic republics in the 1920s.

In the nineteenth century several outstanding scientific schools emerged and worked in Tartu, in particular, that of experimental physiology developing in tight connections with chemists. The university can be viewed as the birthplace of experimental surgery (Nikolai Pirogov, 1810–81); experimental pharmacology (Rudolf Buchheim, 1820–79), and experimental psychiatry (Emil Kraepelin, 1856–1926). Bunge at the time was experimenting in nutritional physiology, and he was one of the founders of the vitamin theory.[6]

Bunge had ceased consuming alcohol during his student years (1863–71), as he had witnessed its devastating effects, especially on educated people. In 1885 Bunge gave a lecture in Tartu on vegetarianism where he attributed the success of the new popular ideology not to the denial of meat products but to its total denial of any alcohol.[7] The latter statement was also central to Bunge's inaugural lecture at the University of Basel in 1886. It discussed physiological topics and was headed "Die Alkoholfrage" (The alcohol question).[8]

In his speech Bunge proved, relying on scientific methods, the harmfulness of alcohol on human physiology. It was mainly because of this presentation that Bunge managed to convince many of his colleagues—physiologists as Robert Adolf Armand Tigerstedt (1853–1923) from Finland, Rudolf Wlassak (1865–1930) from Austria, and Adolf Eugen Fick (1829–1901) from Germany—to become supporters of his anti-alcohol work.[9] At the beginning of the 1890s, the Swiss temperance movement was joined by the famous psychiatrist Auguste-Henri Forel (1848–1931), who later became a prominent anti-alcohol activist in Europe.[10] Bunge also impressed Alfred Ploetz (1860–1940), a German physicist and eugenicist, who coined the infamous term "racial hygiene."[11]

Bunge's "Die Alkoholfrage" was translated into twenty languages, and more than a million copies were issued.[12] Bunge's contribution was especially valuable, as he managed to draw the educated circles not belonging to clergy (i.e., scientists, medical professionals, students, schoolteachers, trade unionists) into the temperance movement.[13] Freeing the movement from clerical dominance guaranteed the movement a broader reception.

The wave of anti-alcoholism also reached the Russian Empire, with its Western provinces pioneering the ideals. The geographic distinction can be explained by the cultural one—the dominant Lutheran faith of the region created an atmosphere favoring civic activity.[14] But there seem to have been even stronger factors that convinced the oppressed Baltic indigenous people to participate in organized abstinence work.[15] A hint toward these factors can be seen in the heading of a study on the history of Finnish abstinence movement: "Temperance as a Civic Religion." In Finland the anti-alcohol movement can be viewed as the first organized popular movement.[16] The same can be said of Estonia as perhaps "the first successful" one.

Centuries under German dominance meant not only economic and individual oppression—declared a seven-hundred-year slavery by Estonian nationalists—but it was also an environment where many cultural traditions were being taken over. Civic activity among Estonians in the nineteenth century mimicked the German pattern and was also a reaction against traditional class society. In the nineteenth century we witness the emergence of different German-style music and agricultural societies, student fraternities, and so on, uniting ethnic Estonians.[17] There was still one phenomenon in local public life where Estonians were pioneering and Germans lagging behind, and that was the establishment of temperance societies.

Our chapter aims to open some aspects in the Baltic temperance movement. The task is to point at the different ways ideas were received by the Baltic ethnic and social groups at the time.[18] Special attention is paid to Gustav von Bunge.

The Estonian Temperance Movement

The beginning of the organized work against alcohol abuse in Estonia can be traced back to the eighteenth century, when the religious sects were acting as pioneers.[19] At the same time there were some local moralists-enlighteners, including members of the medical profession, who spread a similar message. From the beginning of the nineteenth century, there is data on several Lutheran congregations taking abstinence oaths.[20] The nineteenth century witnessed a gradual increase of anti-alcohol literature, and among the authors were some early Estonian activists.[21]

The first modern temperance society in Estonia was established in 1889 and was based on the Finnish example.[22] Its founder, Jüri Tilk (1865–1929), a primary school teacher, was a Fennophile. The same can be said about Matthias Johann Eisen (1857–1934), an Estonian cleric and folklorist who had been a pastor at different Finnish congregations in Karelia and Ingermanland and had established contacts with a Finnish abstinence activist, Aksel August Granfelt (1846–1919).[23] The latter—who had converted to the "abstinence faith" allegedly in 1880 by reading some relevant English literature[24] and later published an international journal, *Internationale Monatschrift zur Bekämpfung der Trinksitten*—suggested to Eisen, who was already abstinent by personal conviction, to publish articles in the Estonian popular calendars with a call to establish anti-alcohol societies.[25] There were already seventy-four societies of this kind in Finland by 1886, all promoting Christian and patriotic values.[26]

The articles suggested by Granfelt and written by Eisen are available in two calendars for the year 1887.[27] The first Estonian temperance society was established two years later. Initially this society, located in rural southwest Estonia, included members all over Estonia and even from St. Petersburg.[28] Soon it had numerous followers. The emerging societies usually covered a rural parish or a town, uniting Estonian-speaking people of different backgrounds, including peasants and schoolteachers, but also women, who had the right to join. Societies were spread out to Estonian communities all over the Russian Empire, including Riga and St. Petersburg.[29] The Finnish and Estonian anti-alcohol societies represented mainly lower social ranks. In Estonia they consisted predominantly of the rural population, while in Finland the ratio of urban laborers was high.[3031]

The rapid spread of anti-alcohol societies in Estonia can be explained by several factors. As abstinence work was perhaps seen as a smaller threat to the state in comparison to the increasing popularity of different cultural societies, they must have been more easily accepted by the officials. Thus, it was one of the easiest ways for the Estonian ethnic minority, belonging predominantly to the peasantry and affiliated with the Lutheran Church (which placed them in a subordinate position in the Baltic for the first reason; for both reasons in the Russian social hierarchy), to organize itself for cultural and patriotic aims.

Such an explanation is confirmed by the fact that the soaring membership in abstinence societies among Estonians correlated with the second rise in Estonian national movement in the last decade of the nineteenth century. In 1885 it was suggested that abstinence work should replace the failed first wave of "national awakening," lasting from 1860s until the middle of 1880s.[32] The person behind this idea, Ado Grenzstein (1849–1916), is usually characterized as a pro-Russian.[33]

The official Russian alcohol policy of the last decade of the nineteenth century, aiming at limiting consumption, supported the emergence of abstinence societies. The temperance societies founded in Russian-inhabited parts of the empire functioned under the auspices of the Orthodox Church and, unlike Finnish and Estonian societies, which were being organized from below, were elitist, constituted mainly of individuals belonging to the middle and upper classes. The same is true of the so-called Guardianships of Public Sobriety (попечительства о народной трезвости), organized by the state and meant to support the official alcohol policy. As the state wanted to avoid losses from alcohol sales, the guardianships propagated the so-called moderate concept in anti-alcohol work. Their aim was to distract people from periodic excessive drinking and cure them of alcoholism.[34]

Such modest goals created disappointment among many Russian teetotalers and resulted in the politicization of the issue in Russia, where in the increasingly revolutionary atmosphere there were heard rather radical demands to start a new era in alcohol politics by remodeling the whole society.[35] As a reaction to the obviously insufficient state-run campaigns against alcohol, private initiatives in the abstinence work emerged in the Russian-speaking parts of the empire.[36] In the Baltic region, Russian policy supported local developments but added some new areas deriving from the socioethnic controversies in the region.

The Politicization and Ideologization of
Estonian Temperance Movement

The peak of the Estonian temperance movement was the year 1903, when a total of sixty-one abstinence societies were active. After the Russian Revolution of 1905, this number started to diminish (with fifty-three in 1914, and the number of active members falling).[37] The decline was, besides the persecution of activists by the counterrevolution, mainly due to the emergence of rather liberal conditions of postrevolutionary Russia, enabling more open activities for the national minorities, including ethnic Estonians. Accordingly, the new educational societies and the first Estonian political party (Rahvameelne Eduerakond, Popular Party of Progress), established in 1905, entered the niche of patriotic activity that had until recently been dominated by abstinence societies. (Later it was acknowledged that abstinence societies had been the first to carry out popular educational work among the broader masses, especially in matters concerning natural sciences and health.[38])

One more reason for the decline may have been the growing alienation within the abstinence work between national elites pretending to see "a broader picture" and the activists at the local level. The latter targeted alcohol itself as a social vice, while the leaders preferred an approach by which the fight against alcohol served broader national goals. This is especially true of the years after the revolution of 1905, when the cover organization of Estonian abstinence societies became a battleground for different wings in Estonian national movement.[39] Among the latter, three main directions can be identified: liberals and socialists, plus a radical party trying to find a "third way" between the first two.

As the anti-alcohol societies in the modern Estonian territory were mainly uniting ethnic Estonians, the fight against alcohol had become a factor in Estonian national emancipation. A comparison of the Estonians' outstanding activity in abstinence work with the inactiveness in the same field of the local German-speaking Baltic elites supports this argument.

As already mentioned, the social division in Estonia in these times paralleled an ethnic one. Indigenous Estonian speakers, predominantly peasant folk, were in the second half of the nineteenth century at the beginning of their national emancipation. The process caused social tension, expressed in a conflict between the Deutsch (Baltic Germans) and the so-called Undeutsch (Estonians and Latvians). The anti-German sentiment among Undeutsch was supported by growing Russian influence in the region during the final decades of the nineteenth century, aiming to abolish the remnants of Baltic autonomy and singularity. Russification in its practical aspects targeted at firsthand the Undeutsch, but it also supported their political struggle against Baltic German domination.[40]

Estonians targeted different privileges of the German upper class. As in rural areas the right to run taverns was mainly a privilege of the predominantly German-speaking landlords, the fight against drinking places was often accompanied by anti-German sentiment.[41] The same Estonian schadenfreude was present when Russian state monopoly for alcohol sales introduced in 1894 came into force in the Baltic provinces in 1900, limiting with it the historic privileges of the local Ritterschaft. Unlike other parts of Russia, where dissatisfaction concerning alcohol policies was channeled into state criticism, the Baltic region saw the local elites being targeted. Such developments, initiated by the Russian state, caused local elites economic harm and were used by Estonian nationalists for propagandistic purposes, and they must be viewed among the factors distancing the local German-speaking elites from the abstinence work.

There seems to have been one more reason that the Baltic German aristocracy misunderstood the ideas of anti-alcohol work and Estonians grasped after it. At this point one has to admit a rather far-reaching biologizing of the concept of nation by Estonian elites in the turn of the past century—the ideas of eugenics and racial theories influencing the national discourse. Historians of eugenics have explained this development with the wish to challenge the existing logics of class society by meritocratic ideas.[42] And as mentioned previously, it must have also been a way, typical to the era, of defining a nation's distinctive character in a context in which it was questioned.

The tendency to biologize the concept of nationality was common in Europe, but in Estonia a special facet has to be taken into account. Estonia could be said to suffer from a national inferiority complex caused by its small population, compared especially to Russians and Germans. Furthermore, according to the theories of the era, without statehood Estonians were seen as a culturally inferior *Naturvolk*, as opposed to the politically developed so-called *Kulturvolk*.[43]

A peasant society with "no history" had to forget about its future as a political nation, a fate not accepted by the leaders of Estonian national movement. Juhan Luiga (1873–1927), a psychiatrist and an early propagandist of eugenics in Estonia, resisted this ideology, declaring that instead of so-called political history, arguments from natural sciences should be implemented to justify the existence and emancipation of Estonians. The "Laws of Nature" became a national challenge.[44] They could not be voted by parliaments nor denied by monarchs.[45] The concept of nation was in Estonian tradition understood mainly through linguistic criteria, but it also included biological aspects.[46]

As a result, different phenomena in social life were pathologized or medicalized; eugenic targets—both the quality and quantity of people—were put forward; and alcohol, as a broadly accepted threat for the "national body," received a central position in national discourse.[47] The main proponents of the threats of alcohol in a eugenic sense were Luiga and Jaan Tõnisson (1868–1940?). The latter, an outstanding national leader of his time, head of the party of liberals and editor of the influential Estonian newspaper *Postimees*, declared that even if people were not receptive to the anti-alcohol sentiment, they ought to support the movement for its eugenic character—the fate of the Estonian nation was at stake.[48] Such an approach was generally welcomed by different Estonian nationalist movements.[49]

The ideologization and politicization of the temperance movement was the context in which the previously mentioned alienation between the national elites and local activists can be seen. Tõnisson, who was to make abstinence work one of the tools of his political work, declared in 1898 that "the whole abstinence ideology seems to be imported, and is lacking understandable goals."[50] In 1907 complaints were already arising—as the Tõnisson's group had won a leading position in the movement—that educated leaders were campaigning against alcohol in a far too complicated way that "ordinary men" found hard to understand and felt themselves diverted from abstinence work.[51]

The increasing involvement of the educated circles in the Estonian temperance movement caused its medicalization.[52] Villem Reiman (1861–1917), a pastor and a leading temperance activist, already described alcohol in Darwinian and hereditarian terms in 1890.[53] Tõnisson, after participating at the International Anti-Alcohol Congress in Vienna in 1901, eagerly spread the ideas of A. Forel and Dumeng Bezzola (1848–1931).[54]

As a result, one might agree with the leftist historian Hans Kruus (1891–1976), who in 1921 wrote that at the turn of the century the ideology of Estonian liberals, the followers of Tõnisson—who were definitely the most idealistic among the nationalist groups—had departed from the metaphysical concept of "national spirit" and was based on a new entity, the allegedly science-based "national body." Kruus, who blamed German influence for making racial theories important for Estonian ideologists, stated that instead of Hegel and Kant, in Estonia the theories of racial hygiene were welcomed.[55] German traces, next to the Finnish ones, can also be seen in the anti-alcohol work. The Estonian abstinence propagandists were also familiar with the texts of Bunge.[56]

Gustav von Bunge and His Abstinence Writings

Bunge must have become interested in the temperance work while working in Tartu. In his booklet *Die Alkoholfrage*, he discussed his own studies concerning the harm of alcohol on organisms and presented his ideas on how to fight the dangers. Bunge based his anti-alcohol message on the theory of degeneration. It saw a broad spectrum of items (including alcohol), as "racial poisons," agents capable of weakening directly or indirectly (i.e., by breastfeeding mothers) the biological quality of present and future generations. In Basel Bunge continued to collect scientific data on the harmfulness of alcohol. He studied breast milk and breastfeeding and in this study Bunge used a questionnaire that he sent to numerous colleagues at home and abroad.[57] Bunge's aim was to collect data on the influence of alcohol consumption on the length and quality of breastfeeding.[58] He included in the questionnaires propagandistic material he prepared himself.

Bunge believed that the fate of his passion was mainly dependent on the good will and attitude of the elites: "It is the duty of educated, rich, influential and reigning, to impinge by their personal example." The final step— prohibition of alcohol—was to be taken by the state, but for that "passing legal acts by the state a path for it has to be prepared by private societies."[59]

Bunge admitted that his dedication to anti-alcohol work hindered his career. His colleagues were suspicious and spread rumors that he had become mentally ill and was hospitalized. The latter rumor emerged because he was not spending time with his friends and drinking beer.[60] In a letter to his sister Elisabeth von Ruckteschell (1850–1948), from the year 1903, Bunge is convinced that he made the right choice, especially as the circle of his supporters was gradually growing.[61] Confirmation for that comes from the year 1900, when the Estonian newspaper *Postimees* informed its readers that the opening of the annual Livonian Doctor's Days was greeted, among others, by the "Society of Abstinent Doctors of Germany."[62] The document was undersigned by E. Kraepelin, a world-famous psychiatrist who had worked in Tartu between 1886 and 1891 and contributed, among other things, to medical anti-alcohol work.

The predominantly German-speaking medical professionals in the Baltic were rather reluctant to accept matters related to alcohol into their agenda. The same applies to the Baltic German community in general, especially the aristocrats. They were acquainted with the abstinence work but reluctant to become involved in the movement. This is reflected in a letter Bunge received from his brother Woldemar (1842–92) in 1891: "Quite a number of people here are interested in the alcohol-issue, but it is not easy for them to make a decision to join an anti-alcohol society."[63]

Gustav von Bunge was very unhappy about the drinking frenzy among the students of his alma mater; these youngsters were after all the future elites of the society. The contacts Bunge had kept in his homeland supported his conviction that the drinking traditions of German Burschenschaften—continuing also among alumni—had spoiled the health of the men involved (he believed that the Baltic German women were still unspoiled).[64] The situation was mocked in the Estonian media. An Estonian anti-alcohol booklet from 1895 includes an ironic comment by which the only reaction of local students to Bunges's propagandistic anti-alcohol speech held in Tartu was to name one popular schnapps after Bunge.[65]

Bunge noticed and was especially annoyed by the fact that Estonians were more active in anti-alcohol work than local Germans. In 1904 he complained to his sister, "This is really disgraceful that our Estonians have more sense than our Germans. It seems that no one is telling the truth in Tartu to our moonshine-soaked members of student fraternities."[66] In 1910 Bunge wrote, "The *Herren* (meaning the Baltic Germans) have no right to complain about the Russification as long as they Russify themselves itself [with alcohol]. My only hope is that Estonians and Latvians shake them awake from their crystallized numbness."[67]

Wishing to bring about changes, Bunge sent temperance literature to the student fraternity he had belonged to (Korp! Livonia). Bunge also provided his sister with the relevant literature, the latter wishing to start a temperance movement among the youth of Tartu in 1910. Bunge advised her to seek support from August Rauber (1841–1917), the professor of anatomy at the University of Tartu, and the teacher of the local private gymnasium, Georg Rathlef (1846–1914).[68] The latter, along with the popular professor of practical theology Traugott Hahn (1875–1919), became actively involved in the temperance movement.[69]

The attitude of Baltic Germans toward the alcohol-issue started to change in parallel with the growing Russification on one hand and the emancipation of Estonians on the other. An important factor sparking German activity in the temperance movement must have been the Russian Revolution of 1905, which affected the urban middle classes. This is also where the Finnish left their marks. A change in Baltic-German attitudes towards alcohol did not take place among the academic circles of Tartu but in the local economic center that was Riga, modern Latvia. In 1906 this town hosted an exhibition dedicated to the living conditions of workers. It included a section about health matters, where the topic of alcohol was discussed through lectures and three spectacles for children, organized by a Finnish doctor Alli Trygg-Helenius (1852–1926). Her approach became highly popular in Riga. As a result, the topic of anti-alcohol work entered the agenda of local German craftsmen's guild.[70]

In 1908 the Riga Society for Promoting People's Welfare (Der Verein zur Förderung der Volkswohlfahrt) was created. The next year a group of teachers and women organized in it a section for a fight against alcohol (Sektion zur Bekämpfung des Alkoholismus). The section propagated the ideology of absolute abstinence. It supported the ideas of Bunge and Kraepelin but also appreciated works by the Finnish professor of hygiene and abstinence activist Taavetti Laitinen (1866–1941). The section handed out literature and leaflets. It included Latvians and Russians as members, and in 1910 a workers' section was attached to it.[71]

In Baltic German-language abstinence work women took on an important role. In Germany the first "abstinence circle" for women had emerged in 1900. The Abstinence Society of Baltic Women (Bund der Baltischen Abstinenten Frauen) was organized in Riga in February 1909 with the support of German agitators and chaired by Elisabeth von Grewingk (?–1930). The society became attached to the Sektion zur Bekämpfung des Alkoholismus. There were attempts to organize similar, German-speaking female abstinence societies in Tallinn (then Reval) and Tartu (both in modern Estonia), but these plans never came to fruition.[72]

The Medical Profession in Anti-alcohol Work

For Bunge the most important challenge seems to have been the task of changing the mentality of local medical doctors. Bunge was a supporter of full abstinence, which he demanded also of the anti-alcohol societies and activists. He stressed that the history of anti-alcohol movement has proved that the societies propagating moderation have been unable to get results.[73]

The problem was that the doctors of his homeland seemed to stand on the opposite side. The protocols from the Tartu and Tallinn medical societies from the end of nineteenth century until the year 1912 show no interest in the alcohol issue, as there were no presentations on alcohol during that time and during the meetings the doctors drank beer.[74] Bunge was convinced that the old-school professionals with their alcohol-friendly attitude did great harm to the reception of abstinence work in society, and there was no hope for improvement until the change of generations had taken place. Bunge believed that the new generation of medical professionals would reason in a different—modern—way.[75]

The local, predominantly German-speaking medical professionals also exposed their old-fashioned attitude by paying rather modest attention to the pleadings of the Estonian anti-alcohol societies. The latter wished the annual local provincial doctors' meetings (so-called doctors' days) to use their authority and denounce the popular belief among people that alcohol was a remedy. There was some reaction as at the Livonian doctors' days in 1900 a commission was elected, whose task it was to work out a position for doctors on the alcohol issue, but the results seem to have remained unsatisfactory.[76]

In 1909 an institution emerged uniting the medical professionals of all three Baltic provinces. The so-called Baltic Congress of Doctors (Baltischer Ärztekongress) was held in Tartu and was once more approached by Estonian anti-alcohol societies with a plea to take a critical position on alcohol. Again there was no immediate official reaction, and Estonian newspapers had a reason to criticize the event.[77] One of the then outstanding

Estonian doctors involved in the national movement, Henrik Koppel (1863–1944), had to admit that the atmosphere of the congress was dominated by German mentality, and a critical topic for every practicing medical doctor was missing from its agenda—the health of his circle, homeland, and nation.[78]

In reaction to the possible negligence of local medical societies toward the concerns of indigenous population, the Estonian-born doctors declared a need to organize on a national basis. Such a standpoint had been confirmed by the visit of some leading Estonian nationalists also participating in the anti-alcohol work to the Eleventh International Abstinence Congress, held in Stockholm in 1907. The visit was reflected in Estonian media with an article by Koppel, headlined "Alcohol, Medical Science and Doctors" ("Alkohol, arstiteadus ja arstid"), in which several Nordic authorities were cited to stress the importance of medical professionals' role in the anti-alcohol movement.[79]

The North Baltic[80] Doctors' Society (Põhja Balti Arstide Selts) was established in 1912, integrating Estonian-speaking doctors and veterinarians. Among other activities, the society took over the publication of the popular Estonian-language journal *Tervis* (Health), established in 1903 by Tõnisson and Koppel, thereby contributing to the temperance movement.

Retrospectively, the split along national lines among Baltic medical professionals was an overreaction caused by national tensions. Relative to the anti-alcohol work, changes were also taking place in German-dominated medical circles. The chairman of the 1909 Baltic Congress of Doctors, Prof. Karl Dehio (1851–1927), had, in fact, declared the pleadings of Estonian anti-alcohol societies very important and made a proposal to discuss the topic during the next congress, scheduled to take place three years later. Despite the skepticism of some of the participants, Dehio's will prevailed. It was decided that the medical profession had an obligation to formulate its position concerning alcohol. In response to Dehio's proposal, a so-called alcohol commission was formed. Its members had to prepare scientific presentations on the influence of alcohol on human organism and to discuss the ways of fighting its harmfulness.[81] At the Second Congress of Baltic Doctors, held in 1912, several presentations were given on the topic. They were published in the journal *St. Petersburger medizinische Zeitschrift*, uniting the German medical professionals of Russia.[82] In addition, a separate booklet was issued with a resolution of the congress on the matters of alcohol.[83]

The presentations held at the congress lauded the abstinence movement but also stressed individual autonomy to decide whether to consume alcohol. There were presentations pro and con absolute abstinence as well as moderation. Knowing the inclination of doctors to support moderation in alcohol consumption, the congress was approached by the Riga Society for

Promoting People's Welfare, which by then had become involved in the treatment of alcoholism, with a public letter to support total abstinence.[84]

As a reaction to complaints that the presentations given at the congress had been too scientific and did not agitate for abstinence, the chair of the commission, Dehio, commented that the aim was not to make propaganda for abstinence but to analyze the severity of the alcohol problem. Dehio also declared that criticism of the principle of moderation in abstinence work is not justified because this method promises results. As an example, he brought data showing that the students in Tartu had quit their practice of drinking beer in the mornings and evidence that sports and hiking were gaining popularity.[85] Not only that, there were also other hints that among students the topic of alcohol had become a matter of interest, and they discussed the issue in their fraternities.[86]

The congress declared alcohol an ultimate social vice, "a poison to the people." It was also admitted that until then the most successful fight against alcohol had been conducted by the abstinence societies. However, the congress did state that adults had the right to decide for themselves whether to consume alcohol.[87] In this way the resolutions of the congress were a compromise that did not demand absolute denial of alcohol, and this angered Bunge greatly.[88]

Bunge's Legacy

Gustav von Bunge died in 1920, in the same year the Estonian Republic was de facto born. The anti-alcohol movement had played an important role in the process of Estonian national emancipation and nation building, serving as one context where political culture was learned.[89] Civic activity remained in the newly independent Estonia. Temperance movements continued to remain active, promoting, among other things, women's emancipation. The Estonian eugenics society, established in 1924, kept alive the discussions on the biological essence of the nation. It was also never agreed among different parties within the abstinence work whether moderation or total abstinence, as was demanded by Bunge, was to be preferred.[90]

It is impossible to say how Bunge would have greeted the emergence of the Estonian state. Perhaps he would have been positively inclined; after all, Estonia came very close to introducing a prohibition law in the early 1920s.[91] The newborn state also introduced a policy somewhat resembling the so-called Gothenburg system, redistributing the profits earned (in Estonia's case, by the state) from alcohol sales for public purposes, including supporting anti-alcohol work. The idea was already propagated in Estonia before independence.[92] The Gothenburg system lasted in Estonia until 1926. Then alcohol sales were liberated in Estonia.[93]

However, the new state expropriated the land of the Baltic-German nobility, an act fitting the general anti-German atmosphere in Europe in the years after the Great War. Bunge's name can be found on the pages of the histories of German nationalism, imperialism, and racial hygiene.[94] Bunge's driving motivation in his fight against alcohol very well might have been Pan-Germanism. In 1904 he wrote to his sister, justifying his campaign, "If Germans in Russia could follow two principles: 1) stop poisoning themselves with alcohol; 2) stop mixing with inferior races, then they could rule not only in Russia, but in the whole world. No race in the world can compete with the pure and healthy German blood."[95]

Historically, the medical justification of abstinence ideology has supported racially biased theories and eugenics. Yet Bunge's case seems to be more complicated, as he personally was inconsistent with regard to biological reductionism. On the one hand, he participated in the increasingly popular nineteenth-century trend of idealizing biological elements in social discourse. On the other hand, some of his scientific theories express discontent with mechanical explanations in some natural sciences. Bunge was one of the founders of biovitalism (neovitalism), a theory that resists reducing life processes to simple physical and chemical mechanisms.[96]

In fact, several representatives of the Baltic scientific community supported theories diverging from the main direction of the natural sciences: Karl Ernst von Baer (1792–1876) supported teleological principles in life sciences, Wilhelm Ostwald (1853–1932) became one of the founders of monist ideology, and Jakob Johann von Uexküll (1864–1944) that of biosemiotics.[97] The theory that the choices made by the mentioned Baltic scholars were accidental, is not credible. It seems, instead, that the local sociopolitical context where the Baltic upper-class society was endangered by modernization, but also where the social Darwinist environment of the Russian Empire was endangering ethnic and cultural minorities, was a catalyst for such defensive ideological inclinations.

Bunge in that way seems to have been in an awkward position concerning his scientific views, understood within the political discourse of his homeland. Representing Baltic aristocracy, Bunge had to witness his aristocratic compatriots clinging to traditional class society and denying the objectification of the members of their social status under any concepts limiting individual autonomy or substituting the traditional social patterns with the reductionist mechanisms of the natural world. The Baltic upper classes felt threatened by the growing pressure from Russian central authorities and were losing ground to the emerging indigenous ethnic groups—Estonians and Latvians. Such developments could cause defensive reactions against modern ideologies. As a result, the anti-alcohol work in the Baltic countries was limited to the middle and lower classes and women, all emerging as the new players on the historical scene.

Notes

This study was funded by the Ministry of Education and Research of the Republic of Estonia (Projects IUT 2-16 and P170021SPTL).

1. Hermann Blocher, *Gustav von Bunge: Eine Gedächtnisrede, gehalten in der am 28. November 1920 vom Basler Abstinentenverband veranstalteten Gedenkfeier* (Lausanne: Alkoholgegnerverlag, 1920), 14, 17.

2. Eduard Graeter, *Gustav von Bunge: Naturforscher und Menschenfreund* (Basel: Schweizerischer Verein abstinenter Lehrer und Lehrerinnen, 1952), 15–16.

3. Gunnar Broberg and Mattias Tydén, "Eugenics in Sweden: Efficient Care," in *Eugenics and the Welfare State*, ed. Gunnar Broberg and Nils Roll-Hansen (East Lansing: Michigan State University Press, 1996), 77–149, esp. 83.

4. Björn Felder, "Introduction: Eugenics, Sterilisation and the Racial State; The Baltic States, Russia, and the Global Eugenics Movement," in *Baltic Eugenics: Biopolitics, Race and Nation in Interwar Estonia, Latvia and Lithuania 1918–1940*, ed. Björn Felder and Paul Weindling (Amsterdam: Rodopi, 2013), 5–29, esp. 9.

5. Paul Weindling, "Race, Eugenics and National Identity in the Eastern Baltic: From Racial Surveys to Racial States," in Felder and Weindling, *Baltic Eugenics*, 33–48, 35.

6. Cristiaan Eijkman and Frederick Hopkins, "The Earlier History of Vitamin Research," in *Nobel Lectures: Physiology or Medicine 1922–1941* (Amsterdam: Elsevier, 1965), http://www.nobelprize.org/nobel_prizes/medicine/laureates/1929/hopkins-lecture.html.

7. Graeter, *Gustav von Bunge*, 17.

8. Gustav von Bunge, *Die Alkoholfrage: Ein Vortrag* (Leipzig: Vogel, 1887).

9. Blocher, *Gustav von Bunge*, 19.

10. Ibid., 26–27.

11. Paul Weindling, *Health, Race and German Politics between National Unification and Nazism, 1870–1945* (Cambridge: Cambridge University Press, 1989), 71–72.

12. Graeter, *Gustav von Bunge*, 18. In 1894 it became available in Estonian.

13. Blocher, *Gustav von Bunge*, 18–19.

14. Patricia Herlihy, *The Alcoholic Empire: Vodka & Politics in Late Imperial Russia* (Oxford: Oxford University Press, 2002), 108.

15. Ibid., 118–19.

16. Irma Sulkunen, *Raittius kansalaisuskontona* (Helsinki: SHS, 1986).

17. Erki Tammiksaar, "Alexander Theodor von Middendorff und die Entwicklung der livländischen Gesellschaft in den Jahren 1860 bis 1865," *Zeitschrift für Ostmitteleuropa-Forschung* 59, no. 2 (2010): 147–85.

18. The article does not discuss in detail the anti-alcohol movement among ethnic Latvians. It has been written that the first Latvian abstinence society, established in 1891 in Riga, followed among others Estonian example—Герман Ассар, "Исторический очеркъ противоалкогольнаго движеия у латышей," in *Труды Перваго Всероссийскаго Съѣзда по Борбѣ съ Пянствомъ: Санкт-Петербургъ, 28 декабря 1909 г.–6 января 1910 г.* (С.-Петербургъ: Типография П. П. Сойкина, 1910), 974.

19. Rudolf Põldmäe, "Eesti vennastekoguduste võitlus rahva joomapahega," *Eesti Kirjandus* 32, no. 6 (1938): 281–93.

20. Otu Ibius, "Eesti karskusliikumise ajalugu," manuscript, Tartu University Library, Department of Rare Books and Manuscripts, booklet I–V. 1939: I; booklet, 131–35.

21. Friedrich Reinhold Kreutzwald, *Wina katk* (Tartu: Lindforsi pärijad, 1840).

22. A feature distinguishing Estonians from other Baltic people was a special relation to Finland. The so-called Finnish Bridge was a romantic euphemism to mark the admiring glance of Estonian elites toward Finland, a nation more developed in social sense with a similar language.

23. It is perhaps worth mentioning that Granfelt also visited Estonia in 1880 to learn from the work of the by then existing Estonian cultural societies, organizing among others national song festivals. Sulkunen, *Raittius kansalaisuskontona*, 49.

24. Mattias Eisen, "Isiklikke mälestusi Soome-Eesti kultuurilisestest kokkupuutumistest 50 aasta eest ja neile järgneval ajal," in *Tervitus lahe tagant*, ed. Friedebert Tuglas (Tartu: Eesti Kirjanduse Seltsi Kirjastus, 1931), 56–72, esp. 68.

25. Ibid.

26. Mattias Eisen, "Karskuse seltsid," in *Isamaa Kalender 1887 aastaks (Lisa)* (Tartu: Schnackenburg, 1886), 24, 26.

27. Ibid.; Eisen, "Joomine ja karskus."

28. Eduard Kubjas, *Eesti Karskusliit 1906–1931* (Tartu: Eesti Karskusliidu Kirjastus, 1931), 7.

29. Ellen Karu, "Pilk Eesti karskusseltside algusaastaisse," in *100 aastat karskusliikumist Eestis*, ed. Erki Silvet (Tallinn: Eesti Raamat, 1989), 8–29, esp. 9–10.

30. Ibid., 12–13.

31. Herlihy, *The Alcoholic Empire*, 118.

32. Grentzstein, "Joomise vastu," 1.

33. Toomas Karjahärm and Väino Sirk, *Eesti haritlaskonna kujunemine ja ideed 1850–1917* (Tallinn: Eesti Entsüklopeediakirjastus, 1997), 276.

34. Herlihy, *The Alcoholic Empire*, 14–17.

35. Ibid., 9–13.

36. Ibid., 111–28.

37. Karu, "Pilk Eesti karskusseltside algusaastaisse," 9.

38. Ernits, "Karskusliikumine ja haridustöö Eestis," 27.

39. Ibius, "Eesti karskusliikumise ajalugu," booklet II, 142.

40. Alexander von Tobien, *Die livländische Ritterschaft in ihrem Verhältnis zum Zarismus und russischen Nationalismus*, vol. 1 (Riga: Löffler, 1925); vol. 2 (Berlin: Walter de Gruyter, 1930); Reinhard Wittram, *Meinungskämpfe im baltischen Deutschtum während der Reformepoche des 19. Jahrhunderts* (Riga: E. Bruhns, 1934); Michael Haltzel, *Der Abbau der deutschen ständischen Selbstverwaltung in den Ostseeprovinzen Russlands: Ein Beitrag zur Geschichte der russischen Unifizierungspolitik 1855–1905* (Marburg a. d. Lahn: Herder-Institut, 1977); Edward C. Thaden, *Russification in the Baltic Provinces and Finland, 1855–1914* (Princeton, NJ: Princeton University Press, 1981).

41. For the sake of truth, it has to be stressed here that there were also landowners who were closing taverns by their own initiative, either for economic or moral reasons.

42. Greta Jones, "Theoretical Foundations of Eugenics," in *Essays in the History of Eugenics*, ed. Robert A. Peel (London: Galton Institute, 1997), 1–19, esp. 7.

43. Ken Kalling, "Application of Eugenics in Estonia 1918–1940," in Felder and Weindling, *Baltic Eugenics*, 49–82, 49–50.

44. Juhan Luiga, "Rahvaste tõus ja langemine" (speech given in 1909), in *Mäss ja meelehaigus*, ed. Hando Runnel, 132–40 (Tartu: Ilmamaa, 1995), 221.

45. Mihkel Pill, "Darwini saja-aastase sünnipäeva mälestuseks," *Eesti Üliõpilaste Seltsi Album* 8 (1910): 24–58, 58.

46. Ken Kalling and Leiu Heapost, "Racial Identity and Physical Anthropology in Estonia 1800–1945," in Felder and Weindling, *Baltic Eugenics*, 83–114.

47. Ken Kalling, "Karskusliikumine sünnitab eugeenikaliikumise," *Mäetagused* 36 (2007): 59–78.

48. Jaan Tõnisson, "Sõnavõtt," in *Kuues Eesti karskusseltside kongress* (Tartu: Eesti Karskusseltside Kesktoimkond, 1907), 7–9.

49. Kalling, "Application of Eugenics in Estonia 1918–1940."

50. Jaan Tõnisson, "Kolmas üleüldine Eesti karskuskoosolek," *Postimees*, January 5/17, 1898, 1–2.

51. *Kuues Eesti karskusseltside congress*, 13.

52. Ken Kalling, "Karskusliikumine ja arstiteadus sõjaeelses Eestis," *Eesti Arst* 91, no 9 (2012): 415–22.

53. Villem Reiman, "Kas elutilk või surnumeri," *Postimees*, February 27, 1890, 1.

54. Jaan Tõnisson, "Alkoholivabast kultuurist," in *Tulev Eesti Jõulualbum 1921* (Tartu: O. Lõhmuspuu, 1921), 9–15, esp. 9–10.

55. Hans Kruus, *Jaan Tõnisson Eesti kodanluse juhina* (Tartu: Odamees, 1921), 89.

56. Villem Ernits, "Villem Reiman karskustegelasena," in *Tulev Eesti Jõulualbum*, 29.

57. Gustav von Bunge, *Die zunehmende Unfähigkeit der Frauen ihre Kinder zu stillen: Die Ursachen dieser Unfähigkeit, die Mittel zur Verhütung* (Munich: Ernst Reinhardt, 1903). The research was published in Estonian in 1904.

58. "Statistisches Material: Eine Anzahl Fragebogen, ausgefüllt von verschiedener Medizinern," in *Öffentliche Bibliothek der Universität Basel, Handschriftenabteilung, Nachlass Gustav von Bunge*, die Mappe 57.

59. Gustav von Bunge, *Alkoholi küsimus* (Jurjew: K. A. Hermann, 1894), 20, 22.

60. Gustav von Bunge to Louise von Bunge, Basel, November 15/27, 1896. In *Öffentliche Bibliothek der Universität Basel, Handschriftenabteilung, Nachlass Gustav von Bunge*, Bestand No 114.

61. Gustav von Bunge to Elisabeth von Ruckteschell, Basel, June 21, 1903. In *Öffentliche Bibliothek der Universität Basel, Handschriftenabteilung, Nachlass Gustav von Bunge*, Bestand No 114.

62. "Liivimaa XII arstidepäeva üle," *Postimees*, September 6/12, 1900, 2.

63. Woldemar von Bunge to Gustav von Bunge, Dorpat, September 14/26, 1891, in *Öffentliche Bibliothek der Universität Basel, Handschriftenabteilung, Nachlass Gustav von Bunge*, Bestand No 114.

64. Gustav von Bunge to Louise von Bunge, Basel, November 27, 1900, in *Öffentliche Bibliothek der Universität Basel, Handschriftenabteilung, Nachlass Gustav von Bunge*, Bestand No 114.

65. "Professor Gustav v. Bunge," in *Eesti Karskuse Seltside Kalender 1895*, ed. Jüri Tilk (Jurjev: A. Grentzsteini trükikoda, 1894), 30.

66. Gustav von Bunge to Elisabeth von Ruckteschell, Basel, October 23, 1904, in *Öffentliche Bibliothek der Universität Basel, Handschriftenabteilung, Nachlass Gustav von Bunge*, Bestand No 114.

67. Gustav von Bunge to Elisabeth von Ruckteschell, Basel, October 25, 1910, in *Öffentliche Bibliothek der Universität Basel, Handschriftenabteilung, Nachlass Gustav von Bunge*, Bestand No 114.

68. Gustav von Bunge to Elisabeth von Ruckteschell, Basel, August 17, 1910, in *Öffentliche Bibliothek der Universität Basel, Handschriftenabteilung, Nachlass Gustav von Bunge*, Bestand No 114.

69. Gustav von Bunge to Elisabeth von Ruckteschell, Basel, March 21, 1913, in *Öffentliche Bibliothek der Universität Basel, Handschriftenabteilung, Nachlass Gustav von Bunge*, Bestand No 114.

70. Alexander Selenkoff, *Eine Skizze der Alkoholfrage (Nach einem am 12. April d. J. im Gewrbeverein gehaltenen Vortrage)* (Riga: Paul Kerkovius, 1907), 3.

71. Carl W. Schmidt, "Bericht über die Tätigkeit der Sektion zur Bekämpfung des Alkoholismus für das Jahr 1910," in *Verein zur Förderung der Volkswohlfahrt in Riga. Berichte über die Tätigkeit des Vereins, abgestattet auf dem 4. öffentl. Versammlung am 9. Febr. 1911* (Riga: G. Löffler, 1911), 5–14; Schmidt, "Über Trinkerfürsorge," *Hefte der Gesellschaft für kommunale Sozialpolitik in Riga* 3, no. 20 (1910): 117–52.

72. "Balti Naiste Karkusliidu tööst," *Eesti Naine* 7, no 8 (1926): 171.

73. Bunge, "Alkoholi küsimus," 22.

74. "Dörptsche medizinische Gesellschaft," Estonian Historical Archives 3576-1-13, Tartu, Estonia; "Die Gesellschaft der practischen Ärzte in Reval, 1911–1918," Estonian Historical Archives 5042-1-14.

75. Gustav von Bunge to Elisabeth von Ruckteschell, Basel, October 10, 1908, in *Öffentliche Bibliothek der Universität Basel, Handschriftenabteilung, Nachlass Gustav von Bunge*, Bestand No 114.

76. "Liivimaa XII arstidepäeva üle," 2.

77. Aadu Lüüs, "Ons eesti arstide ühing tarvilik?," *Postimees*, August 31, 1909, 1.

78. Henrik Koppel, "Mõni seletuse sõna eilase juhtkirja kohta: 'Ons eesti arstide ühisus tarvilik?,'" *Postimees*, September 1, 1909, 1.

79. Henrik Koppel, "Alkohol, arstiteadus ja arstid: XI üleilmlisel karskuse kongressil Stockholmis," *Tervis* 5, no. 1 (1907): 49–62.

80. Euphemism for Estonia, a word not acceptable for the then czarist authorities.

81. *Protocolle des I. Baltischen Aerztekongresses in Dorpat, 23.–25. August 1909* (St. Petersburg: Wienecke, 1910), 66.

82. Karl Dehio, "Der Alkohol und menschliche Organismus," *St. Petersburger medizinische Zeitschrift* 37, no. 20 (1912): 295–300; Christian Siebert, "Vorschläge zur Bekämpfung des Alkoholmissbrauches," *St. Petersburger medizinische Zeitschrift* 37, no. 20 (1912): 300–301; Hugo Hirsch, "Alkohol und Nerven," *St. Petersburger medizinische Zeitschrift* 37, no. 21 (1912): 311–15; Roderich von Engelhardt, "Die Alkoholfrage in individual- und sozialhygienischer Beleuchtung," *St. Petersburger medizinische Zeitschrift* 37, no. 21 (1912): 316–20.

83. Karl Dehio, *Der Alkoholmissbrauch und seine Bekämpfung. Vier Vorträge, gehalten auf dem II. baltischen Aerztekongress zu Reval 1912* (Jurjew: Krüger, 1912).

84. Carl W. Schmidt and Burchard von Schrenck, *An die vom Baltischen Aerztekongress gebildete ärztliche Kommission zur Begutachtung der Alkoholfrage* (Riga: Müllersche Buchdruckerei, 1912).

85. Dehio, *Der Alkoholmissbrauch und seine Bekämpfung.*

86. Werner Gruehn, "Was hat der Dorpater Student mit der heutigen Alkoholfrage zu tun? Gehalten im Theologischen Verein zu Dorpat am 14. November 1912," Estonian Historical Archives 1867-1-452.

87. Dehio, *Der Alkoholmissbrauch und seine Bekämpfung*, 52.

88. Gustav von Bunge to Elisabeth von Ruckteschell, Basel, March 14, 1913, in *Öffentliche Bibliothek der Universität Basel, Handschriftenabteilung, Nachlass Gustav von Bunge*, Bestand No 114.

89. Lauri Vahtre, "Karskusseltsid Eesti riikluse sünnis," *Akadeemia* 9, no. 5 (1997): 957–71.

90. Kalling, "Application of Eugenics in Estonia 1918–1940."

91. Jüri Ant, "Alkoholipoliitikast ja karskusliikumisest Eestis 1920–1940," in *100 aastat karskusliikumist Eestis 1889–1989*, ed. Erki Silvet (Tallinn: Eesti Raamat, 1989), 38–60, esp. 41–42.

92. "Göteborgi süsteem," *Tallinna Teataja*, nos. 68–69 (1910).

93. Ant, "Alkoholipoliitikast ja karskusliikumisest Eestis 1920–1940," 53.

94. Weindling, *Health, Race and German Politics between National Unification and Nazism, 1870–1945*.

95. Gustav von Bunge to Elisabeth von Ruckteschell, Basel, October 23, 1904, in *Öffentliche Bibliothek der Universität Basel, Handschriftenabteilung, Nachlass Gustav von Bunge*, Bestand No 114.

96. Gustav von Bunge, *Vitalismus und Mechanismus Ein Vortrag* (Leipzig: Vogel, 1886); Gerhard Schmidt, *Das geistige Vermächtnis von Gustav von Bunge: Inaugural-Dissertation zur Erlangung der Doktorwürde der gesamten Heilkunde vorgelegt der Medizinischen Fakultät der Universität Basel* (Basel, 1973), 72–77; Schmidt, *Das geistige Vermächtnis von Gustav von Bunge*, 26–37.

97. Tammiksaar Kalling, "Descent versus Extinction: The Reception of Darwinism in Estonia," in *The Reception of Charles Darwin in Europe*, ed. Eve-Marie Engels and Thomas F. Glick (London, New York: Continuum, 2008), 1:217–29.

Part Two

Bridging the Baltic

Comparative Studies

Chapter Six

Network Transfer

Paul Ehrlich and German-Scandinavian Scientific Relationships around 1900

AXEL C. HÜNTELMANN

The Statens Serum Institut in Copenhagen was inaugurated on September 9, 1902. Life scientists from Sweden, Great Britain, Germany, Italy, and the United States traveled to Copenhagen for the official ceremony, which lasted more than two days. Several Danish ministers attended the festivities. The accompanying program included official speeches, an eight-course gala dinner, a guided tour through the new institute and, as is customary on these occasions, excursions to tourist sites in Copenhagen and the surrounding area, and other scientific institutions in Copenhagen. Among the visitors were Julius Morgenroth from the Royal Prussian Institute for Experimental Therapy in Frankfurt, the institute's director, Paul Ehrlich, and his cousin, Carl Weigert, professor of pathological anatomy at the Senckenberg Foundation in Frankfurt. Ehrlich was placed prominently at the head of the table between the council president (the prime minister of Denmark), Johann Henrik Deuntzer, and the director of the Statens Serum Institute, Carl Julius Salomonsen.[1]

Despite having the character of an official ceremony, the inauguration also had elements of a private (family) celebration. Ehrlich and Deuntzer were bookended by the Salomonsens: Ellen Salomonsen sat next to Deuntzer. Next to her husband sat the minister of war, Vilhelm Hermann Oluf Madsen, the father of Thorvald Madsen. As Salomonsen's scientific

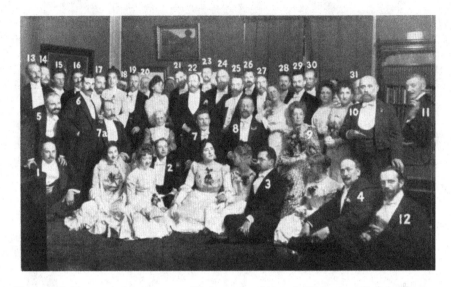

Figure 6.1. First grand Serumparty (Første store Serumfest). Source: E. Schelde-Møller, *Thorvald Madsen. I Videnskabens og Menneskehedens Tjeneste* (Copenhagen: Nyt Nordisk Forlag, 1970), 62–63.

assistant and a member of the new institute, the younger Madsen was also in attendance. Thorvald Madsen had spent some time as a guest researcher in Frankfurt at the Royal Prussian Institute for Experimental Therapy and the Pasteur Institute in Paris. Besides these family ties, there were other, quasi-genealogical ties. Scientists worked within the traditions of a certain field of research, and they defined themselves as scholars of someone else; for instance, Thorvald Madsen defined himself as a disciple of Salomonsen and Ehrlich. As a whole, members of an institution—a research institute, but also a thought community—could form a close network, as Sandra Legout describes the "famille pasteurienne."[2] During the inauguration ceremony, visitors were photographed in Thorvald Madsen's private rooms (fig. 6.1). Paul Ehrlich is placed at the center of the picture (7), framed by Vilhelm Hermann Oluf Madsen (8), and his wife, Albertine Henriette Madsen (maiden name Petersen, unnumbered on the photograph). At Ehrlich's feet were the three Madsen daughters (unnumbered) and Thorvald Madsen (2). Directly behind Ehrlich stood Carl Julius Salomonsen (25) and the Swedish physicochemist Svante Arrhenius (22). The above-mentioned Julius Morgenroth (3) sat on the floor, and Carl Weigert (10) stood at the right edge of the group.[3]

The photograph not only captures a joyful moment during the social events of the inauguration celebration; it also allegorizes the close community of a family-like thought collective,[4] taking place in the private rooms of one of its members, with true biological family members participating. Furthermore, the photograph allegorizes the idea of research networks—in this case, the international (research) network of Paul Ehrlich. In this chapter I will discuss the prehistory of this photograph and explain why Ehrlich played such a prominent role during the inauguration ceremony of the Statens Serum Institute. I analyze his (personal) networks with Scandinavian scientists like Thorvald Madsen, Carl Julius Salomonsen, and Svante Arrhenius. Alongside the relationships between German and Scandinavian life scientists, scientific networks provide an insight into knowledge production and the (international) spread of scientific ideas and practices through networks and, as such, the generation and workings of thought collectives.

This chapter stems from a biography of Ehrlich,[5] in which I characterize his work as network "management,"[6] analyzing the procedures and economies of communication and relationship. Mainly on the basis of Paul Ehrlich's personal papers (and his German perspective), I describe the different levels of networks, and the multiple transfers within these networks, that were an essential precondition of network building. First, I outline Paul Ehrlich's relationship to Carl Julius Salomonsen and, subsequently, the transfer of this personal exchange to Salomonsen's assistant Thorvald Madsen—described as generational network transfer. The personal relationship had been stabilized by the exchange of letters, mutual visits, meetings at conferences, and hosting scientists from abroad. Consequently, I describe the knowledge transfer that resulted from these personal relationships. Personal networks are not isolated entities but entangled frameworks, combining to build a (thought) collective of scientists: Just as Salomonsen and Madsen were important partners in Ehrlich's network(s), he was one of many partners in the networks of Salomonsen and Madsen. I follow the "post-history" of the photograph and summarize the developments after the inauguration ceremony. Along with the knowledge transfer through networks via personal relationships, there is a mutual transfer of credit expressed in official awards like prizes, titles, and honorary memberships in the national academies (of science). I emphasize the different layers within the network construction and trace the mutual transfer of recognition between Paul Ehrlich and his Scandinavian colleagues, which can be analyzed from the viewpoint of reciprocity.[7] As I show, all these different, multiple transfers built the (strong) ties of scientific networks.[8] The networks were not limited to life scientists but also included natural scientists such as Swedish physical chemist Svante Arrhenius. Using the example of Paul Ehrlich's relationship with Svante Arrhenius, I sketch the problems and misunderstandings that might occur in international and interdisciplinary collaborations and thus disrupt the network.

How Everything Started—
the Emergence of Personal Networks

Carl Julius Salomonsen

Carl Julius Salomonsen, born in 1847 in Copenhagen, son of physician Martin S. Salomonsen,[9] finished his medical studies in 1871. Beginning in 1873, he worked as a physician at the municipal hospital in Copenhagen, where he started carrying out bacteriological research.[10] In 1876, he published an article on the isolation and breeding of bacteria in a German botanical journal, referring to German publications of the Wroclaw scientists Julius Cohnheim and Ferdinand Cohn.[11] In his dissertation,[12] Salomonsen observed that the changing color of putrid blood was caused by microbes that had begun to putrefy. He developed a method to conserve blood in *capillaries*—very small glass tubes—which could then be used to isolate and cultivate microbes and analyze them under the microscope. Furthermore, he developed a method for staining bacteria in a water-fuchsine dilution.[13] In his early work, Salomonsen shared Ferdinand Cohn's view that bacteria were distinct species. Adopting Cohn's position, he sided against the view, mainly championed by the influential surgeon Theodor Billroth and his school, that microbes were only variants of one unspecific ubiquitous form of microorganism.[14]

After Salomonsen had finished his medical dissertation in 1877, he went to Wroclaw for several months to deepen his studies in "pathological anatomy" and "experimental pathology," as the emerging field of bacteriology was labeled at that time. It was not necessarily foreseeable that Salomonsen would choose to go to Wroclaw. Since the beginning of the nineteenth century, the previously close relationship between Prussia and Denmark had become increasingly strained, changing from that of friendly neighbors to rivals and cumulating in the military conflict of 1848–51, and the Danish-German War in 1864 (also known as the First and Second Schleswig Wars). Even thirteen years after the German-Danish War, there was still resentment toward the new German Empire in Denmark.[15]

Ferdinand Cohn and Julius Cohnheim were professors in Wroclaw, however, and it was only reasonable that Salomonsen, since he shared their scientific views, wanted to collaborate with them personally. According to Madsen, Salomonsen "was never in doubt of his destination: he wanted to go to Breslau [now Wroclaw] in order to work under Cohnheim, the greatest experimental pathologist of the time."[16] In Wroclaw, Salomonsen entered a close-knit community of researchers working on pathological and bacteriological problems, where he met, among others, Carl Weigert, Paul Ehrlich, Robert Koch, and the American William Welch. At this time, Koch was an unknown district physician in the West Prussian district town of Wollstein, and he had presented his first scientific results to Ferdinand Cohn in 1876.

Since then, Koch had collaborated with Cohn and Cohnheim, traveling to Wroclaw from time to time.[17] During his stay in the summer of 1877, Salomonsen became close friends with Carl Weigert and William Welch, who was also a guest researcher. Weigert was Julius Cohnheim's research assistant and the first person to stain bacteria in the early 1870s.[18] For the next few months, Salomonsen continued his bacteriological studies. Under the supervision of Julius Cohnheim, he inoculated the eye chamber of a rabbit with tubercular material to produce the typical symptoms of tuberculosis of the iris. The experiment was intended to prove the specificity of diseases, especially tuberculosis.[19] Furthermore, Salomonsen carried out Cohnheim's "frog experiments on inflammation, stasis, embolism, etc., which he later turned to such good account in his courses on experimental pathology."[20]

Decades later, in March 1914, Carl Julius Salomonsen published an article in the *Berliner Klinische Wochenschrift*, a well-known German medical journal, on the occasion of the sixtieth birthday of Paul Ehrlich. In a witty speech, Salomonsen traced a line back to the summer of 1877, remembering his time in Wroclaw.[21] His "closest friend," William Welch, shared similar memories:[22] the discussion of "the newest medical ideas" and current problems and developments in medicine, the open and intense working atmosphere in the laboratories, the teaching and development of new methods and bacteriological techniques, the participation in lectures and practical courses, the friendliness of their German colleagues. Together, they made excursions in and around Wroclaw: they joined the local botanical society on trips in the immediate vicinity, they attended meetings of the medical society in Wroclaw, they were invited to picnics and to private dinners by their colleagues and introduced into Wroclaw society.[23] As a Jew,[24] Salomonsen probably felt even more comfortable in Wroclaw, one of Germany's Jewish centers,[25] and in the company of Weigert, Cohnheim, Cohn, Ehrlich, and others. The different activities on multiple private and scientific levels built their ties and the personal relationships of Welch, Salomonsen, and Weigert. Madsen said that the travels to Wroclaw and Paris "were to influence the whole of his life."[26]

As was customary at that time, after his visit to Wroclaw, Salomonsen continued his educational tour. While Welch went to Vienna and Strasbourg,[27] Salomonsen traveled to Prague and Paris, where he continued his studies in the laboratories of Louis Pasteur during the following months.[28] The visit in Pasteurs institute became "an encounter that later proved to be of great significance for young Danish bacteriologists."[29] Back in Copenhagen, he introduced bacteriological methods to his Danish colleagues, and, on being appointed lecturer in bacteriology in 1883, he became the driving force behind the establishment of bacteriology as a scientific discipline in Denmark.[30] In 1893, he was appointed professor of pathology at the University of Copenhagen, and two years later, in 1895, Salomonsen established a bacteriology laboratory.

Paul Ehrlich and Carl Julius Salomonsen

In the summer of 1877, Salomonsen remembered, Paul Ehrlich was still a medical student, though preparing for his final examinations. Salomonsen was a few years older, and, because of that, he had a much closer relationship to Weigert.[31] Weigert was Ehrlich's older cousin, and he became his mentor and lifelong friend; in many ways, Ehrlich was his successor. In the photograph of Cohnheim's "pathology group" in the summer of 1877 (fig. 6.2), Ehrlich is standing alongside Julius Cohnheim behind the table—in the center of the photograph. According to Arthur M. Silverstein, William Welch is seated on the far left, with Weigert next to him, and Carl Julius Salomonsen is seated on the far right.[32] Paul Ehrlich, born in 1854 in the small city of Strehlen near Wroclaw, studied medicine in Wroclaw, Strasbourg, and Freiburg. His student days in Strasbourg, from September 1872 to spring 1874,[33] must have been an important link he shared with Welch, who had been in Strasbourg (and then Leipzig) before he came to Wroclaw. Both attended the same courses in anatomy, pathology, chemistry, and histology; both knew the same professors, such as Wilhelm von Waldeyer, Ernst von Leyden, and Friedrich Daniel von Recklinghausen.[34] As a student, Ehrlich was known as a passionate "dyer"—staining and differentiating tissue. While still a student, he published an article in the prestigious journal *Archiv für mikroskopische Anatomie* on the use of aniline dyes in microbiology, in which he reported the identification of a new type of cell (i.e., mast cells).[35] He finished his studies in Wroclaw, and, when Julius Cohnheim became professor of pathology at Leipzig, Ehrlich and his cousin, Weigert, followed him. In Leipzig, Ehrlich wrote his dissertation on the theory and practice of histological staining.[36] After his graduation from medical school, Ehrlich became a ward physician under Friedrich Theodor Frerichs at the Charité Hospital in Berlin. In addition to his clinical work as a hospital physician, he conducted scientific research in a small laboratory. Within a few years, he became a well-known expert in the fields of histology, hematology, and microbiology. By 1882, he had already been named a professor.[37]

Just like Welch, Salomonsen often returned to Germany. Salomonsen kept in touch with Koch by letter,[38] and he traveled to Berlin in the early 1880s after Koch had been appointed medical officer at the Imperial Health Office.[39] Salomonsen might have participated in one of the practical bacteriological courses held at the Imperial Health Office.[40] In his memoirs, Salomonsen mentions that he visited Koch in his laboratory at the Imperial Health Office in Berlin, where he also met his assistants Georg Gaffky and Friedrich Löffler. On this occasion, Salomonsen also visited Paul Ehrlich at the Charité Hospital in Berlin, which was practically across the street from the Imperial Health Office. Subsequently, Salomonsen traveled to Berlin

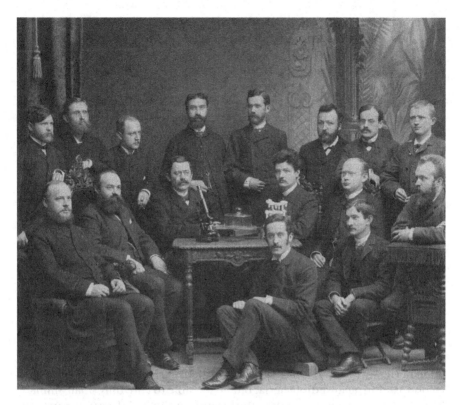

Figure 6.2. Cohnheim's pathology group in Wroclaw, summer 1877. Courtesy of Johns Hopkins Medical Archives.

many times, meeting Koch and Ehrlich;[41] for instance, he visited them during his stay at the Tenth International Congress of Medicine in August 1890.[42]

In addition to memories, Ehrlich and Salomonsen now shared several mutual research interests: the staining of tissues and pathogens, as well as their practical work in a hospital setting. Furthermore, in the 1880s they were both pioneers in a new, specialized research field—called "experimental pathology," bacteriology or microbiology—at the interface between medicine and chemistry, and the interspace between laboratory and bedside. And insofar as they shared similar views and experiences as specialized experts and interdisciplinary researchers in everyday life, they could have demonstrated and discussed their research results; new developments in medicine; and new practices, devices, and techniques in their common field of research, such as the tinctorial power of (new) dyestuffs or innovations in the optical industry. As members of a distinct thought collective, they perceived themselves as leaders in medical research and engines of progress. However, they also experienced similar problems and conflicts with "old" and established institutions: the struggle for financial and personal resources and the need to perform extra work to become accustomed to interdisciplinary research techniques, practices, and codes (a precondition so that research results are accepted and recognized by the relevant scientists of a discipline that is not "your own").[43] The possibility of misunderstanding often made it necessary to "translate" their research ideas and outcomes for scientists outside their own thought collective—which many times resulted in a lack of recognition and a reputation as outsiders[44] (according to their own perceptions).

After Koch had developed tuberculin in the autumn of 1890, Ehrlich assisted in the clinical trials at the Moabit Community Hospital in Berlin, and, after Koch became director of the newly founded Royal Prussian Institute for Infectious Diseases in 1891, he offered Ehrlich a laboratory and work space. At the institute in Berlin, Ehrlich worked with Emil Behring. Between 1890 and 1894 they developed—first in competing, and then in collaborating, work groups—a serum against diphtheria. Behring observed that certain species of animals were immune to specific diseases and, in contrast, that other species of animals were susceptible to a specific pathogen and, after recovering from the infection, developed an immunity to the disease.[45] Furthermore, he found that this immunity could be transferred—even interspecies—via blood transfusion. Emil Behring successfully developed a (blood-)serum against diphtheria, but he was able to cure only small animals. Ehrlich was able to increase the effectiveness of the blood serum: a precondition for its use as a remedy for humans, as well as for the industrialization of serum therapy. Now, large animals like horses were used as serum hosts. The emerging pharmaceutical industry was also an important cooperative partner, and, in August 1894, antidiphtheritic serum became available in German pharmacies. Both referring to and in competition with the research group at the Institute for Infectious Diseases, Émile Roux and other life scientists at the Pasteur Institute in Paris were also working on the development of a serum to cure diphtheria. In September 1894, Roux announced at the Eighth International Congress of Hygiene and Demography in Budapest that he too was able to produce antidiphtheritic serum.[46]

Like many bacteriologists of his time, Salomonsen must have followed developments in the medical journals carefully,[47] and we may also take for granted that he repeated the experiments he read about. Salomonsen remembered that after Roux's publication "the production of anti-diphtheric serum was eagerly taken in hands everywhere" and in "Denmark, too, the first introductory steps were made. . . . As the director of the University Laboratory of Medical Bacteriology I felt it my duty to study more thoroughly the technique of the production of antidiphtheric serum."[48]

Building on his previous research visit in the autumn of 1877, Salomonsen contacted Louis Pasteur. In September 1894, he visited the "production site" for the manufacture of serum at the Pasteur Institute, where members of the institute shared "the experience they had gained."[49] Back in Copenhagen, Salomonsen sent a petition to the Danish Ministry of Cultural Affairs asking for extra money to enable his laboratory to perform serotherapeutic experiments. Salomonsen wanted to install a special serotherapeutic department like those in Paris and Germany, to produce large quantities of antidiphtheritic serum. The serum would be provided free of charge to Danish hospitals and doctors. Moreover, in the new facility "some young medical men would be thoroughly trained in the technique" of serum production.[50]

The manufacture of serum in large quantities involved various difficulties at all levels of production: the production was spread out all over Copenhagen,[51] the serotherapeutic department was far too small, and the different strains of diphtheria bacteria produced toxins of varying strengths. Last but not least, the "individuality of the horse" also affected serum production.[52] Salomonsen contacted serum laboratories in Europe and the United States that were dealing with similar problems, remarking gratefully that some of them had "placed their experience at our disposal." In Salomonsen's 1902 statement about current methods of serum production and evaluation, he pointed to his ramified working network:

> I will only state that our method of immunization follows very closely upon that applied by Dr. Dean at the Jenner Institute for Preventive Medicine. It is Dr. Dean, too, whom we have to thank for so kindly supplying us with the strain of diphtheria bacillus (Parke & Davis no. 8) which we are using now. The methods of measuring are, of course, those of Ehrlich. This eminent pathologist has, during the whole existence of the Department assisted us in every possible way, and I take this opportunity to express to him my heartfelt gratitude.[53]

Whereas in France and Denmark serum had been produced mainly in scientific laboratories and provided free of charge to hospitals, in Great Britain and Germany serum was produced by private companies and available on the pharmaceutical market. In Germany, the new serum therapy attracted intense interest from the state, and a system of state control was implemented in hopes of minimizing any associated public health risks. In February 1895, a so-called control station was established as a department of the Institute for Infectious Diseases, where every serum that was sold on the German market had to be tested and proved harmless and effective. In 1896, the department was converted into a separate institute, the Royal Prussian Institute for Serum Research and Serum Survey (ISRSS), with Paul Ehrlich as its director. The new name emphasized the shift from testing to research: in addition to testing serum, members of the institute conducted research to improve methods and techniques of serum evaluation, thus helping to standardize the production process.[54]

Salomonsen visited Ehrlich at the institute in Steglitz, near Berlin,[55] where Ehrlich demonstrated the complex procedure of serum evaluation. We may also assume that he visited the Jenner Institute for Preventive Medicine in London. Salomonsen's history with the State Serum Institute demonstrates the entanglement, networks, cooperation and knowledge, and object transfer between the Danish and the German, French, British, and North American institutes. In addition, members of the London institute had visited the German institute. Dealing with the same problems described by Salomonsen—varying serum quality and effectiveness—German Sims Woodhead contacted Ehrlich in the summer of 1896 for help. He asked Ehrlich for a standard toxin to use as a basis on which to compare the different British sera.[56] And, in October 1897, Woodhead asked for permission "to study the methods in use at the government laboratory for the preparation and testing of serum at Steglitz."[57] Subsequently, Ehrlich maintained close contact with Woodhead and George Dean[58] and other members of the Institute for Preventive Medicine. However, when Salomonsen mentioned that the method of immunization followed "closely upon that applied by Dr. Dean" at the Institute for Preventive Medicine, he overlooked that the British method was mainly based on German-Franco research (and the literal exchange of research results) and on knowledge Woodhead had exchanged and collected in Steglitz. In return, Ehrlich received a stronger strain of bacteria cultures (as the basis for diphtheria toxin) from the Danish laboratory that had traveled originally from the United States via London and Copenhagen to Steglitz. Together, this represents a transfer of knowledge and objects as part of a closely intertwined network, a network that stretched beyond the Baltic Sea, connecting and bridging German, Danish, and British scientific institutions.[59]

Generational Networks—Madsen's "Inheritance" of Salomonsen's Networks

Over the years Ehrlich and Salomonsen visited each other several times and corresponded regularly. Ten or twelve letters spanning several years have survived in Paul Ehrlich's personal papers. Although not all his letters have survived, we can assume that in one of his letters Salomonsen may have asked whether his assistant, Thorvald Madsen, could visit the laboratories in Steglitz. Beyond their personal relationship, these men initiated an exchange of their students and coworkers to expand (and "hand down") their networks. Hence, Salomonsen transferred his networks to Thorvald Madsen.

As mentioned above, Thorvald Madsen was the son of Danish general and war minister (1901–5) Vilhelm Hermann Oluf Madsen. Born in 1870, he was a generation younger than Ehrlich (b. 1854) and Salomonsen (b. 1847). Madsen studied medicine in Copenhagen, and he was fascinated by the new microbiological and bacteriological sciences taught by Salomonsen. He finished his medical education in 1893 and, after a year as practitioner, entered Salomonsen's bacteriological laboratory, becoming his assistant in the serotherapeutic department.[60] The tiny department consisted only of Madsen and two assistants, and he was mainly responsible for producing serum to meet Danish demand. As Salomonsen mentioned, it was difficult to produce serum that was consistent in quality. The serum's quality, which mainly means its effectiveness, was determined according to immunization units. Different methods were used for measuring these immunization units and for evaluating the serum, leading to inconsistent results. This led to discrepancies in and doubts over the effectiveness of antidiphtheritic serum and serum therapy in general—in Denmark and elsewhere.[61] In this context, Madsen began a medical dissertation on diphtheria toxin, in which he compared the French, English, and German methods of serum evaluation.[62]

In his thesis, he concluded that the German method of evaluation had advantages over the French, since it was more precise and seemed to be cheaper and more convenient.[63] Madsen ended his comparative study with the suggestion that, because of the extraordinary importance of serotherapy, "the serum's potency should be evaluated based on an *international* scale unit because only in such a way is it possible to compare and to correctly appreciate the successes achieved."[64] As the basis for an international scale unit, Madsen favored the German method, which was reliable and easily accessible. Madsen also published his research results in a German journal, the prestigious *Zeitschrift für Hygiene*—edited by Robert Koch—summarizing his results in German.[65] Alongside his comparative study, he and Salomonsen were involved in clinical trials introducing antidiphtheritic serum at the Blegdamshospitalet that confirmed the effectiveness of the new therapy.[66] At this time, Madsen remembered, he began a lively correspondence with Paul Ehrlich.[67]

But the German method did not function exactly as expected either, and the results of the serum evaluations varied. It emerged that the "test toxin" used as a reference unit attenuated over time and was not as fixed and stable as Ehrlich originally assumed. This led to conflicts with the serum producers and the state-run test institute, and threatened to discredit serotherapy as a whole.[68] As a consequence, Ehrlich searched for a serum evaluation method that would produce clearer results, independent of place, time, and the person executing it. Between the summer of 1896 and spring of 1897, he worked on modifying the German method.

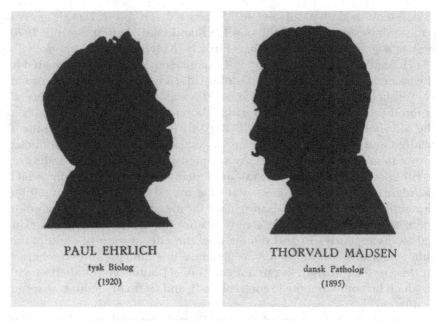

PAUL EHRLICH
tysk Biolog
(1920)

THORVALD MADSEN
dansk Patholog
(1895)

Figure 6.3. Left: Paul Ehrlich, silhouette made by Carl Julius Salomonsen in 1908. Right: Thorvald Madsen, silhouette made by Carl Julius Salomonsen in 1895. Source: Carl Julius Salomonsen, *Medicinske Silhouetter* (Copenhagen: Levin & Munksgaard, 1921), plates XXXV and XV.

The method was a relational system based on a defined vacuum-dried standard serum and standard toxin, and a serum that was tested on guinea pigs as bioindicators. One test run, including observation of the laboratory animal's reaction, took several days; carrying out a series of experiments with the calibration of the standard serum and standard toxin took weeks. For the test procedure, a guinea pig was injected with a mixture of a specified quantity of antidiphtheritic serum labeled by the manufacturer and a corresponding quantity of diphtheria toxin. If the guinea pig died on the fourth day, the number of immunization units was exactly as stated on the label; if the guinea pig died earlier, the serum was weaker than labeled and, conversely, if the guinea pig was still alive after four days, the serum was stronger than labeled.[69] While Ehrlich was working out a new method of evaluation, he was also developing a theory to explain immunological processes: the side-chain theory.[70]

In early 1899, Salomonsen and Madsen traveled to Berlin. Madsen wanted to learn more about the new evaluation method and Ehrlich's thoughts about immunological processes, and Salomonsen introduced him to Koch.[71] After his visit to Berlin, Madsen went to Marburg to visit

Emil Behring and, like his teacher Salomonsen, to Paris.[72] Only a few months later, Salomonsen returned to Germany, but this time he traveled to Frankfurt on Main, where the renamed ISRSS—now called the Royal Prussian Institute for Experimental Therapy—had moved. Salomonsen had been invited to celebrate the official inauguration of the institute. On his way back, he stopped by Dyestuff Industries in Hoechst and visited Behring in Marburg. Ehrlich was curious about Salomonsen's impressions of Behring's institute and the production site at Hoechst, and asked Salomonsen for his opinion.[73] Just half a year later, they met again in Paris at the Thirteenth International Medical Congress, where Ehrlich gave a talk about his side-chain theory.[74] Their relationship was closest between 1896 and 1902, and they met nearly every year—sometimes even twice a year—frequently sending letters between Berlin or Frankfurt and Copenhagen. Additionally, in 1902, Ehrlich was invited to the official inauguration of the Statens Serum Institute in Copenhagen.

Reciprocal Networks—Building Strong Ties:
The Maintenance of Networks

Establishment and Maintenance

In the years between 1899 and 1902, Carl Julius Salomonsen and Paul Ehrlich shared—in addition to many other things—one common experience in particular: the establishment and maintenance of a new institution. Salomonsen saw—as had Ehrlich before—that unforeseen difficulties might emerge during the establishment of an institution: in this case, doubts about the effectiveness of serotherapy, political turbulence, and financial difficulties. In March 1900, Salomonsen mentioned in a letter that the prospects for the planned serum institute were not good.[75] In the correspondence between Ehrlich and Salomonsen, as well as between Ehrlich and Madsen, various matters with private, scientific, and institutional aspects were inextricably entwined—just like their relationship. This multilayered entanglement explains why the ties between Ehrlich and his friends in Copenhagen were so strong. Furthermore, on the basis of their correspondence, we can analyze the underlying gift relationship—the reciprocal relationship of "give and take"[76]—that was necessary to establish and maintain a network.

As a starting point for an analysis of their gift relationship, I will single out an arbitrary event. Salomonsen employed Madsen as an assistant in his bacteriological laboratory, where he managed the production of antidiphtheritic serum. In the context of his work, Madsen began his dissertation on the differences in quality of antidiphtheritic serums and methods of evaluation. As mentioned, the comparison concluded that the German evaluation method was superior to the French. We can assume that Ehrlich was grateful to Madsen, but also to Salomonsen, and happy about this positive appraisal. Although this seems obvious, it had practical consequences. A member of the ISRSS, Wilhelm Dönitz, summarized the results of Madsen's dissertation. Ehrlich used the report for his own benefit and sent it to the Prussian Ministry of Cultural Affairs, which had authority over the ISRSS. In the cover letter, he pointed out that his work had been recognized by foreign scientists.[77] We can assume that Ehrlich was satisfied and had a positive impression of Madsen and, as a consequence, started a lively correspondence with Madsen. For Madsen, in return, Ehrlich's positive reception of his work had positive effects: Assuming that the reputation of the quality of a scientist's work depends on the confirmation of a third party—mainly members of the scientist's own thought collective—we can further suppose that Ehrlich's positive recognition of Madsen's work confirmed Salomonsen's good opinion of his assistant, Madsen. In general, Madsen's recognition in the scientific community increased. As we will see, he could now profit not only from Salomonsen's but also from Ehrlich's network. In the following years, they corresponded regularly; the letters addressed mainly scientific issues. In 1898, for instance, Ehrlich and Madsen extensively discussed the composition of diphtheria toxin and the quantitative determination of its elements. Ehrlich was satisfied that Madsen had proved and confirmed his findings.[78] In another letter, Ehrlich gave advice on one of Madsen's prospective publications.[79]

From January to April 1899, Madsen visited the ISRSS, where he was received with open arms. During that time, Ehrlich continued his work on the constitution of toxins and antitoxins, and Madsen became involved in these theoretical questions—and their experimental validation—as well as in the practical work of serum evaluation. In some ways, Madsen seemed a bit disappointed that Ehrlich was so involved with his side-chain theory and less involved with practical aspects. In an interview decades later, he remembered that he practically witnessed the "construction" of the side-chain theory: When visitors came to the institute, Ehrlich always explained his theoretical ideas. And if the visitor did not understand his explanations or objected, Ehrlich started all over again, sharpening his arguments. Madsen observed that Ehrlich's account had now changed and realized (at least in retrospect) that in the course of these constant discussions, Ehrlich had developed and fine-tuned his own theory.[80] Soon, Madsen became close friends with Julius Morgenroth, Ehrlich's assistant. Despite Ehrlich's strict work regime, Madsen remembered that Ehrlich was always very kind to him. Sometimes Madsen was invited to have tea or coffee in Ehrlich's private home, and he was invited to private dinners and evening gatherings,[81] in the course of which he was introduced to Berlin's scientific community and into society. In fact, Madsen's experiences in Berlin were similar to Salomonsen's twenty years earlier in Wroclaw.

After his visit to Berlin, the correspondence between Madsen and Ehrlich changed. Their letters now contained the same mixture of scientific and private topics as Ehrlich's correspondence with Salomonsen: constant inquiries about family and the exchange of greetings with them, congratulations on engagements and invitations to weddings,[82] congratulations when awards were received,[83] and invitations for private visits.[84] Furthermore, Ehrlich's letters now sometimes had a paternal tone. Soon after Madsen left the institute, he received a letter from Ehrlich. Ehrlich wrote to Madsen—almost as though Madsen would be returning soon—that Morgenroth was traveling and he was alone at the institute. He thanked Madsen for a gift of flowers and asked whether Madsen would write him with his impressions of his journey from Berlin, via Marburg and Frankfurt, to Paris.[85] Madsen replied immediately and in detail. First, he thanked Ehrlich for the training he had received in the previous months. He wrote that he had traveled to Marburg, where he visited Behring's Institute of Experimental Therapy, reporting that he had found the laboratories to be splendidly equipped but too small. In Frankfurt, Madsen met Carl Weigert and he had visited Dyestuff Industries in Hoechst, where Arnold Libbertz—the director of the new biological department, and a friend of Robert Koch—had shown him the laboratories, which he found unimpressive. Finally, he reported from Paris that nobody at the Pasteur Institute had really understood Ehrlich's theory prior to that point. Madsen had explained both Ehrlich's theory and the German method of serum evaluation, and the head of the serotherapeutic department, Louis Martin, had been very interested. Martin ask whether he could also contribute German standard serum and standard toxin. Madsen assured him that he would monitor the execution of serum evaluation à la Ehrlich.[86]

Ehrlich was delighted. Immediately upon receiving Madsen's letter, he replied. He emphasized that he was very happy and grateful to have worked with Madsen. He would always have good memories of their productive partnership, and he expressed the hope that the close connection between him and Madsen would prove to be long lasting. Besides their good personal relationship, Ehrlich added, it was important for him to have Madsen as a fellow campaigner aboard.[87] Further letters followed. In early July, Madsen must have sent another report. In his reply, Ehrlich expressed his thanks, and he, in return, informed Madsen about the developments at the ISRSS and the turmoil over the forthcoming move to Frankfurt. He encouraged Madsen to publish a planned article in German in "Koch's journal," *Zeitschrift für Hygiene und Infektionskrankheiten* (Journal for hygiene and infectious diseases, edited by Robert Koch and Carl Flügge). Finally, Ehrlich invited Madsen to participate in the ceremonial inauguration of the new institute in Frankfurt[88]—an honor for the young scientist and a clear sign of their emerging friendship. In return, Madsen campaigned on behalf of Ehrlich's side-chain theory in Paris.[89]

Maintenance—Reciprocity within Networks

The "give and take" referred to above includes not only letters of gratitude, direct and indirect expressions of mutual esteem, and the sending of gifts in return for a favor (not to mention the expected expression of gratitude for the gift received).[90] Give and take means a continuous flow of exchange: in words, in objects, and in actions. Not every exchange needs to be acknowledged, but, overall and in the long run, the give and take within a relationship (and within a network) need to be in balance.[91] Just as Madsen had championed Ehrlich's side-chain theory, Ehrlich advocated for Madsen. After publishing an article in the *Annales de l'Institut Pasteur* explaining Ehrlich's theory, Madsen was criticized by Jean Danysz, a member of the Pasteur Institute. Ehrlich reacted immediately. He praised Madsen's clearly written article and assured him of his full support.[92] To others, he commended Madsen's article, and he criticized and spoke ill of Danysz.[93] After Madsen complained that his manuscript was ill managed at the Pasteur Institute—the publication took too long and parts of the text had been shortened and changed without his permission—Ehrlich suggested that Madsen should publish his article in a German journal. Ehrlich offered to make linguistic corrections[94] and promised to contact the publisher and put in a good word to ensure speedy publication.[95]

Ehrlich wrote to Salomonsen that the delay he had experienced in France was inconceivable in a German journal and speculated that Metchnicov wanted to obstruct scientific results.[96] We cannot presume that Madsen's publication was delayed in Paris because the article favored the German method of serum evaluation, but we can take for granted that Ehrlich supported the article because he had a personal interest in its publication. If we accept that science is not the outcome of pure research and that scientific results are influenced by cultural factors and social relationships, then the publication is the result of a fruitful collaboration and positive for both sides.

After Madsen's residence in Steglitz, the frequency of their letters increased, and the topics and tone changed. They continued to discuss scientific results of Ehrlich's side-chain theory; Madsen informed Ehrlich about his experiments, which were verified by Ehrlich's assistants, and different findings were discussed. When a dispute arose with Emil Behring and members of the Pasteur Institute, Salomonsen and Madsen supported their friend Ehrlich in articles and simply by speaking ill of and gossiping about Behring, Émile Duclaux (director of the Pasteur Institute) and Metchnicov.[97] Alongside scientific matters, the private sphere was also accorded great importance. Madsen had been a guest in Ehrlich's home (so had Salomonsen), and he knew Ehrlich's wife and children. In letters to Salomonsen and Madsen, Ehrlich wrote about his children's marriages, medical conditions, and friends in common. In another letter, Ehrlich expressed his gratitude for the hospitality shown to him by the Salomonsens and for a postcard Salomonsen sent that brought back enjoyable memories.[98] Ehrlich and Salomonsen (and later Madsen) referred to each other as "my dear friend" and, very unusually, "du," and they closed their letters with "Julius" and "Paulus." This informal salutation was reserved for very close and old friends (from university days).

This mix of scientific and personal issues, and of personal and scientific friendships, characterizes the communication between Ehrlich and his Scandinavian colleagues. In a letter to Ehrlich in 1903,[99] Salomonsen congratulated him on the marriage of his oldest daughter, Stefanie, and then shifted directly to reporting about his move to a home in the countryside outside of Copenhagen. In the next paragraph, he thanked Ehrlich for the offprint of an article he had sent him, in which Ehrlich discussed an article by Max von Gruber. Salomonsen encouraged Ehrlich and harshly criticized Max von Gruber, who had attacked Ehrlich's side-chain theory.[100] In four other paragraphs, Salomonsen wrote about Madsen's visit to Brussels, expressed relief that Ehrlich—finally—had received some tumor mice from Carl O. Jensen,[101] and discussed the failed appointment of their common friend, Almroth Wright, in Great Britain. He then asked after Carl Weigert, wondering whether he was alright, since he had written him a letter some time ago but had not yet received an answer. Finally, he gave his regards to Julius Morgenroth and "other common friends" and to Ehrlich's family.[102]

I have quoted this letter extensively because it includes all the elements of an entangled and reciprocal network relationship. The letter refers to their common network partners in Great Britain,[103] to the entanglement of private and scientific issues as an example of strong ties, and to the mutual exchange of information and the need for reciprocity—the (moral) economy of give and take. As Salomonsen's inquiry about Weigert demonstrates, every letter had to be answered. It was expected that the recipient of an offprint sent one of his own offprints—or something else—in return, or, at the very least, that the recipient expressed his gratitude in recognition of the gift, and, as a sign of their close relationship, that he commented on the article (for instance, expressing agreement or validating research results). Ehrlich always ordered a large number of offprints and sent them to colleagues and friends.[104] The sending of offprints was also used to express thanks for a previous collaboration or exchange of thoughts and, especially, if someone was explicitly mentioned in the article (in the acknowledgments or as confirming the research).[105] For several of these reasons, Ehrlich sent offprints, and even copies of the voluminous *Handbook of Microscopic Techniques*, to Copenhagen,[106] while in return, he received offprints from Madsen and Salomonsen.[107] Just as in the exchange of offprints, the cyclical economy of give and take could be very "material" and could include specimens or preparations. Ehrlich, for example, received mice tumors and cultures of a certain strain of bacteria. In return, he organized a certain cobra toxin to be sent to the Danish institute and sent quantities of preparation "606"—a new preparation to treat syphilis—to Copenhagen as well.[108] The currency of this reciprocal give and take were bacteria and tumor cultures, blood samples, newly developed chemotherapeutic preparations, case histories, offprints, recommendations, invitations, and information.

Information was an important item of exchange. As Ehrlich shared his knowledge with Madsen, Madsen in return informed him about the working procedures, processes, and organization at the Pasteur Institute. Later, Madsen circulated information about the bacteriological institutes in Louvain (Leuwen) and Brussels,[109] and he reported on his experiences during his journey to North America, describing the production sites and laboratories of the serum manufacturers in Detroit (Parke & Davis) and Philadelphia (Mulford).[110] All of the information about the internal structure, organization, and research performed at other institutions—even if it was partly gossip—was valuable to Ehrlich. For instance, Madsen reported that everybody he met in the United Stated paid tribute to Ehrlich's work and that he enjoyed great acclaim. As a "disciple of Ehrlich," he was welcomed warmly everywhere, especially in Baltimore, where William Welch recounted his memories of the wonderful summer term he spent in Wroclaw in 1877.[111] Again, in the conferral of support[112] and patronage (Madsen defined himself as a disciple of Ehrlich) and, in exchange, the communication of information (and recognition), we find another example of the give-and-take economy between German and Scandinavian scientists.

Just as Madsen went to Berlin and the United States, in return, Paul Ehrlich's assistant Julius Morgenroth visited Copenhagen. On Ehrlich's recommendation, he went to the Statens Serum Institute for several months.[113] And after Madsen became a member of Ehrlich's scientific network, Ehrlich became an essential part of Madsen's scientific network. Madsen recommended a colleague to Ehrlich, Niels Muus, asking whether he could work as a guest researcher at the Institute for Experimental Therapy.[114] Recommendations were not limited to life scientists. Christian Bohr, a physiologist in Copenhagen, was a close friend of Carl Julius Salomonsen. During one of his stays in Copenhagen, Paul Ehrlich made his acquaintance. Bohr's son Harald (the brother of Niels Bohr[115]), studied mathematics in Copenhagen and wanted to visit Göttingen—one of the leading centers for mathematics at that time[116]—for a term. After Ehrlich's son-in-law, Edmund Landau, was appointed professor of mathematics at Göttingen, Salomonsen recommended Bohr and asked whether Ehrlich could put in a good word for Bohr with Landau in Göttingen. Immediately, Ehrlich asked Landau whether he would take care of Bohr and introduce him into Göttingen society (or whether he could "take him [Bohr] under his wing").[117] Apparently, the collaboration was successful, and the German-Scandinavian network expanded: in 1910, Harald Bohr finished his dissertation under the supervision of Landau.[118]

Meeting at conferences and mutual visits and scientific guest stays at institutes in Frankfurt, Berlin, and Copenhagen, were essential parts of network building and maintenance. But the exchange of young scholars during their "training," in particular, was more than networking: first, these exchanges strengthened the ties between the institutes and "old" network partners; second, these exchanges strengthened the ties between Salomonsen and Madsen and between Ehrlich and Morgenroth—between master and disciple. The network was "reproduced" and transferred from one generation of researchers to the next, and the "cultural" and "social capital" handed down from "teacher" to "student."[119] Third, these exchanges enlarged the network (of each network partner) as a whole. And finally, knowledge of "experimental pathology" and immunological and bacteriological knowledge was transferred via personal exchange. This knowledge transfer provided the basis for an international thought collective.

The status and reputation of a scientist depended (and still depends) on the recognition of other scientists and the broader scientific community. Around 1900, that status came—just as it does today—in the form of honorary memberships, academy memberships, awards such as the Nobel Prize, or, especially in Prussia, orders and titles. Receiving a prize is not "natural" but the result of successful networking.

I will illustrate how the economy of give and take functions by using the example of awards in the German-Scandinavian context. Awards had consequences for the reputation (and career) of a scientist. After Ehrlich had been appointed member of the Swedish Society of Medicine, he thanked Madsen, assuming that his nomination was related to Madsen's recent visit to Stockholm.[120] And, after Ehrlich had been awarded a Danish-Norwegian order, the Commander Cross, he speculated about Madsen's and Salomonsen's influence on this honor.[121] After Ehrlich was informed that he would be awarded the Nobel Prize, he wrote directly to Salomonsen, thanking him for his long-standing loyalty.[122]

I could continue with several other examples, but now let us trace the further effects of an award. To accept the Commander Cross mentioned above from the Danish king, Ehrlich, who was a medical official and privy councillor to the Prussian state, had to ask for permission from the higher authorities. The head of the ministerial department, on being informed of this award, noted that Ehrlich would have to be given a Prussian honor in the near future and that, furthermore, this honor needed to be superior to the Danish one.[123] Moreover, in celebration of the official inauguration of the Statens Serum Institute in September 1902, Ehrlich submitted a petition to the Prussian government for Salomonsen and Madsen to be awarded Prussian orders for their merits in the field of immunology and in honor of the German-Scandinavian collaboration.[124]

The Limits of Networks and Networking

Nothing lasts forever. Although the relationships between Ehrlich and his Scandinavian colleagues had been very close between 1896 and 1902, their ties weakened after 1902 for several reasons. The good relationship between Ehrlich and Salomonsen was based on their regular personal contact and friendship. Their ties were strengthened after Madsen visited the ISRSS. After Madsen returned to Copenhagen, they kept in touch by letter, discussing scientific questions that resulted from their personal collaboration. Further links (and common interests) resulted from the establishment of the ISRSS and the Statens Serum Institute and their experiences working in institutional settings. The institutes provided the possibility of inviting guest researchers and offering research stays, which not only provided opportunities to strengthen network relationships but also served as "currency" in the exchange of give and take. But after 1902, because of the geographical distance between Copenhagen and Berlin or Frankfurt, as well as the growing temporal distance caused by Madsen's research stay and personal dealings in Berlin in 1899, their ties weakened little by little. Furthermore, Madsen himself enlarged his "own" network: he collaborated with Swedish physical chemist Svante Arrhenius, and he traveled to Paris and the United States. According to Mark Granovetter, the maintenance of strong ties is very time consuming, and without regular personal renewal of the relationship, the ties weaken;[125] or, to the same extent to which Madsen's network expanded, his ties to Ehrlich became weaker.

Another reason for Ehrlich's and Madsen's shrinking network relationship was Madsen's collaboration with Svante Arrhenius.[126] When Madsen returned to Copenhagen 1899, he did not fully agree with all aspects of Ehrlich's side-chain theory. He especially called Ehrlich's notion of the toxin-antitoxin-binding into question. Madsen began a collaboration with Svante Arrhenius in Stockholm. He traveled to Stockholm, and Arrhenius visited Madsen in Copenhagen several times over the following years. Arrhenius was interested in the nature of immunological processes. While Madsen taught Arrhenius the practices and techniques of serotherapy, Arrhenius, in return, interpreted, discussed, and transformed the results of their experiments into mathematical equations and curves. According to Elisabeth Crawford, Arrhenius tried to make "serotherapy and immunity studies more scientific, using the concepts and methods of physical chemistry."[127]

Arrhenius crossed the Baltic Sea in various directions, building bridges between Sweden, Germany, and Denmark. Born in 1859, he studied physics and mathematics in Uppsala and Stockholm, graduating in 1876. He wrote his dissertation on the conductivity of electrolytes. His thesis drew the attention of physical chemists in Germany, among them Wilhelm Ostwald, who traveled to Stockholm specifically to meet Arrhenius. Between 1886 and 1891, Arrhenius traveled to Germany, Austria, and the Netherlands to work in the laboratories of Wilhelm Ostwald (Riga, later Leipzig), Friedrich Kohlrausch (Würzburg), Ludwig Boltzmann (Graz), and Jacobus H. van 't Hoff (Amsterdam). Working mainly in the emerging field of physical chemistry, Arrhenius also published various articles and books on geophysics, meteorology and astrology,[128] and immunology and immunochemistry.[129]

Madsen and Arrhenius published their research results in the *Festskrift* on the occasion of the official inauguration of the Statens Serum Institute.[130] Ehrlich became acquainted with Arrhenius during the inauguration ceremony, and he invited him to Frankfurt to discuss their differing views. In spring 1903, Arrhenius stayed for six weeks as a guest researcher at the Institute for Experimental Therapy, where he worked on the hemolysis of red blood cells by antibody and complement.[131] They must have discussed their differing views on toxin-antitoxin interaction. Arrhenius continued his scientific journey, and in December 1903 he delivered a speech at the Imperial Health Office in Berlin on the application of physical chemistry on serotherapy.[132] Despite Arrhenius and Madsen acknowledging that to Ehrlich "belongs the honour of the first theoretical foundation of the science of immunity,"[133] they did not confirm all of Ehrlich's research results. While Ehrlich postulated on the basis of his experiments that the toxin-antitoxin binding was irreversible, Arrhenius and Madsen had observed that the binding of tetanolysin and antitetanolysin took place in the same way as a chemical reaction of weak acids and bases, and this interaction was in fact reversible. Since hemolysis, the rupturing of erythrocytes, could be followed in vitro (and the intensity of the process measured using colorimetric analysis), Arrhenius criticized Ehrlich's method of in vivo experiments. In vivo experiments involved too many factors that might invalidate the scientific results. The conflict between Arrhenius and Madsen, on one side, and Ehrlich on the other side, was embedded in a broader discussion about hemolysis and the nature of toxins and antitoxins and their interaction.[134] In reference to the discussion of the German-Scandinavian network, I will not trace the scientific debate in detail. It is also irrelevant, since Ehrlich might not have fully understood the article written in English by Arrhenius and Madsen in the *Festskrift*, as Silverstein assumes,[135] and Ehrlich would have discovered the full extent of their differences only after a German translation of the article was published. However, we can presume that Ehrlich knew of the differences in their scientific views and for this reason invited Arrhenius to discuss the issue with him in hopes of changing his mind. Although they did not solve their scientific differences, they parted as friends—at least for the present.[136] But, in the summer of 1903, their scientific differences gained a momentum of their own. After Arrhenius and Madsen's article was published in German, it was taken up by Max von Gruber, a German hygienist. Gruber attacked Ehrlich and his side-chain theory viciously, describing Ehrlich as "Dr. Phantastus" and referring to Jules Bordet, Madsen, and Arrhenius. Ehrlich, in return, responded in sharp words. He also asked Arrhenius for his support,[137] but, after he did not respond, Ehrlich began to attack his position in several papers. In return, Arrhenius defended himself in a series of lectures he gave in Bonn, the Netherlands, Paris, Great Britain, and the United States.[138] Beyond their differences in terms of specific details, one might argue that they followed different approaches: Ehrlich followed a biochemical approach, while Arrhenius adhered to a physicochemical approach to the understanding of immunological processes. In this respect, they were proponents of different ways of thinking about and understanding organic processes.[139] According to Cay-Rüdiger Prüll, "Ehrlich had to defend his biological point of view against the physico-chemical interpretation of antitoxin-binding. Arrhenius and Madsen applied basic chemical laws to processes of life, which, according to Ehrlich, could not be expressed in such rigid formulas."[140] The reduction and transfer of life processes to test tube or in vitro experiments, as Arrhenius favored, did not reflect the complexity of living organisms and processes. In a note for a lecture, Ehrlich emphasized that these things cannot be thought of simplistically, and, in a side blow to Arrhenius and his preference for processing large amounts of data, he noted that it is necessary first to do biological research before one can start to make calculations.[141] During the broader conflict, Ehrlich began to separate his colleagues and (network partners) into supporters and opponents or, in other words, into friends and enemies (of his theory).[142] In this conflict (and in Ehrlich's binary separation), Madsen's position in Ehrlich's network changed from that of a close friend to a scientific opponent. Ehrlich did not classify him as an "enemy"—he blamed Arrhenius for their social alienation[143]—but their relationship cooled, and, as a consequence, their correspondence diminished.

During this time, Ehrlich continued his correspondence with Salomonsen. And, overall, the conflict interrupted their exchange of letters only for a short while. Madsen regretted their scientific differences and especially regretted that they were not discussed in private but coram publico (publicly). Madsen expressed his hope of bridging the scientific gap and was eager to maintain good relations.[144] In return, Ehrlich assured Madsen that the scientific differences did not affect their personal relationship, and that Ehrlich held Madsen in high regard.[145] The fact that they had to reassert their mutual respect, however, demonstrates that the relationship had changed. It seems that it was easier to bridge the Baltic Sea than to bridge different disciplines or different conceptual approaches[146] and different thought collectives.

Along with their relationship, Ehrlich's field of work also changed. In the letter, Ehrlich reassured Madsen of his personal respect and informed him that, in addition to the directorship of the Institute for Experimental Therapy, he was to become head of a new chemotherapeutic institute.[147] A year later, Madsen must have informed Ehrlich that a new book by Arrhenius had been published, and that Ehrlich's theory came off well in it. Ehrlich was delighted, hoping that the "old conflicts" were over. However, Ehrlich no longer seemed very interested in the topic itself, mentioning that he was no longer interested in immunity: "I am now doing cancer research and working on (the control of) trypanosomes."[148] And so, at least, their ties weakened after 1902 because Ehrlich moved into the new field of chemotherapy.

Network Transfer—Concluding Remarks

The photograph taken during the celebration of the inauguration of the Statens Serum Institute in Copenhagen showed Ehrlich sitting in the center. This was not coincidental. Ehrlich knew most of the scientists present personally or at least via the exchange of letters: Madsen's and Salomonsen's families, as well as the German and the British visitors. He already knew several of the Scandinavian visitors, or he became acquainted with them during the inauguration ceremony and stayed in contact, enlarging his network.

The photograph does not just portray a scientific event or a scientific network. As I have shown, the scientists present were related to each other on multiple levels: family ties, friendship, scientific (and economic) collaborations. The different kinds of ties were the basis for their relationships and for the foundation of their mutual network, as well as being characteristic of stable networks. The networks were secured at multiple levels. And, just as Salomonsen was part of Ehrlich's international scientific network, Ehrlich was part of Salomonsen's network and the networks of the other participants. Ehrlich's network, in particular, is characterized by this degree of multiplexity on various levels. These close relationships were an indispensable condition for the success of Ehrlich's work.

Every network has an implicit give-and-take economy that has to maintain a certain equilibrium. If not, the network will fall apart over time. This reciprocal process of give and take within a network can be illustrated by using the example of Ehrlich and Salomonsen (and Madsen). I have demonstrated how this network was established and maintained, how it was handed down (as the inheritance of social and cultural capital) to a succeeding generation of young scholars, and how knowledge was transferred (and distributed)—in both directions—within these network structures. I have described the pre-history of Ehrlich's network, starting with Salomonsen's summer term in 1877 in Wroclaw, and the long-lasting friendship between him and Ehrlich, including the emergence and maintenance of this relationship via letters and personal visits—in the beginning, mainly from Copenhagen to Berlin. Salomonsen had good reasons for traveling to Berlin—medical conferences, scientific collaborations in the field of bacteriology, and continuing his studies—and, by doing so, he transferred bacteriological knowledge from Berlin to Copenhagen. His unique position in Denmark as a pioneer in bacteriology resulted from his relationships with German bacteriologists and his access to the German/international bacteriological scientific community. The German (and French) supremacy in bacteriology (microbiology) resulted, however, in scientists like Salomonsen going to Berlin to receive training in bacteriological methods (which in turn means he accepted the German/French interpretational sovereignty). In the end, both sides benefited from this situation. This reciprocal interrelatedness continued on several different levels. After Salomonsen's assistant Madsen was trained in Berlin and the knowledge transferred to Copenhagen, Madsen (at first) supported Ehrlich's theory explaining immunological processes. On the other side, German (and French) knowledge influenced the establishment of the serum institute in Copenhagen. The Danish institute took the best parts from both the German and French systems: it produced and tested serum for purity and effectiveness as in France, and it adopted the German method of serum evaluation.

Finally, it must be emphasized that networks are about mutual relationships and moral economies. "Thank you" is one of the most commonly used terms in society. No one provides or demands a service without some sort of payment being involved: the sending of offprints to each other; supporting and recommending staff members; (positively) evaluating colleagues; or by favors such as invitations to dinner, recommendations for honors or awards, and, most of all, sharing information. These networks are less concerned with immediate exchange than with the overall economic balance of give and take, including future expectations. Though networks helped scientists cross the Baltic Sea, Ehrlich's network could not bridge disciplinary borders and conceptual approaches. When Arrhenius did not meet Ehrlich's expectations (and vice versa), the ties were cut, leaving a hole in this particular network.

Ehrlich's network can be characterized by its multitude of ties and the dense entanglement of these ties. Ehrlich did not strategically and purposefully organize these relationships aiming to "construct" a network, nor do people in general. Networks are characterized by their, so to speak, natural growth, with the individual knots resulting from historically contingent situations. Ehrlich was a master of networking, just as he was of organizing and administering these networks and balancing the give and take of the entangled relationships. Networks are important most of all in this context because science is part of a societal process of knowledge production (and construction), and because network partners must acknowledge, confirm, evaluate, and verify each other's scientific results within a thought collective.

Notes

1. Cf. seating plan September 9, 1902, Collection Hüntelmann, Berlin.
2. Sandra Legout, "La famille pasteurienne: Le personnel scientifique permanent de l'Institut Pasteur de Paris entre 1889 et 1914" (diss. rer. soc., Paris: EHESSS, 1999).
3. The photograph is reproduced in E. Schelde-Møller, *Thorvald Madsen: I Videnskabens og Menneskehedens Tjeneste* (Copenhagen: Nyt Nordisk Forlag, 1970, 62–63).
4. Thought collective in the sense of Ludwik Fleck, *Entstehung und Entwicklung einer wissenschaftlichen Tatsache. Einführung in die Lehre vom Denkstil und Denkkollektiv* (Frankfurt: Suhrkamp, 1980; 1st ed., 1935).
5. Cf. Axel C Hüntelmann, *Paul Ehrlich: Leben, Forschung, Ökonomien, Netzwerke* (Göttingen: Wallstein, 2011).
6. This is an ahistorical term, but it describes best how Ehrlich formed, maintained, administered, stabilized, and enlarged his personal networks.
7. For networks see in general Johannes Weyer, ed., *Sozial Netzwerke: Konzepte und Methoden der sozialwissenschaftlichen Netzwerkforschung* (Munich: R. Oldenbourg, 2000); Jürgen Barkhoff et al., eds., *Netzwerke: Eine Kulturtechnik der Moderne* (Cologne: Böhlau, 2004); Heiner Fangerau and Thorsten Halling, eds., *Netzwerke: Allgemeine Theorie oder Universalmetapher in den Wissenschaften? Ein transdisziplinärer Überblick* (Bielefeld: Transcript, 2009); Mark E. J. Newman, *Networks: An Introduction* (Oxford: Oxford University Press, 2010); for an overview, see Guido Caldarelli and Michele Catanzaro, *Networks: A Very Short Introduction* (Oxford: Oxford University Press, 2012).
8. Cf. Mark Granovetter, "The Strength of Weak Ties," *American Journal of Sociology* 73 (1973): 1360–80.
9. Cf. "Salomonsen, Carl Julius" (and thereafter Martin), s.v., *The Jewish Encyclopaedia*, vol. 10 (New York: Wagnalls, 1909), 657.
10. Cf. *Dansk Biografisk leksikon 20* (Copenhagen: J. H. Schultz, 1941), 516–19; Thorvald Madsen, "Obituary—Carl Julius Salomonsen," *Journal of Pathology and Bacteriology* 28 (1925): 702–8; E. Snorrason, "Salomonsen, Carl Julius," *Dictionary of Scientific Biography*, vol. 10 (New York: Scribner, 1981), 87–89.
11. Cf. Carl Julius Salomonsen, "Lebenserinnerungen aus dem Breslauer Sommersemester 1877," *Berliner Klinische Wochenschrift* 51 (1914): 485–90, esp. 486.
12. Cf. Carl Julius Salomonsen, "Studier over Blodets Forraadnelse" [Studies in the Decomposition of Blood[(diss. med., Copenhagen, 1877). Snorrason, "Salomonsen," 87, evaluated his dissertation as the "fundamental starting point for the study of bacteriology in Denmark."
13. Cf. Madsen, "Obituary Salomonsen," 703; Snorrason, "Salomonsen," 87.

14. Cf. Madsen, "Obituary Salomonsen," 703–4; Christoph Gradmann, *Krankheit im Labor: Robert Koch und die medizinische Bakteriologie* (Göttingen: Wallstein, 2005), 69.

15. Cf. Bo Steen Frandsen, *Dänemark: Der kleine Nachbar im Norden* (Darmstadt: Wissenschaftliche Buchgesellschaft, 1994).

16. Cf. Madsen, "Obituary Salomonsen," 704.

17. Cf. Thomas D Brock, *Robert Koch: A Life in Medicine and Bacteriology* (Madison, WI: Science Tech, 1988); Bernhard Möllers, *Robert Koch: Persönlichkeit und Lebenswerk, 1843–1910* (Hannover: Schmorl & von Seefeld Nachf., 1950), 104–7.

18. Cf. Robert Rieder, "Carl Weigert in seiner Bedeutung für die medizinische Wissenschaft unserer Zeit," in *Carl Weigert: Gesammelte Abhandlungen*, vol. 1, ed. Robert Rieder (Berlin: Julius Springer, 1906), 1–132, esp. 14; Paul Ehrlich, "Weigerts Verdienste um die histologische Wissenschaft," in *Carl Weigert*, 1:138–41, esp. 138; Georg Dhom, *Geschichte der Histopathologie* (Berlin: Springer 2001, 289.

19. Cf. Madsen, "Obituary Salomonsen," 704–5; for specificity see Pauline M. H. Mazumdar, *Species and Specificity: An Interpretation of the History of Immunology* (Cambridge: Cambridge University Press, 1995).

20. Madsen, "Obituary Salomonsen," 705.

21. Cf. Salomonsen, "Lebenserinnerungen."

22. Cf. Simon and James Thomas Flexner, *William Henry Welch and the Heroic Age of American Medicine* (New York: Viking Press, 1941), 99, 103.

23. Cf. Salomonsen, "Lebenserinnerungen"; Flexner, *Welch*, 103–4.

24. Cf. the article about Carl Julius Salomonsen in the *The Jewish Encyclopaedia*, 10:657; see also Jette Kristiansen et al., "Briefe des Nobelpreisträgers Paul Ehrlich an Thorvald Madsen, Direktor am dänischen Staatlichen Serum-Institut (Statens Serum Institut)," *Chemotherapie Journal* 16 (2007): 143–51, esp. 144.

25. Cf. Till van Rahden, *Jews and Other Germans: Civil Society, Religious Diversity, and Urban Politics in Breslau, 1860–1925* (Madison: University of Wisconsin Press, 2008).

26. Cf. Madsen, "Obituary Salomonsen," 704.

27. Cf. Flexner, *Welch*, 106–10.

28. Madsen, "Obituary Salomonsen," 705; Snorrason, "Salomonsen," 87.

29. Snorrason, "Salomonsen," 87.

30. Madsen called him the "father of Danish bacteriology," cf. Madsen, "Obituary Salomonsen," 701; Snorrason, "Salomonsen."

31. Cf. Salomonsen, "Lebenserinnerungen," 490. Weigert was also able to communicate in Danish, or at least he could read Danish. Letters from Salomonsen and Madsen to Weigert (dating between 1899–1901), were written in Danish, while letters to Ehrlich were written in German. The letters to Weigert are stored at the Staatsbibliothek Berlin, Collection Darmstädter (henceforth SB CD), 3 d 1897 (Madsen); and 3 d 1890 (Salomonsen); Hüntelmann, *Paul Ehrlich*, 40.

32. Cf. Arthur M Silverstein, *Paul Ehrlich's Receptor Immunology: The Magnificent Obsession* (San Diego: Academic Press, 2002), 107.

33. Cf. Hüntelmann, *Paul Ehrlich*, 30–32.

34. Ibid., 30–32; Flexner, *Welch*, 77–82.

35. Cf. Paul Ehrlich, "Beiträge zur Kenntniss der Anilinfärbungen und ihrer Verwendung in der mikroskopischen Technik," in *Paul Ehrlich: Gesammelte Arbeiten in vier Bänden einschließlich einer vollständigen Bibliographie*, vol. 1, *Histologie, Biochemie und Pathologie*, ed. Fred Himmelweit (London: Pergamon Press, 1956), 19–28.

36. Cf. Paul Ehrlich, "Beiträge zur Theorie und Praxis der histologischen Färbung" (diss. med., Leipzig, 1878). Ehrlich did not follow Cohnheim personally, but he was affiliated with the University of Leipzig, where he officially finished his dissertation.

37. He was awarded the title professor by the Prussian Ministry of Cultural Affairs as an honorary degree, not as a (full) university professorship. For Ehrlich's years at the Charité, see Hüntelmann, *Paul Ehrlich*, 45–73.

38. See, for instance, the letter Koch wrote to Salomonsen in April 1879, describing his current research; the letter is quoted in Möller, *Robert Koch*, 687.

39. Cf. Salomonsen, "Lebenserinnerungen," 486.

40. Welch, for instance, attended a bacteriological course in 1885, cf. Flexner, *Welch*, 143–49.

41. Cf. Salomonsen, "Lebenserinnerungen," 490.

42. Cf. the list of participating members in *Verhandlungen des X. Internationalen Medicinischen Congresses: Berlin, 4.–9. August 1890* (Berlin: August Hirschwald, 1891), cxii; Kristiansen et al., "Briefe," 144.

43. Pierre Bourdieu has expressed these efforts as the "accumulation" of "scientific capital," which means the acquisition of the proper competence, scientific knowledge, training, habits, and reputation, cf. Pierre Bourdieu, *Science of Science and Reflexivity* (Cambridge: Polity, 2004), 33–34, 55–62.

44. Regarding the difficulties of interdisciplinary research, see Klaus Nathaus and Hendrik Vollmer, "Moving Inter Disciplines: What Kind of Cooperation are Interdisciplinary Historians and Sociologists Aiming For?," *InterDisciplines: Journal of History and Sociology* 1 (2010): 64–93.

45. See Mazumdar, *Species*.

46. Cf. Derek S Linton, *Emil von Behring, Infectious Disease, Immunology, Serum Therapy* (Philadelphia: American Philosophical Society, 2005), 41–196; Axel C Hüntelmann, "Diphtheriaserum and Serumtherapy—Development, Production and Regulation in Fin de Siècle Germany," *Dynamis: Acta Hispanica ad Medicinae Scientiarumque Historiam Illustrandam* 27 (2007): 107–31; Jonathan Simon, *Diphtheria Serum as Technological Object: A Philosophical Analysis of Serotherapy in France 1894–1900* (Lanham, MD: Lexington, 2017).

47. Detailed information on the development of antidiphtheritic serum was freely available in well-known medical publications; a health professional trained in bacteriology would have been able to reconstruct the experiments and produce serum without encountering legal problems, since antidiphtheritic serum was unpatented.

48. Cf. Carl Julius Salomonsen, "The Rise and Growth of the State Serum Institute," in *Festskrift ved indvielsen af Statens Serum Institut 1902: Contributions from the University Laboratory for Medical Bacteriology to Celebrate the Inauguration of the State Serum Institute* (Copenhagen: O. C. Olsen, 1902), 1–20, esp. 3.

49. Salomonsen, "Rise and Growth." Salomonsen visited Paris because the Pasteur Institute was the only laboratory where research and the large-scale production of serum were unified in one institution. This was not the case in Germany, where serum was produced at private companies like Dyestuff Industries in Hoechst.

50. Ibid., 3–4.

51. Ibid.

52. Ibid., 5. The difficulties of serum production, esp. the establishment of a stable production process and the "calibration" of the actors involved, are described in Axel C. Hüntelmann, "The Dynamics of *Wertbestimmung*," *Science in Context* 21 (2008): 229–52; Hüntelmann, "Evaluation and Standardisation as a Practical Technique of Administration: The Diphtheria-Serum Example," in *Evaluations: Standardising Pharmaceutical Agents 1890–1960*, ed. Christoph Gradmann and Jonathan Simon (Basingstoke: Palgrave, 2010), 31–51.

53. Cf. Salomonsen, "Rise and Growth," 6.

54. Cf. Hüntelmann, "Dynamics"; Hüntelmann, "Evaluation."

55. Cf. Salomonsen, "Lebenserinnerungen," 490.

56. Cf. the correspondence between Ehrlich and the Prussian Ministry of Cultural Affairs (as superior authority of the ISRSS), June 27, 1896. Ehrlich asked for permission to send test toxin to the British institute. See also copies of the request of Woodhead and Joseph Lister, GStA PK (Prussian Secret Archive), 1. HA, Rep. 76 Vc, Sekt 1, Tit. XI, Part II, No. 18, Vol. 1.

57. Cf. the request of Woodhead to the German authorities, October 7 and 26, 1897, and the following correspondence in GStA PK, 1. HA, Rep. 76 Vc, Sekt 1, Tit. XI, Part II, No. 18, Vol. 1.

58. Who were both present at the inauguration ceremony in 1902, see on the photograph (fig. 1) No. 7a (George Dean) and 21 (German Sims Woodhead).

59. See also the report about the inauguration of the Danish Institute and the *Festskrift* in the *British Medical Journal* no. 2183, November 1, 1902: 1453; and no. 2191, December 27, 1902: 1965–66.

60. Cf. Kristiansen et al., "Briefe," 143; Schelde-Møller, *Thorvald Madsen*, 10–40.

61. Cf. Anne Hardy, "Actions Not Words: Thorvald Madsen, Denmark, and International Health, 1902–1939," in *Of Medicine and Men: Biographies and Ideas in European Social Medicine between the World Wars*, ed. Iris Borowy and Anne Hardy (Frankfurt: Peter Lang, 2008), 127–43.

62. Cf. Thorvald Madsen, "Experimentelle undersøgelser over difterigiften" [Experimental investigations on diphtheria toxin] (diss. med., University Copenhagen, 1896).

63. Cf. ibid; Madsen, "Forskere omkring Århundredskriftet: Koch, Ehrlich og Metchnikoff" [Researchers around 1900: Koch, Ehrlich and Metchnikoff], *Medicinsk Forum* 18, no. 5 (1964): 140–44; Schelde-Møller, *Thorvald Madsen*, 41. I want to express my thanks to Anne Hardy, who sent me an English translation of Madsen's text.

64. Report summarizing Thorvald Madsen's article by Wilhelm Dönitz, member of the ISRSS, March 11, 1897, Paul Ehrlich Institute (henceforth PEI), Dept. Va, No. 1, Vol. 1, emphasis in original.

65. Cf. Thorvald Madsen, "Ueber Messung der Stärke des antidiphtherischen Serums," *Zeitschrift für Hygiene und Infektionskrankheiten* 24 (1897): 425–42.

66. Cf. Hardy, "Actions Not Words," 131.

67. Cf. Madsen, "Forskere omkring Århundredskriftet."

68. Cf. Wilhelm Dönitz, "Bericht über die Thätigkeit des Königl. Instituts für Serumforschung und Serumprüfung zu Steglitz Juni 1896–September 1899," *Klinisches Jahrbuch* 7 (1899): 1–26, esp. 3.

69. Cf. in detail Hüntelmann, "Diphtheriaserum"; Hüntelmann, "Dynamics"; Hüntelmann, "Evaluation." The procedure is described in Richard Otto, "Die staatliche Prüfung der Heilsera," *Arbeiten aus dem Königlichen Institut für experimentelle Therapie zu Frankfurt a. M.* 2 (1906): 1–86.

70. Cf. Paul Ehrlich, "Die Wertbemessung des Diphtherieheilserums und deren theoretische Grundlagen," *Klinisches Jahrbuch* 6 (1898): 299–326.

71. Cf. Salomonsen, "Lebenserinnerungen," 486.

72. Cf. Kristiansen et al., "Briefe," 144; E. Gotfredson, "Dr. Thorvald Madsen fortaeller," *Medicinsk Forum* 6 (1953): 197–217. I want to express my thanks to Anne Hardy, who sent me an English translation of this article.

73. Ehrlich to Salomonsen, November 14, 1899, Rockefeller Archive Center, Paul Ehrlich Collection 650 Eh 89 (henceforth RAC PEC), Box 6.

74. Cf. Salomonsen, "Lebenserinnerungen," 490.

75. Cf. Salomonsen to Ehrlich, March 17, 1900, RAC 650.3 Eh 89 Martha Marquardt Collection (henceforth MMC), Box 2.

76. Cf. Marcel Mauss, *Die Gabe: Form und Funktion des Austauschs in archaischen Gesellschaften* (Frankfurt: Suhrkamp, 1990; originally published 1923/1924); Frank Adloff and Steffen Mau, eds., *Vom Geben und Nehmen: Zur Soziologie der Reziprozität* (Frankfurt: Campus, 2005); Stephan Moebius and Christian Papilloud, eds., *Gift— Marcel Mauss' Kulturtheorie der Gabe* (Wiesbaden: Verlag für Sozialwissenschaften, 2006); Alain Caillé, *Anthropologie der Gabe* (Frankfurt: Campus, 2008).

77. Ehrlich to the Prussian Ministry of Cultural Affairs, March 14, 1897, PEI, Dept. Va, No. 1, Vol. 1.

78. Ehrlich to Madsen, November 8, 1898, RAC PEC Box 4.

79. Ehrlich to Madsen, undated (November 14, 1898); and Dec. 15, 1898, RAC PEC Box 4.

80. Cf. Gotfredson, "Thorvald Madsen fortaeller."

81. Cf. Madsen, "Forskere omkring Århundredskriftet"; Gotfredson. "Thorvald Madsen fortaeller."

82. Cf. Ehrlich to Madsen, January 5, 1906, RAC PEC Box 69 Folder 13.

83. Madsen congratulated Ehrlich on the bestowal of an order, September 13, 1899, RAC MMC Box 2; Madsen congratulated Ehrlich on the bestowal of a Swedish order, March 3, 1900, ibid.; Ehrlich expressed his thanks for Madsen's congratulations (on winning the Nobel Prize), Ehrlich to Madsen, November 27, 1908, RAC PEC Box 25, Copy Book XXV.

84. The notice of a private visit to Copenhagen to Madsen (Nov. 27, 1908) and to Salomonsen (November 12, 1908), both letters in RAC PEC Box 25, Copy Book XXV.

85. Ehrlich to Madsen, undated (before May 21, 1899), RAC PEC Box 5.

86. Madsen to Ehrlich, May 21, 1899, RAC MMC Box 1.

87. "Für mich wird Ihr Steglitzer aufenthalt in unsrer armen aber doch gemüthlichen bude stets eine liebe erinnerung sein, und hoffe ich, dass sich das zwischen uns geknüpfte band als ein dauerhaftes erweisen wird. Ganz abgesehen von der persönlichen seite ist es ja auch für die ganze wissenschaftliche seite von der grössten bedeutung, dass grade <u>Sie</u> mitkämpfer geworden sind." Ehrlich to Madsen, undated (between May 22 and 24, 1899), RAC PEC Box 5.

88. Ehrlich to Madsen, undated (ca. July 12 and 14, 1899); and July 18, 1899, RAC PEC Box 5.

89. Ehrlich to Madsen, July 27, 1899, RAC PEC Box 5.

90. For instance, Ehrlich's expression of gratitude for a vase that Madsen must have sent him, cf. Ehrlich to Madsen, August 4, 1899, RAC PEC Box 6.

91. Cf. Mauss, *Die Gabe*; Adloff and Mau, *Geben und Nehmen*; Caillé, *Anthropologie der Gabe*.

92. Ehrlich to Madsen, August 4, 1899 and undated (mid-August 1899), RAC PEC Box 6.

93. "Haben Sie schon die arbeit von Danycz in den Annalen gelesen? Der artikel ist von einer verblüffenden unverschämtheit u dummheit, dann auch noch äusserst commun gegen Madsen. Ich werde mir wohl bald diesen jüngling kaufen." Ehrlich to Aaser, Kristiania (now Oslo), undated (c. August 4, 1899), RAC PEC Box 6. Overlœge Aaser from Kristiania had also been present at the official inauguration of the Statens Serum Institute in 1902, see photograph no. 27.

94. Ehrlich to Madsen, August 4, 1899; two undated letters from August 1899, RAC PEC Box 6.

95. Ehrlich's offer to Madsen, August 4, 1899; Ehrlich to Carl Flügge, editor of the *Zeitschrift für Hygiene und Infektionskrankheiten*, undated (early August 1899), requesting speedy publication of Madsen's article; both letters in RAC PEC Box 6; Madsen to Ehrlich, August 17, 1899, RAC MMC Box 2.

96. Ehrlich to Salomonsen, February 24, 1899, RAC PEC Box 5.

97. Cf. Madsen's letters to Ehrlich from June to August 1899, RAC PEC Box 5 and 6.

98. PE to Salomonson, May 7, 1908, RAC PEC Box 25 Copybook XXIIII.

99. Salomonsen to Ehrlich, September 8, 1903, SB CD, 3 d 1890 (Salomonsen).

100. "Besten Dank für Ihre letzte Publication gegen Gruber. Natürlich hat auch mich die unverschämte Form seiner Polemik sehr geärgert, und seine Harlekinade in der Wiener Klinischen war ja grade zu unanständig. . . . Gruber scheint überhaupt gar nicht die Tragweite Ihrer Immunitäts-Arbeiten zu <u>verstehen</u>, sonst würde er gewiss nicht—selbst als fanatischer Gegener—diesen frechen Ton anschlagen." Salomonsen to Ehrlich, September 8, 1903, SB CD, 3 d 1890 (Salomonsen).

101. Jensen was also present during the official inauguration of the Statens Serum Institute in 1902; see photograph no. 15.

102. Salomonsen to Ehrlich, September 8, 1903, SB CD, 3 d 1890 (Salomonsen).

103. In another letter Salomonsen mentioned, for instance, William Bulloch had asked after Marianne, Ehrlich's youngest daughter, cf. Salomonsen to Ehrlich, December 25, 1904, Salomonsen to Ehrlich, September 8, 1903, SB CD, 3 d 1890 (Salomonsen).

104. Cf. the order for three hundred offprints of Ehrlich, undated (c. May 1899), RAC PEC Box 5; concerning the moral economy of gift exchange see Hüntelmann, *Paul Ehrlich*, 233–38. Offprints and so-called separata were also used to indicate precedence on an issue or an innovation.

105. Ehrlich is mentioned explicitly in Salomonsen, "Rise and Growth," 6.

106. Madsen and Salomonsen each received the two-volume Paul Ehrlich et al., eds., *Encyklopädie der mikroskopischen Technik mit besonderer Berücksichtigung der Färbelehre* (Berlin: Urban & Schwarzenberg, 1903); cf. list of recipients, around March 11, 1903, RAC PEC Box 22.

107. Cf., for instance, Ehrlich thanking Madsen for offprints received in Ehrlich to Madsen, undated (c. August 1899), RAC PEC Box 6; and in return, Madsen thanking Ehrlich for offprints received in Madsen to Ehrlich, March 3, 1900, RAC MMC Box 2.

108. For the tumor mouse, see Salomonsen to Ehrlich, September 8, 1903, SB CD, 3 d 1890 (Salomonsen). On Madsen's request Ehrlich sent 15 to 20 ampoules of "606" to Dr. Rasch, Ehrlich to Madsen, July 27, 1910, RAC PEC Box 69 Folder 13.

109. Madsen to Ehrlich, June 21, 1901, SBCD, 3 d 1897 (Madsen).

110. Madsen to Ehrlich, January 23, 1902, RAC MMC Box 2.

111. Madsen to Ehrlich, January 23, 1902, RAC MMC Box 2.

112. When Madsen went to Great Britain and the United States in 1901, Ehrlich wrote letters of recommendation and contacted his friends in London, Liverpool, Cambridge, and Netley, as well as in New York, Baltimore, and Boston.

113. Morgenroth thanks Ehrlich for his recommendation, January 30, 1908, RAC MMC Box 1.

114. Madsen to Ehrlich, March 7, 1900, SB CD, 3 d 1897 (Madsen).

115. Niels Bohr received the Nobel Prize for physics in 1922. For his family history, see Abraham Pais, *Niels Bohr's Times: In Physics, Philosophy and Polity* (Oxford: Clarendon Press, 1994).

116. With Hermann Minkowski, David Hilbert, Felix Klein, and Minkowski's successor, Edmund Landau, the most important mathematicians of that time were located in Göttingen.

117. Ehrlich to Edmund Landau, April 14, 1909; Ehrlich informed Salomonsen the same day that everything had been arranged, both letters, RAC PEC Box 25, Copybook XXVI.

118. Cf. Børge Jessen, "Harald Bohr," s.v., *Complete Dictionary of Scientific Biography*, 2008 (Encyclopedia.com) (August 16, 2015).

119. And insofar as "cultural" and "social capital" were transferable and not "bound" to only one person, as Bourdieu argues; for the different forms of capital, see Pierre Bourdieu, "Forms of Capital," in *Handbook of Theory of Research for the Sociology of Education*, ed. John E Richardson (New York: Greenwood Press, 1986), 241–58.

120. Ehrlich to Madsen, undated (between February 27 and March 1, 1900), RAC PEC Box 6.

121. Correspondence around 1900 in Personal File, PEI, Dept. III, No. 1, Vol. 1.

122. "Du wirst es ja längst wissen, dass diesmal ich der Glückliche bin, der im Verein mit Metschnikoff den Nobelpreis erhalten soll. . .! Ich weiss ja, dass diese Erteilung, um die Du seit Jahren für mich gekämpft hast, Dir die grösste Freude bereitet, und es ist mir ein Herzenswunsch, Dir für die mir allezeit und ganz besonders in dieser Hinsicht erwiesene Freundschaft herzlichst zu danken!" Ehrlich to Salomonsen, November 12, 1908, RAC PEC Box 25, Copybook XXV.

123. Ehrlich was later awarded the "Goldene Medaille der Wissenschaft" (the Golden Medal of Science), the highest scientific honor of the Prussian state.

124. Cf. they had been awarded the Roter Adler-Orden Vierter Klasse (Order of the Red Eagle, 4th class), PEI, Dept. III, No. 1, Vol. 1.

125. Cf. Granovetter, "Strength."

126. Arrhenius had also been invited to the official inauguration ceremony of the Statens Serum Institute, cf. no. 22 behind Paul Ehrlich in Schelde-Møller, *Madsen*, 62–63.

127. Elisabeth Crawford, *Arrhenius: From Ionic Theory to the Greenhouse Effect* (Canton: Science History, 1996), 170.

128. Cf. Crawford, *Arrhenius*.

129. Cf. Svante Arrhenius, *Immunochemistry: The Application of the Principles of Physical Chemistry to the Study of the Biological Antibodies* (New York: Macmillan, 1907). Ehrlich held a copy of this book in his library, see Ehrlich's library list in RAC PEC Box 2, Folder 5.

130. Cf. Svante Arrhenius and Thorvald Madsen, "Physical Chemistry Applied to Toxins and Antitoxins," in *Festskrift ved indvielsen af Statens Serum Institut 1902: Contributions from the University Laboratory for Medical Bacteriology to Celebrate the Inauguration of the State Serum Institute*, ed. Carl Julius Salomonsen (Copenhagen: O. C. Olsen, 1902), 1–111.

131. Cf. Silverstein, *Paul Ehrlich's Receptor Immunology*, 64.

132. Cf. Svante Arrhenius, "Die Anwendung der physikalischen Chemie auf die Serumtherapie," *Arbeiten aus dem Kaiserlichen Gesundheitsamte* 20 (1904): 559–66.

133. Cf. Arrhenius and Madsen, "Physical Chemistry," 3.

134. Cf. Arthur M. Silverstein, *A History of Immunology* (San Diego: Academic Press, 1989); Silverstein, *Paul Ehrlich's Receptor Immunology*, 55–75; Cay-Rüdiger Prüll, "Part of a Scientific Master Plan? Paul Ehrlich and the Origins of his Receptor Concept," *Medical History* 47 (2003): 332–56; Cay-Rüdiger Prüll, Andreas-Holger Maehle, and Robert F. Halliwell, *A Short History of the Drug Receptor Concept* (Basingstoke: Palgrave, 2009), 16–40; and Lewis P. Rubin, "Styles in Scientific Explanation: Paul Ehrlich and Svante Arrhenius on Immunochemistry," *Journal of the History of Medicine and Allied Sciences* 35 (1980): 397–425.

135. Cf. Silverstein, *Paul Ehrlich's Receptor Immunology*, 64.

136. Cf. Crawford, *Arrhenius*, 194.

137. Julius Morgenroth, who was friends with Arrhenius, wrote a letter to him, urging Arrhenius to dissociate himself from Gruber's attack.

138. Cf. Silverstein, *Paul Ehrlich's Receptor Immunology*, 65–68.

139. Cf. Rubin, "Styles"; Franz Luttenberger, "Arrhenius vs. Ehrlich on Immunochemistry: Decisions about Scientific Progress in the Context of the Nobel Prize," *Theoretical Medicine* 13 (1992): 137–73; for a broader context, Silverstein, *History*; Joseph S. Fruton, *Contrasts in Scientific Style: Research Groups in the Chemical and Biochemical Sciences* (Philadelphia: American Philosophical Society, 1990).

140. Prüll, "Part of a Scientific Master Plan?," 349.

141. Ehrlich, notes for a lecture in London, April 17, 1907, RAC PEC Box 28, p. 263.

142. Cf. Prüll, "Part of a Scientific Master Plan," 347–49.

143. Cf. Ehrlich to Ludwig Darmstädter, February 15th, 1910, reflecting retrospectively on the conflict: "Madsen is a nice guy (ein lieber und netter Mensch) and Ehrlich regrets that Arrhenius "der faule Kopf" ("faul" could mean lazy as well as ill-minded) was able to place them in opposing positions, see RAC PEC Folder 1 Box 8.

144. Madsen to Ehrlich, copies of two letters in 1903 and 1904, RAC PEC Box 2, Folder 4.

145. Ehrlich to Madsen, May 5, 1905, RAC PEC Box 24, Copybook XVII. In another letter, Ehrlich reassured him that the scientific conflict had not affected his personal feelings; Ehrlich to Madsen, June 14, 1906, RAC PEC Box 69, Folder 13.

146. While Ehrlich and Madsen found common ground, the situation was completely different with Ehrlich and Arrhenius. They attacked each other for some time, and Arrhenius, as part of the Nobel Committee, opposed Ehrlich's nomination as Nobel Laureate, cf. Crawford, *Arrhenius*, 227–29; Silverstein, *Paul Ehrlich's Receptor Immunology*, 69; Luttenberger, "Arrhenius vs. Ehrlich"; Ulf Lagerkvist, *Pioneers of Microbiology and the Nobel Prize* (River Edge, NJ: World Scientific, 2003), 109–65.

147. Ehrlich to Madsen, May 5, 1905, RAC PEC Box 24, Copybook XVII.

148. Ehrlich to Madsen, June 14, 1906, RAC PEC Box 69, Folder 13.

Chapter Seven

Dorpat University in the Late Nineteenth Century as a Transit Space for Psychiatric Knowledge

The Example of Emil Kraepelin and His Conceptualization of Melancholia

MAIKE ROTZOLL AND FRANK GRÜNER

An Estonian Peasant

He felt "like a wheel on a wagon that has to roll along submissively." A "melancholic" patient of German psychiatrist Emil Kraepelin (1856–1926) made this statement, and Kraepelin quoted it in several editions of his powerful textbook on psychiatry. The patient, referred to as a "simple farmer" and an example of melancholia simplex, found his way into the text[1] during Kraepelin's time in Dorpat (Tartu). Later editions called him an "Estonian peasant" and used his case history as an example of melancholy as a disease related to old age.[2] In the same way that physical regions are first part of one state and then another—a not too far-distant historical experience in the Baltics—melancholy symptom complexes were switched from one category to another in the eight editions of *Psychiatry* published in Kraepelin's lifetime. As the classification processes evolved throughout the editions, some disease entities earned their sovereignty while others lost it, and some turned into nosological categories while others were dropped, transformed, or absorbed into other categories.

Such was the case for age-related melancholy, which dissolved into manic-depressive insanity by the eighth edition in 1913.[3] The "Estonian farmer" also disappeared in this process. He had already lost his identity in the seventh edition of 1904 and was by then recognizable only to initiates by his statement. The author had included him in a downright baroque description of a type that contained the contributions of many individuals: "The patient is 'discouraged and submissive' as a wheel on the wagon that just rolls along, internally frozen and petrified, hardly speaks a word, often sits for days, puts his hands in his lap, dully brooding, unable to pull himself together for any action. The slightest accomplishment costs him an outrageous effort."[4] This characterization did not actually describe the melancholy of advanced age—a category that still existed in this edition—but rather the depressive stages of manic-depressive insanity. Thus, like a wheel on a wagon, the Estonian peasant became a nonparticipating wanderer between Kraepelin's categories.[5]

This chapter examines how Kraepelin's concept of melancholy changed over the time he was working on his psychiatric textbook. Particularly in view of Kraepelin's five-year stay in Dorpat, which represented a contact zone for exchange processes between Western and Eastern Europe during the nineteenth century,[6] the question arises whether and how this location influenced the development of his nosological constructions.

The Baltic Sea region—in particular, the Baltic area that belonged to the Russian Empire—was historically shaped by German culture and housed its leading academic institution, the University of Dorpat. The Estonian city of Tartu represented itself as a transnational place and cultural contact zone at the end of the nineteenth century. Founded as a Russian fortress with the name Jur'ev around 1030, the Baltic town developed under the rule of the German *Schwertbrüderorden* during the thirteenth century into the Hanseatic city of Dorpat. It became part of the Russian Empire in 1721 as a result of the Great Northern War between Sweden and Russia (1700–21), and it was given the Russian name Jur'ev again in 1893 in the context of the Russification of the Baltic region. Only after Estonia became independent in 1918 was the city officially called Tartu. Thus, Tartu served as a contact zone and "transit space" between Germany and Russia from the 1880s until the early 1900s. This period in particular was characterized by intensive cross-cultural encounters and processes of exchange between the two nations in the fields of medicine and science. This chapter presents one concrete example of how these cultural entanglements and exchange processes impacted the conceptualization of melancholy. It focuses particularly on the role of Emil Kraepelin—a leading figure in the systematization and treatment of emotional disorders and mental illnesses—in these transnational processes of knowledge production and the circulation of concepts of melancholy.

As was the case in central Europe, modern psychiatry began to develop gradually in Russia during the second half of the nineteenth century. The first chair of psychiatry was established in 1859 at the St. Petersburg Academy of Medicine and Science, followed by chairs in Moscow and Dorpat. In the following years, psychiatric hospitals were also set up in Kazan, Kiev, and Kharkov. At around the same time, as part of the social reforms of the 1860s, new organs of local self-government were established in the Russian Empire, and these became responsible for taking care of mentally ill people in the cities and provinces. The number of psychiatric asylums in Russia remained comparatively low, however, and working and living conditions were relatively poor.[7] Beginning in the 1880s, the professionalization of Russian psychiatrists developed more dynamically.[8] Several independent psychiatric clinics were founded during this time, and the professional education of psychiatrists through the establishment of special academic institutions and professorships filled a serious deficit. The total number of psychiatrists in Russia, however, increased slowly at first.[9] Transfers of knowledge from Europe, particularly France and Germany, played a crucial role in the formation of Russian psychiatry during this period. The adaption of Emil Kraepelin's nosological system was fundamental to the formation of a scientifically based, medical understanding of melancholy.

This chapter operates on two interrelated premises: first, that epistemological and ontological transfers in the fields of science and medicine between Germany and Russia shaped the understanding, redefinition, and experience of melancholy and gloom in various cultures in central, northern, and Eastern European countries; and, second, that the Baltic Sea region, in particular, the area belonging to the Russian Empire, served as a contact zone between Germany and Russia and thus played an important role in the formation of a modern, scientifically based understanding of melancholy.

Kraepelin's Research Program at Dorpat

Whether or not Kraepelin set out to be a full professor by the age of thirty, he achieved it with his appointment to Dorpat in 1886. This possibility had seemed inconceivable to him just a short time before. After his medical studies, Kraepelin went first to Wurzburg, then worked for several years at the Upper Bavarian District Mental Hospital in Munich with Bernhard von Gudden (1824–86). He seemed to be on the verge of a promising academic career with his move to the Psychiatric University Clinic in Leipzig in 1882, but he was soon embroiled in tense disagreements with neuroanatomist Professor Paul Flechsig (1847–1929), which finally ended in Kraepelin's "scandalous departure."[10]

If it is true that Kraepelin had predicted to his wife early on that Dorpat was the only university that might eventually appoint him,[11] this feeling may have been caused by the setback in Leipzig, leading him to believe that his chances of obtaining a professorship within the Reich itself were slim.[12] Several friends and colleagues also seem to have considered Dorpat a viable "transitional stage" between his pursuits of a career within the German Reich.[13] A correspondent advised Kraepelin that the post be "certainly accepted without hesitation, even though at the moment the circumstances over there may not be exactly tempting."[14] But why was he chosen by the University of Dorpat? It seems that, despite his youth and minimal professional experience, the decision was greatly influenced by the recommendation of his former teacher and predecessor, Hermann Emminghaus (1845–1904).[15]

Were the conditions really so uninviting in Dorpat? The university, originally founded in 1632 under Swedish rule and then reopened in 1802 by Czar Alexander I (1777–1825), had experienced significant improvements in the decades before Kraepelin's arrival.[16] Its psychiatric clinic, founded as a private institution in 1877, was taken over by the state and the university in 1880. Hermann Emminghaus, its first professor, left in 1886 to assume an appointment as chair in Freiburg.[17] According to Kraepelin's recollections and those of his student Heinrich Dehio (1861–1928), both the clinic and the professor's home were located in an old park and enjoyed a wonderful view.[18] Initially, however, the financial and structural conditions there required serious work from the newly appointed professor.[19] Apparently, though, Kraepelin found these problems modest in comparison with the challenges of developing the university's educational policy.[20]

Although Latin and German were initially the exclusive teaching languages, Russification began in the 1880s under Czar Alexander III (1845–94) and would reach its climax soon after Kraepelin's departure.[21] Restrictions on the use of the German language had been imposed since 1884.[22] Like many of his German colleagues (forty out of forty-six professors were German), Kraepelin strove to return to the German Reich.[23] The "increasingly unedifying political conditions in Dorpat" had led him to hope for an appointment in Heidelberg[24] since the summer of 1890, according to the reminiscences he wrote later in life. In retrospect, his years in Dorpat seemed like an "exile": Reflecting on his appointment to Heidelberg, Kraepelin wrote, "Only those who have lived as we for nearly five years in a kind of exile, can appreciate what this day meant for us, especially since the professorship in Heidelberg, next to Munich always appeared as the most desirable even if unattainable goal to me. . . . I left Dorpat in a light-hearted manner at the end of March 1891." [25] From this "exile" a "kind fate brought him back to the homeland."[26]

But Kraepelin expressed these opinions only in hindsight. On arriving at his new place of work five years before, he found that "the first impressions were friendly."[27] The new professor actively dedicated himself not only to the organization and material conditions of his clinic but also to the science and teaching of psychiatry. In his inaugural lecture, he spoke programmatically about the "different schools in psychiatric research." According to qualified opinion, this lecture, published later, was one of "the most incisive presentations in the contemporary medical research landscape in Germany of the last third of the nineteenth century."[28] The lecture's "guidelines" offered an advanced perspective for a new audience and an ambitious program for a new field.

Kraepelin distanced his views from both "speculative approaches" and neuropathology.[29] Kraepelin saw a way forward in experimental psychology, which was the focus of both his inaugural lecture and his scientific work in Dorpat. From his point of view, psychological experiments—for example, the measurement of reaction times—could raise psychiatric diagnosis to a scientific level.[30] Supported by his teacher Wilhelm Wundt (1831–1920), Kraepelin had high hopes of changing psychiatric science by introducing this new method—hope that led to some disappointment later. Kraepelin enthusiastically advocated psychological experimentation at Dorpat; he founded a Psychopathological Society and worked diligently with his colleagues and students.[31] In part, the focus on this method rather than clinical research had to do with the language situation at Dorpat. Since Kraepelin could not understand some of his patients without an interpreter, it was easier to adopt a nonverbal experimental approach.[32] After several years without satisfactory results from his psychiatric research, however, Kraepelin turned more and more to a clinical approach.

The relationship between experimental psychology and nosological research, and the references to them in Kraepelin's work, has been assessed in varying ways by researchers. While the experimental approach was certainly predominant in Kraepelin's work,[33] he also took a decisive turn toward nosology during his time in Dorpat.[34]

Kraepelin engaged in nosological research from the very beginning of his career in Dorpat. At a key moment, at the end of his inaugural lecture, Kraepelin spoke about classification as a significant task for the psychiatrist, despite all the understandable resignation concerning the then current state of knowledge about nosology. The "real subject" for clinical psychiatry seemed to Kraepelin to be able to deal with "mental disorders" immediately without requiring any additional tool; it was all about "the uninhibited view and indefatigable pursuit of the individual cases of psychiatric illness."[35] For him, the focus was on different, naturally occurring "illness processes"—that is, disease entities—although he did not yet emphasize the importance of the courses or development of these disease entities as strongly as he did in later writings.[36] Kraepelin actually admitted that "a way out of the labyrinth of clinical pictures cannot be seen for the moment."[37] But the objective was to be reached by means of the classification of "mental disorder symptoms" based on sober observation, a monographic treatment of "all those little variations and intermediate forms, which today, well known to the individual practitioner, are brought together indiscriminately in the oversized and therefore devoid of meaning categories of popular nomenclature."[38] Only afterward would it be possible to delimit each of the clinical pictures at a higher level and ascribe them in a final step to their pathological causes.

In following years, Kraepelin dealt simultaneously in his textbook with both the almost overabundant description of observed details and the demarcation of categories. Observations made in Dorpat were also included in this process, as demonstrated by the introductory example of the melancholic Estonian farmer. In the inaugural lecture, however, melancholy played only a minor role.[39]

Out of the nine doctoral theses supervised by Kraepelin during his time in Dorpat, none were dedicated to melancholy; seven dealt with experimental psychology. Only two were dedicated to clinical subjects: catatonia (Albert Behr, 1860–1919) and hebephrenia (Leon Daraszkiewicz, 1866–post-1926), both of which were important for Kraepelin's later conception of dementia praecox.[40] He recalls later in his memoirs that it was only in the last years of his stay in Dorpat that he was able to determine "more clearly the more or less rapid forms of mental enfeeblement from the incoming cases."[41]

Kraepelin delivered a lecture on clinical psychiatry each semester during his time in Dorpat. The role played by melancholy in them is unknown. Kraepelin published his lectures for the first time in 1901, and they very likely refer to Heidelberg patients. All editions of his *Introduction to Clinical Psychiatry* start with "cases" of melancholy; these were apparently the same ones contained in the series of lectures, possibly because they seemed to be the easiest for students to understand.[42] Perhaps Kraepelin was already applying this pattern in Dorpat. In any case, tradition has it that Kraepelin did his best to deliver interesting lectures at Dorpat, and that he succeeded in doing so—students traveled long distances to attend them.[43] Kraepelin reported in his memoirs that the number of attendees amounted to about fifty and consisted of different groups. The majority was made up of "actual Balts," and the remainder was Polish and Jewish students, the latter coming from both Poland and Russia (523 of the 1,578 students at the University of Dorpat came from different parts of the Russian state).[44]

Although his teaching was also hampered by language difficulties, the "eagerness" of the attendees was nonetheless "quite satisfactory."[45] Therefore, the cross-border diffusion of Kraepelin's lectures was already ongoing at that time. Language barriers impacted his interaction not only with students but also with patients. In this respect, it was only in Heidelberg that "more favorable conditions than ever before"[46] came along in his clinical research. It was probably here also that Kraepelin began to work with the famous scorecards.[47] As Kraepelin stated in his memoirs regarding the Dorpat editions of his textbook, "Due to the unfavourable conditions under which my clinical activity was exercised, I was only able to stay on the beaten track without making any particular progress." But he also stated that it was during those years that "the ever-increasing conviction of the importance of the development of the disease for the classification of insanity" imposed itself on his thinking.[48]

The Fate of Melancholy in the Various Editions of the Textbook

"Nobody will expect anything new from a Compendium,"[49] Kraepelin wrote in the preface to the first edition of his textbook. Although he was addressing the reader, it almost seems that Kraepelin was trying to reassure himself with this sentence. Since he himself came from the field of research, the assignment to write the *Compendium* was helpful to him as well, especially in light of the difficult situation after his dismissal from the university clinic in Leipzig.[50] He then named the authors on whom he based his work: Wilhelm Griesinger (1817–68) and Richard von Krafft-Ebing (1840–1902).[51] In addition, Kraepelin cited his teacher (and predecessor at Dorpat) Hermann Emminghaus as informing the general section of the *Compendium*, and he acknowledged the groundwork of his teacher Wilhelm Wundt, as well. Kraepelin also drew on these authors for the other clinical subjects covered in the first edition of this small, thin book, and his treatment of melancholy was no exception.

Few medical concepts have fascinated and been adorned with as many epithets through the centuries as melancholy. Although the psychiatric term had already been separated from the "ancient humoral pathology views" of Greek antiquity, it definitely still carried vestiges from past eras.[52] "Since times immemorial," wrote Griesinger, "individual kinds and varieties of melancholy" have been theorized.[53] The spectrum of his representations of melancholy ranges from simple depression (i.e., religious melancholy) to the feeling of being possessed (i.e., demonic melancholy). In principle, Griesinger considered melancholy to be the initial stage of unitary psychosis. According to this concept, there is ultimately only one form of "insanity," manifesting as different disorders in its various stages. For example, these include manic states after an initial melancholy and, eventually, a permanent "mental enfeeblement." At the symptomatic level, he cited three basic forms: "melancholy with stupor," "depression with destructive impulse," and "depression with persistent mental excitement."[54]

Krafft-Ebing also distinguished several forms in his textbook, the main ones being melancholia simplex, melancholia cum stupore sive attonita, and, in another section under the heading "Periodic Insanity," melancholia periodica.[55] In Kraepelin's *Compendium*, what first stands out is the "fragmentation" of melancholy and its subordination to various broader concepts. In this respect, Kraepelin differed from the above authors, in consistence with the goal of "a certain independence of representation" that he announced in the preface.[56] Forms of melancholy were to be found not only among the "depressive conditions" (melancholia simplex and melancholy with delusions) but also among the "twilight conditions" (melancholia attonita), the "excitement conditions" (melancholia activa), and the "periodic psychoses."[57]

Ever since the first edition, Kraepelin had tended toward extensive juxtapositions in his descriptions of clinical pictures, and thereby the formation of types. He gave an example of melancholy with delusions: "The patient is afraid of becoming seriously ill, of being impoverished; therefore he has no money to pay for food and suddenly believes that something terrible has happened to his wife, his children, that his house was burned down, that the apocalypse is imminent and similar occurrences."[58] He continually referred to "the patient," "the person who is ill," meaning the typical patient, not a specific individual. Although Kraepelin had already worked in psychiatry as a resident, he appears to have described three-dimensional, concrete, personal observations only after his rise to professorship in Dorpat: "Then I saw a young melancholic bursting into bitter tears while listening to merry music."[59]

Might this development also correspond to Kraepelin's growing clinical experience, considering the fact that he summarized melancholy in the following editions again as an independent disease? In any case, it is significant that melancholy gets a separate chapter in the second and third editions. The author distinguished three forms: melancholia simplex as a sort of basic form, melancholia activa with fear and anxiety in the foreground, and melancholia attonita as a depressive stupor.[60] Nothing changed in the basic classification in the fourth edition, which was developed in Heidelberg but still largely based on Kraepelin's clinical experience in Dorpat.[61] It was the fifth edition that marked the "decisive transition from the 'symptomatic to the clinical approach,' but also the momentous redefinition of the term melancholy,"[62] whose development over the years was now in the foreground. Melancholy was now reduced to a depressive disease in old age, while depressive insanity included manic, depressive, and circular forms.

Kraepelin held on to age-related melancholy in the sixth (1899) and seventh editions (1903/4), while decisive changes concerning depressive insanity occurred between the fifth and sixth editions. Manic-depressive insanity appeared as a category at the same time as the final shaping of his understanding of "dementia praecox."[63] Only afterward, between the seventh and the eighth editions, did Kraepelin decide—based on the criticism of his contemporaries, including the Russian psychiatrist Sergei Alekseevich Sukhanov (1867–1915)[64]—to eliminate the notion of melancholy as being related to old age or to integrate it into manic-depressive insanity.

Kraepelin had apparently kept melancholy as an independent clinical category for so long to preserve the "independence of the oldest psychiatric illness concept."[65] He could have rebaptized "manic-depressive insanity" as "manic-melancholic insanity" after abandoning it as an age-related category in the eighth edition. Because he failed to do so, melancholy largely disappeared from psychiatric terminology and was replaced by the term "depression."[66]

The development of the concept of melancholy and manic-depressive insanity within the "gigantic enterprise" of Kraepelin's textbook was, in general (though with significant exceptions), similar to that of dementia praecox. The concept underwent multiple phases: a preliminary phase of its formation could be found up to the fourth edition in 1893, a phase of reformulation or definition from 1893 to the sixth edition in 1899, and a consolidation phase from 1902 until 1927.[67] However, the consolidation parallel with dementia praecox was valid only for manic-depressive insanity. As mentioned, melancholy was not consolidated at all at this stage but rather disappeared from Kraepelin's nosology. The textbook itself, however, developed from a thin, small-scale compendium, to a multivolume textbook comprising several thousand pages containing numerous photographs and tables, providing a central "place for systematization and the transfer of knowledge."[68]

Kraepelin's time in Dorpat coincided with the beginnings of psychiatric concept formation, a phase in which, above all, the clarity of clinical observation began to be reflected increasingly in the textbook.[69]

Depression: Melancholy in Patient Records

Before patients can be used as "cases" for a textbook, medical notes recorded in case histories document their statements, as well as the "symptoms" and behaviors observed. These sources, which are essentially for the use of medical colleagues, usually explain little, relying on the reader to draw the conclusions intended by the author from the written observations. While diagnostic conclusions are rare, case histories have been used as an auxiliary tool for nosological classification.[70] It is doubtful, however, that the actual construction of disease entities can be identified in the files.

The Dorpat files from Kraepelin's time have been preserved (the German psychiatrist Kurt Schneider (1887–1967), one of Kraepelin's successors at

Heidelberg, seems to have consulted some files written by Kraepelin during World War II).[71] Until now, it was not possible to trace the file of the melancholic Estonian farmer cited above, but files of other patients with this diagnosis survived.[72] Case histories can also be found in Heidelberg, where Kraepelin's clinical research intensified because of the elimination of the language barrier.

The case history of Johann Faulhaber (1864–1940) is one such example. Faulhaber was admitted to the Heidelberg clinic for the first time in 1889, two years before Kraepelin's appointment.[73] During one of his subsequent admissions, he made "a lot of very interesting notes," which have been preserved.[74] His work became part of the Prinzhorn Collection at Heidelberg, which was established approximately a decade later and remains a world famous collection of asylum art.[75] Faulhaber's depictions of skulls are especially fascinating even today, since they seem to come from a more characteristically sinister sphere of depression.[76] In any case, the subject of the human skull was often used in art exhibitions as a meaningful element in the representation of melancholy.[77] Faulhaber also saw himself as an artist: "He is very proud of the results of his drawing activity; he claims that it will be difficult to find something as good." His doctors, however, suspected megalomania in the "manic, excited" patient.[78]

No diagnosis was entered on the cover of the 1889 case record. At the end of his stay, there was only a note about the former soldier having been discharged in improved condition.[79] Maybe the doctors were unable to do anything with this "changing clinical picture." At the time of admission, the patient was "generally cheerful, boisterous." He laughed, danced, and sang "erotic songs," but he also talked about figures speaking to him and expressed hypochondriacal and melancholic ideas, stating, for example, that "it would have been better had he died immediately after birth."[80]

Between his first and second stays, Faulhaber had recovered and "remained healthy since"; this detail was highlighted in the records.[81] States of agitation occurred just shortly before he was newly admitted, and elation and "flight of ideas" were present once again. A letter written by Faulhaber's wife in 1896, and filed in the case history, proves just how important the long-term course of the illness was to the Heidelberg hospital in Kraepelin's time: it was interesting to know and to document in the file whether the patient showed symptoms after his releasement and how the illness developed. Mrs. Faulhaber tells the clinic director in "polite reply to your letter" that the condition of her husband had been very good so far.[82]

But, in the following years, change was a constant reality for the patient. In 1908, the hospital discerned "constantly changing moods" in Faulhaber and issued a "manic-depressive psychosis" diagnosis. It is not possible to determine the precise date of the corresponding entry on the cover of the case history. However, this diagnosis was clearly recorded by a different person post-1899—the date of the introduction of "manic-depressive insanity" into psychiatric nosology.[83]

Despite his good prognosis, the asylum's gates closed permanently behind Faulhaber in 1926. Although he had been readmitted under his old diagnosis, it soon became apparent that he was now considered a "final case," a designation usually attributed to dementia praecox or schizophrenia. This judgment eventually led to Faulhaber's murder during the national socialist extermination of asylum inmates ("T4") in 1940.[84] In 1926, Faulhaber struck the asylum doctors as cranky and neglected; he also expressed a number of ideas about persecution and impairment.[85] He said that he felt like a "fifth wheel on a wagon, relegated, made fun of and slandered everywhere."[86]

"Like a wheel on a wagon"—this image was introduced decades before by the melancholic Estonian peasant and found its way into psychiatric nosology. Faulhaber may also have been intensively observed during his manic periods from a nosological point of view and thus become a part of the textbook in some way. When he began to feel "like a fifth wheel on a wagon," something that seemed now to fit a rather different diagnostic classification, no one in the asylum was interested in the implications of his psychopathological portrait any longer, and the drawings he still made were no longer preserved.

The Conceptualization of Melancholia as an Example of Psychiatric Knowledge Exchange

"Like a wheel on a wagon" is perhaps an appropriate image for understanding how patients became part of psychiatry textbooks, and not just in Kraepelin's case. They seem to have played a rather passive role, but, nonetheless, their experiences, including their regional, historical, and cultural backgrounds, found their way into books and scientific tradition. Since Kraepelin first had the opportunity to observe patients and the courses of their illnesses for longer periods of time during his stay in Dorpat, it can rightly be inferred that Dorpat's patients impacted the development of his classification system, perhaps even more decisively than his later patients at Heidelberg and Munich.

Kraepelin's experience at the University of Dorpat also had a definite impact on Russian psychiatry.[87] Kraepelin took the teaching of future physicians very seriously, well aware that they would spread their newly acquired knowledge throughout many parts of the Russian Empire. Kraepelin recognized his own role in this process. A former student reported that, in the process of their professors' rigorously examination, aspiring psychiatrists became real specialists in their area.[88]

But it would be one sided to speak only about a "classic" transfer of knowledge from West to East, from Europe to Russia, traveling in only one direction like a wheel on a wagon. In fact, the most important research Russian scientists received from Germany was critically discussed, modified, and filtered through their own background and clinical research. Such was the case with Suchanov's (partial) criticism of Kraepelin. Russian research on melancholy, such as that performed by Suchanov, was also published promptly in leading German, French, and English journals. It appears more appropriate, therefore, to view the production and movement of concepts of melancholy in Western Europe and Russia around 1900 in the context of the medicalization of melancholy as an aspect of the circulation of knowledge. The Baltic region of the Russian Empire, with its leading university, Dorpat, played a central role in this process of conceptual exchange between the West and East in medicine and science.

Notes

1. Emil Kraepelin, *Psychiatrie: Ein kurzes Lehrbuch für Studierende und Ärzte*, 4th ed. (Leipzig: Abel Verlag, 1893), 287. In the edition published after moving to Heidelberg, the patient appears for the first time as an "Estonian peasant." Emil Kraepelin, *Psychiatrie: Ein kurzes Lehrbuch für Studierende und Ärzte*, 4th ed. (Leipzig: Abel Verlag, 1893), 294. Kraepelin was not the only one to bring up "melancholia simplex" in the context of "simple" Estonian peasants: Cf. Hermann Emminghaus, *Die psychischen Störungen des Kindesalters* (Tübingen: Verlag der Laupp'schen Buchhandlung, 1987), 144–46. Emminghaus describes the case history of Minna Rosinale, a fourteen-year-old girl ("esthnisches Bauernmädchen von kindlichem Habitus") diagnosed with "melancholia simplex."

2. Emil Kraepelin, *Psychiatrie: Ein Lehrbuch für Studierende und Ärzte*, 5th ed. (Leipzig: Ambrosius Barth, 1896), 572; Emil Kraepelin, *Psychiatrie: Ein Lehrbuch für Studierende und Ärzte*, 2 vols., 6th ed. (Leipzig: Ambrosius Barth, 1899), 328.

3. Michael Schmidt-Degenhard, *Melancholie und Depression: Zur Problemgeschichte der depressiven Erkrankungen seit Beginn des 19. Jahrhunderts* (Stuttgart: Kohlhammer, 1983), 97.

4. Emil Kraepelin, *Psychiatrie: Ein Lehrbuch für Studierende und Ärzte*, 2 vols., 7th ed. (Leipzig: Ambrosius Barth, 1903/1904), 531. The "type" has already been created in the third edition, cf. Kraepelin, *Psychiatrie: Ein kurzes Lehrbuch für Studirende und Aerzte*, vol. 3 (Leipzig: Abel, 1889), 287. Immediately after the sentence about the "simple peasant," it reads, "The patient is flaccid, lacking in energy and unable to rouse himself, besides, his inner dullness has suppressed his courage and propensity for energetic activities."

5. In the eighth edition, Kraepelin explains why he has abandoned the category of (age-related) melancholy. Emil Kraepelin, *Psychiatrie: Ein Lehrbuch für Studierende und Ärzte*, 2 vols., 8th ed. (Leipzig: Ambrosius Barth, 1909/1913), part 2, 1379–81. The description originally associated with the "Estonian peasant" ("The patient is

'discouraged and submissive' as a wheel on a wagon that just rolls along, internally frozen and petrified") can be found in this volume on p. 1261 in the characterization of "depressive states" in their basic form. Kraepelin includes this description on p. 1265 with the comment, "The picture of simple depression, somehow corresponding to the former 'melancholia simplex' can be multiply enriched by the quite frequent development of hallucinations and delusions; perhaps we could speak in this case of 'melancholia gravis.'" In the end, the "Estonian peasant" is once again conceptually close to his original classification as "Melancholia simplex."

6. Especially in the natural sciences, e.g., chemistry and medicine, the University of Dorpat was a regionally and internationally renowned academic institution during the nineteenth century that served as a hub for knowledge and knowledge exchange between East and West. Cf., among others, Erik Amburger, "Die Bedeutung der Universität Dorpat für Osteuropa: Untersucht an der Zusammensetzung des Lehrkörpers und der Studentenschaft in den Jahren 1802–1889," in *Die Universitäten Dorpat/Tartu, Riga und Wilna/Vilnius 1579–1979: Beiträge zu ihrer Geschichte und ihrer Wirkung im Grenzbereich zwischen Ost und West,* ed. Gert von Pistohlkors, Toivo U. Raun, and Paul Kaegbein (Cologne: Böhlau, 1987), 163–82; Erich Donnert, *Die Universität Dorpat-Jur'ev 1802–1918: Ein Beitrag zur Geschichte des Hochschulwesens in den Ostseeprovinzen des Russischen Reiches* (Frankfurt a. M. [wt al.]: Lang, 2007); Dieter Lenoir, "Eliteuniversität des 19. Jahrhunderts," *Nachrichten aus der Chemie* 57, no. 11 (2009), 1100–103; Ilo Käbin, *Die medizinische Forschung und Lehre an der Universität Dorpat/Tartu 1802–1940: Ergebnisse u. Bedeutung für d. Entwicklung d. Medizin* (Lüneburg: Verlag Nordostdt. Kulturwerk, 1986).

7. Holger Steinberg and Matthias C. Angermeyer, "Emil Kraepelin's Years at Dorpat as Professor of Psychiatry in Nineteenth-Century Russia," *History of Psychiatry* 12 (2001): 297.

8. Cf. Julie Vail Brown, "The Professionalization of Russian Psychiatry: 1857–1911" (PhD diss., Sociology, University of Pennsylvania, 1981); Irina Sirotkina, *Diagnosing Literary Genius: A Cultural History of Psychiatry in Russia, 1880–1930,* Medicine & Culture (Baltimore: Johns Hopkins University Press, 2002); Gregory Zilboorg, "Russian Psychiatry—Its Historical and Ideological Background," *Bulletin of the New York Academy of Medicine* 19, no. 10 (1943), 713–28; Mark D. Steinberg, "Melancholy and Modernity: Emotions and Social Life in Russia between the Revolutions," *Journal of Social History* 41, no. 4 (2008): 813–41.

9. Zilboorg, "Russian Psychiatry," 719. Among the 140 doctors who participated in the First All-Russian Psychiatric Meeting in Moscow in 1887, only 86 specialized in the examination and treatment of mental illness.

10. Wolfgang Burgmair et al., "Menge und Verschiedenheit der Themata," in *Emil Kraepelin: Briefe I. 1868–1886,* ed. Wolfgang Burgmair, Eric J. Engstrom, and Matthias M. Weber, Edition Emil Kraepelin 3 (Munich: Belleville, 2002), 15–25, esp. 23; Cf. Emil Kraepelin, *Lebenserinnerungen* (Berlin: Springer, 1983), 25. Kraepelin returned to Munich and worked in Leubus and Dresden until his appointment to Dorpat.

11. Emil Kraepelin, *Lebenserinnerungen,* 39. Cf. Wolfgang Burgmair et al., "Die Dorpater Klinik ist keineswegs schlecht," in *Kraepelin in Dorpat 1886–1891,* ed. Wolfgang Burgmair, Eric J. Engstrom, Albrecht Hirschmüller and Matthias M. Weber (Munich: Belleville, 2003), 22–23.

12. According to the memoirs of Heinrich Dehio, Kraepelin's assistant in Dorpat, "it was clear to him that he should expect adverse reactions that were not to be underestimated if he were to return to Germany" due to his previous history in Leipzig. Heinrich Dehio, "Meine Erinnerungen an Professor E. Kraepelin in Dorpat u. Heidelberg," in Burgmair et al., *Kraepelin in Dorpat 1886–1891*, 311.

13. Cf. Reginald Pierson's letter to Kraepelin of June 17, 1886, in Burgmair et al., "Menge und Verschiedenheit der Themata," 357n.

14. Wilhelm Moldenhauer's letter to Kraepelin of July 7, 1886, in Burgmair et al., "Menge und Verschiedenheit der Themata," 361n.

15. Steinberg and Angermeyer, "Emil Kraepelin's Years at Dorpat," 300.

16. Burgmair et al., "Die Dorpater Klinik ist keineswegs schlecht," 21n. It was founded in 1632, closed in 1710, and reopened in 1802.

17. Ibid.

18. Kraepelin, *Lebenserinnerungen*, 41.

19. Ibid., 42–45. Cf. Burgmair et al., "Die Dorpater Klinik ist keineswegs schlecht," 28–29nn. The clinic in Dorpat was significantly in debt, but Kraepelin achieved a consolidation. In addition, he restored the clinic to profitability and expanded it. Establishing sufficient fire protection measures was particularly important to him because of its wood construction. Steinberg and Angermeyer, "Emil Kraepelin's Years at Dorpat," 313.

20. Cf. Florian Mildenberger, "Emil Kraepelin (1856–1926) in Dorpat: Psychiatriereform im panslawistischen Daseinskampf," in *Naturwissenschaft als Kommunikationsraum zwischen Deutschland und Russland im 19. Jahrhundert*, ed. Ortrun Riha and Marta Fischer, Relationes 6 (Aachen: Shaker-Verlag, 2011), 219–32.

21. Burgmair et al., "Die Dorpater Klinik ist keineswegs schlecht," 21–22nn.

22. Steinberg and Angermeyer, "Emil Kraepelin's Years at Dorpat," 302.

23. "On the other hand, these conditions had to have a special effect on his yearning for Germany, and so he probably praised the kind fate which led him to the vacant professorship in Heidelberg, after the appointment of Fürstner in Strasbourg." Dehio, "Meine Erinnerungen," 316. Dehio refers here to the preface to the fourth edition of the textbook. For the number of German professors, cf. Steinberg and Angermeyer, "Emil Kraepelin's Years at Dorpat," 302.

24. Kraepelin, *Lebenserinnerungen*, 64. At the end of his summer trip that year, Kraepelin visited the International Medical Congress in Berlin. There, he gathered from conversations with professional colleagues that "the appointment to Heidelberg did not lie beyond the realm of possibility." According to Burgmair et al., Russification directly impacted the faculty circa post-1890. Burgmair et al., "Die Dorpater Klinik ist keineswegs schlecht," 36–39nn.

25. Kraepelin, *Lebenserinnerungen*, 64.

26. Kraepelin, *Psychiatrie* ([4]1893), preface (unpaginated).

27. Kraepelin, *Lebenserinnerungen*, 42.

28. Burgmair et al. "Die Dorpater Klinik ist keineswegs schlecht," 43n. See also Eric. J. Engstrom and Kenneth S. Kendler, "Emil Kraepelin: Icon and Reality"; Engstrom, "Emil Kraepelin's Inaugural Lecture at Dorpat: Contexts and Legacies," *American Journal of Psychiatry* 172 (2015): 1190–96.

29. Emil Kraepelin, "Die Richtungen der Psychiatrischen Forschung," in Burgmair et al., *Kraepelin in Dorpat 1886–1891*, 57, 62, 65–66.

30. Burgmair et al., "Die Dorpater Klinik ist keineswegs schlecht," 46n.; Kraepelin, "Die Richtungen," 68–70.

31. In 1887, Kraepelin founded the Dorpat Psychological Society. Cf. Steinberg and Angermeyer, "Emil Kraepelin's Years at Dorpat," 305, 315.

32. Steinberg and Angermeyer, "Emil Kraepelin's Years at Dorpat," 302.

33. Burgmair et al., "Die Dorpater Klinik ist keineswegs schlecht," 49–53nn.

34. Steinberg and Angermeyer, "Emil Kraepelin's Years at Dorpat," 308–10. Kraepelin continued the psychological experiments throughout his lifetime, but only as a contribution to psychology, not as a part of psychiatric research.

35. Kraepelin, "Die Richtungen," 75. Cf. Volker Roelcke, "Unterwegs zur Psychiatrie als Wissenschaft: Das Projekt einer 'Irrenstatistik' und Emil Kraepelins Neuformulierung der psychiatrischen Klassifikation," in *Psychiatrie im 19. Jahrhundert: Forschungen zur Geschichte von Psychiatrischen Institutionen, Debatten und Praktiken im deutschen Sprachraum*, ed. Eric. J. Engstrom and Volker Roelcke, Medizinische Forschung 13 (Basel: Schwabe-Verlag, 2003), 182.

36. Kraepelin, "Die Richtungen," 75. Cf. Burgmair et al., "Die Dorpater Klinik ist keineswegs schlecht," 53n. Neither in his inaugural lecture nor in the early editions of the textbook did Kraepelin attribute a specific nosological value to the progression of mental illnesses.

37. Kraepelin, "Die Richtungen," 76.

38. Ibid., 77.

39. Kraepelin mentions the ancient humoral pathology that gave origin to the concept of melancholy. He also addresses unknown psychic disease processes, including melancholy. Kraepelin, "Die Richtungen," 58, 60.

40. Burgmair et al., "Die Dorpater Klinik ist keineswegs schlecht," 42n. Dehio reports that Behr's thesis was dedicated to mania with inhibition phenomena, which were later called mixed forms by Kraepelin and were significant to the conception of manic-depressive insanity. Evidently, Dehio's recollection is incorrect in this instance. Dehio, "Meine Erinnerungen," 309.

41. Kraepelin, *Lebenserinnerungen*, 49. He then interpreted this in terms of Hecker's hebephrenia, in which his assistant Daraszkiewicz was particularly interested.

42. Four versions of the *Introduction* appeared in Kraepelin's lifetime (Kraepelin, *Einführung in die psychiatrische Klinik*, [Leipzig: Barth, 1901, 1905, 1916, and 1921]). In the preface to the first edition he states that he was trying "to follow the presentation with the real progress of lessons." In the 1916 and 1921 editions, the first lecture is still named "Melancholy," but now the words "manic-depressive insanity" are added between brackets. Included are three "cases": "common melancholy," melancholy with delusions, and melancholy with stupor. The last category can already be partially found in the first edition (fifty-nine-year-old farmer, an example of melancholia simplex). While in the early editions the distinction between age-related melancholy (severe restlessness) and "circular" states of depression (inhibition phenomena) is foregrounded, the last "case" with recurrent depressive and manic states presents an opportunity to discuss manic-depressive insanity in later editions. The fourth edition of the *Introduction* grew to three volumes: a general volume, the "classical" lecture volume, and a volume with cases for advanced students (derived from the clinical conferences for more or less advanced psychiatrists working in the clinic). Kraepelin mentions here that the order in this case does not follow a progression from simple

to complex, as seemed appropriate for beginners. Thus, it can be assumed that Kraepelin considered melancholy to be something relatively easy to be taught, as it is always at the start of his *Introduction* conceived for beginners.

43. Dehio, "Meine Erinnerungen," 304.

44. Steinberg and Angermeyer, "Emil Kraepelin's Years at Dorpat," 302. Among the students, 552 were Livonians, 335 came from Courland, 145 from Estonia, and 23 were "foreigners."

45. Burgmair et al., "Die Dorpater Klinik ist keineswegs schlecht," 32n.

46. Ibid., 49n.

47. Eric J. Engstrom. "Ökonomie klinischer Inskription: Zu diagnostischen und nosologischen Schreibpraktiken in der Psychiatrie," in *Psychographien*, ed. Cornelius Borck and Armin Schäfer (Zürich: Diaphenes, 2005), 219–40. Cf. Roelcke, "Unterwegs zur Psychiatrie als Wissenschaft," 171.

48. Kraepelin, *Lebenserinnerungen*, 49.

49. Emil Kraepelin, *Compendium der Psychiatrie: Zum Gebrauch für Studierende und Ärzte* (Leipzig: Abel Verlag, 1883), viii.

50. Kraepelin, *Lebenserinnerungen*, 28. Burgmair et al., "Menge und Verschiedenheit der Themata," 24n.

51. Kraepelin, *Compendium*, viii.

52. Cf. Kraepelin, "Richtlinien," 58: "Without resorting to the old humoural pathology views, which are for example the origin for the still common name of melancholy." The idea of a "melancholic temperament" seems to have lasted longer than the notion of an unfavorable mix of the four humors (with a predominance of black bile) as the cause of melancholy. This concept was explicitly taken up again later by Hubertus Tellenbach. Cf. Hubert Tellenbach, *Melancholie: Zur Problemgeschichte, Typologie, Pathogenese und Klinik* (Berlin: Springer, 1961). For the influence of older scientific views on "modern" research developments, cf. Ludwik Fleck, *Entstehung und Entwicklung einer wissenschaftlichen Tatsache: Einführung in die Lehre vom Denkstil und Denkkollektiv* (Frankfurt/M.: Suhrkamp, 1980).

53. Wilhelm Griesinger, *Die Pathologie und Therapie der psychischen Krankheiten für Ärzte und Studierende*, 4th ed. (Braunschweig: Wreden, 1876), 214.

54. Ibid., 250–52. For the classification of unitary psychosis, cf. 213–15.

55. Richard von Krafft-Ebing, *Lehrbuch der Psychiatrie auf klinischer Grundlage für praktische Ärzte und Studierende*, 3rd ed. (Stuttgart: Enke, 1888), 324, 482–83.

56. Kraepelin, *Compendium*, viii. Cf. Schmidt-Degenhard, *Melancholie*, 88.

57. "Periodic insanity," a category that already appears in Krafft-Ebing and in the introduction of the dimension of "progression" in the nosological classification, is by no means insignificant and has its own history, which cannot be discussed further here. Cf. inter alia Esther Fischer-Homberger, *Das zirkuläre Irresein*, Zürcher medizingeschichtliche Abhandlungen 53 (Zürich: Juris Druck und Verlag, 1968).

58. Kraepelin, *Compendium*, 204.

59. Kraepelin, *Psychiatrie* (³1889), 284.

60. Schmidt-Degenhard, *Melancholie*, 88.

61. For more detail on the changes, cf. Schmidt-Degenhard, *Melancholie*, 89. In the fourth edition of Kraepelin, *Psychiatrie* (1893), melancholia simplex is found on pp. 288–304, anxiety melancholy or melancholia activa on pp. 304–10, melancholia attonita on pp. 310–17, and periodically recurrent depression states on pp. 379–83.

62. Schmidt-Degenhard, *Melancholie*, 89.

63. Yvonne Wübben, *Verrückte Sprache: Psychiater und Dichter in der Anstalt des 19. Jahrhunderts* (Konstanz: Konstanz University Press, 2012), 67–68.

64. Cf. Sergei A. Sukhanov and Petr B. Gannushkin, "K ucheniiu o melankholii," *Zhurnal nevropatologii i psikhiatrii im. S. S. Korsakova* [Journal of Neuropathology and Psychiatry named Korsakova] 6 (1902): 1170–87. For a French translation, cf. Serge Soukhanoff and Pierre Gannouchkine, "Étude Sur La Mélancolie," *Annales médico-psychologiques* 18 (1903): 213–38. See also Sergei A. Suchanov, *O Melankholii* (St. Petersburg: Izd. Zhurnala "Prakticheskaia Meditsina," 1906).

65. Schmidt-Degenhard, *Melancholie*, 91.

66. Ibid., 97.

67. Wübben, *Verrückte Sprache*, 66, 68. For the term "dementia praecox," Wübben believes the preliminary stage of concept formation covers the first three editions, i.e., until 1889; the phase of term definition therefore starts earlier. Cf. also Paul Hoff, *Emil Kraepelin und die Psychiatrie als klinische Wissenschaft: Ein Beitrag zum Selbstverständnis psychiatrischer Forschung*, Monographien aus dem Gesamtgebiete der Psychiatrie 73 (Berlin [wt al.]: Springer, 1994).

68. Wübben, *Verrückte Sprache*, 64. Wübben refers to Ludwik Fleck and his considerations about "text book science."

69. For "Cases in Dorpat" in the textbook editions of 1889 and 1893, cf. Wübben, *Verrückte Sprache*, 84–89.

70. Wübben, *Verrückte Sprache*, 89–103. Cf. Maike Rotzoll, "Krankheit schreiben in der Psychiatrie um 1900? Diagnosen, Kranken- und Patientengeschichten von Opfern der nationalsozialistischen 'Euthanasie'-Aktion, 'T4,'" in *Krankheit schreiben: Aufzeichnungsverfahren in Medizin und Literatur*, ed. Yvonne Wübben and Carsten Zelle (Göttingen: Wallstein, 2013), 109–28.

71. According to Wübben, the Kraepelin files are lost. Wübben, *Verrückte Sprache*, 89. According to Steinberg and Angermeyer, however, "many of them can still be found in the Estonian National Archives." Steinberg and Angermeyer, "Emil Kraepelin's Years at Dorpat," 318. The files have been preserved, instead, in the archive of the psychiatric clinic of Tartu. They could be traced with the help of Erki Tammiksaar and Ken Kalling, to whom the authors of this article are deeply indebted.

72. Maike Rotzoll and Frank Grüner, "Emil Kraepelin and German Psychiatry in Multicultural Dorpat/Tartu, 1886–1891," *TRAMES—Journal of the Humanities and Social Sciences* 20 (2016): 351–67.

73. Thomas Röske, "Johann Faulhaber—Ein Gefühl von außerordentlicher Leistungsfähigkeit auf allen Gebieten," in *Todesursache: Euthanasie; Verdeckte Morde in der NS-Zeit*, ed. Bettina Brand-Claussen, Thomas Röske, and Maike Rotzoll, Catalogue Prinzhorn Collection (Heidelberg: Wunderhorn, 2002), 67–69.

74. Case history Johann Faulhaber 93/51, Prinzhorn Collection, University of Heidelberg, University Archives, Heidelberg, Germany (on permanent loan by the University archive), page 2.

75. Thomas Röske, "The Prinzhorn Collection—Psychiatric Art with International Standing," in *Wissenschaftsatlas of Heidelberg University*, ed. Peter Meusburger and Thomas Schuch (Knittlingen: Bibliotheca Palatina, 2012), 244–45.

76. Maike Rotzoll, "Über den Totenköpfen: Johann Faulhaber und Edgar Schmandts Kopf für Prinzhorn 2," in *Ungesehen und unerhört: Künstler reagieren auf*

die Sammlung Prinzhorn, ed. Ingrid von Beyme und Thomas Röske, vol. 1 of Bildende Kunst/Film/Video (Heidelberg: Wunderhorn, 2013), 226–31.

77. Jean Clair, ed., *Melancholie Genie und Wahnsinn in der Kunst* (Ostfildern-Ruit: Hatje Cantz Verlag, 2005), 256–64.

78. Case history Johann Faulhaber, Prinzhorn Collection, page 2.

79. Ibid., page 5.

80. Ibid., page 6. Only toward the end of his stay is it recorded that Faulhaber could now "be recognised as a typical maniac: flight of ideas, typical cheerful mood" (page 8).

81. Ibid., page 11.

82. Ibid., page 16.

83. Ibid., page 1. The third admission to Heidelberg was in 1908, the fourth and fifth in 1917. It seems to have been the usual practice in Heidelberg of recording diagnoses not in the case files but in a separate diagnosis book, cf. Wübben, *Verrückte Sprache*, 92. The author draws the conclusion that the "separate recording of diagnosis and case history in two different locations" was probably done on purpose in Heidelberg (to make a definite diagnosis after observation of the course of the disease).

84. Faulhaber was moved in February 1940 from the asylum in Wiesloch to the regional nursing home in Weinheim, and from there he was transported on October 15, 1940, to the Grafeneck killing center. This date must be considered the date of his death, as patients were usually murdered in the gas chamber on the day they arrived.

85. Röske, "Johann Faulhaber," 68.

86. Case history Johann Faulhaber, Prinzhorn Collection, excerpt on Faulhaber's stays in the Wiesloch asylum, page 6.

87. Kraepelin's first short textbook on psychiatry was translated into Russian as early as 1891. This year marked also the end of his stay as a professor of psychiatry at the University of Dorpat. For this first Russian translation of Kraepelin's textbook (*Psychiatrie: Ein kurzes Lehrbuch für Studierende und Ärzte*, von Dr. Emil Kraepelin, professor in Dorpat) see E. Krepelin, *Kratkoe rukovodstvo po psikhiatrii dlia vrachei i studentov* (St. Petersburg: Prakticheskaia meditsina, 1891). Further works by Kraepelin and new editions of his textbooks on psychiatry were translated into Russian from the late 1890s onward. His works were also regularly reviewed in leading medical journals in Russia. See, e.g., Aleksandr Nikolaevich Bernshtein (reviewer), "Emil Kräpelin. Einführung in die Psychiatrische Klinik. Dreissig Vorlesungen. Leipzig: J. A. Barth, 1901," *Zhurnal nevropatologii i psikhatrii imeni S. S. Korsakova* 1, no. 2 (1901): 487–89; Aleksandr Nikolaevich Bernshtein (reviewer), "Prof. E. Kräpelin. Vvedenie v psikhiatricheskuiu kliniku. 30 klinicheskikh lektsii. Pereveli s nemeckago vrachi Ia. F. Kaplan I S. A. Kaplan. Ufa 1901," *Zhurnal nevropatologii i psikhatrii imeni S. S. Korsakova* 2, no. 5 (1902), 1104–5.

88. Steinberg and Angermeyer, "Emil Kraepelin's Years at Dorpat," 315.

Chapter Eight

Sanatorium Narratives from the Baltic Sea Region and Early Signs of the Pathographical Genre

The Case of Harriet Löwenhjelm

Jonatan Wistrand

On the basis of my own experience, I shall never be able to understand, never manage to understand, that an otherwise cheerful and essentially untroubled person can be destroyed by consumption alone.[1]

Franz Kafka to Hugo Bergmann, August 1923,
Graal-Müritz by the Baltic Sea

In April 1914, the twenty-seven-year-old Swedish poet and painter Harriet Löwenhjelm arrived in Vejlefjord, Denmark, for her first stay at a large, modern, institutional sanatorium. In a letter addressed to her cousin, Marianne Mörner, she wrote enthusiastically, "I arrived in excellent weather . . . and was examined by three doctors, one more distinguished than the next. I seem very healthy, and I hope they will let me return home soon."[2]

Harriet Löwenhjelm's journey to the Baltic Sea coastline was—like Franz Kafka's nine years later—taken in hopes of finding a cure for her tuberculosis. Before too long, however, the initial enchantment had faded. In a letter

from June 1914 to her friend Elsa Björkman, she enclosed a poem expressing, more than anything, a sense of despondency:

> Come and help me for God's sake,
> for my sake,
> for your sake,
> you alone can do it!
> Sorrow fills the world with ache,
> glittering gold is mostly fake.
> For God's sake,
> for my sake,
> help, you who can do it![3]

Like many of her fellow patients, Harriet Löwenhjelm, with her artistic soul
and obstinate manner, apparently found it difficult to adjust to life in the
sanatorium. She would grow accustomed to the setting only gradually. But
despite a four-year odyssey in which she traveled between the finest sanatoriums in Scandinavia, Harriet Löwenhjelm passed away in May 1918, at the
age of thirty-one.

***

The aim of this chapter is twofold.

- First, to illustrate that in the early twentieth century, in addition to a
  transfer of scientific opinions and medical observations, there was also
  an indisputable circulation of illness experiences across the national
  borders of the Baltic Sea region. One category of individuals seems to
  have been particularly active in this experience transfer: the itinerant
  tuberculosis patients at the sanatoriums.
- Second, to contribute to the academic discourse concerning the emergence of pathography—that is, the emergence of the biographical sub-
  genre centering on individual illness experiences. By suggesting that
  this genre was preceded in the early twentieth century by a growing
  number of semistructured narratives I will call "pre-pathographical testimonies," this chapter traces some of the roots of pathography.[4]

After an introductory outline on the characteristics of the pathographical
genre, a theoretical position regarding the emergence of pathography is presented. Next, this theory is examined and illustrated using the specific case
of Harriet Löwenhjelm (1887–1918). While for example Sheila Rothman's
study *Living in the Shadow of Death* (1995) provides the reader with a multitude
of voices from different sanatoriums, this chapter thus seeks to highlight the
experiences of one individual.[5] Focusing on the single story might intuitively

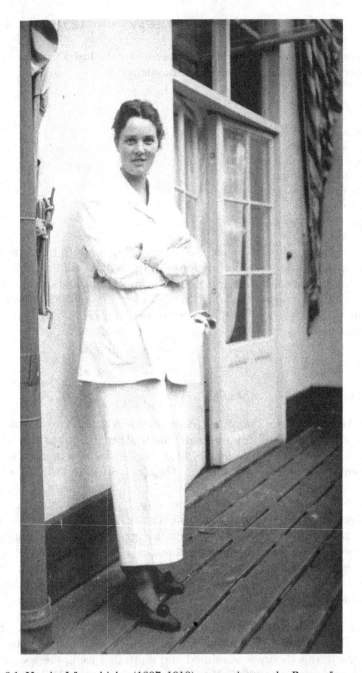

Figure 8.1. Harriet Löwenhjelm (1887–1918) as a patient at the Romanäs sanatorium in southern Sweden. Löwenhjelm wrote some of her most beloved poems here during her last years of life. Photograph taken by her fellow patient Ulf von Konow, on August 25, 1917, nine months prior to Löwenhjelm's death. Courtesy of the National Library of Sweden in Stockholm.

seem less informative, but, as I will show, it also provides an opportunity to reconstruct a more nuanced illness narrative, penetrating deeper into the chosen individual's world of ideas. For that purpose, Harriet Löwenhjelm, as a young and financially privileged sanatorium patient of the early twentieth century, appears as a suitable representative of the individuals most typically involved in the pre-pathographical writing taking shape at the turn of the century. Furthermore, she is a valuable example because her literary work has until now been largely ignored by historians outside of Sweden and thus, despite the clear and perceptive way it describes illness experience, remains more or less unknown to an international audience. In that sense, this chapter provides an opportunity to introduce the poignant writing and intriguing character of Harriet Löwenhjelm to a wider readership.[6] Finally, since Harriet Löwenhjelm traveled between sanatoriums in Denmark, Sweden, and Norway, her illness writing provides an opportunity for a comparative approach on sanatorium experience, spanning the national borders of the Scandinavian countries.

Introducing the Pathographical Genre

As historians, we rely predominantly on one specific mode of expression, the *written* word—an obvious yet disappointing fact for any narrative-based historical researcher, since the overwhelming majority of narratives have always been oral. Any medical historian interested in narratives of illness must therefore be aware that most material has already been filtered out for no other reason than its form of presentation. What remains is, first and foremost, a mishmash of written diaries, letters, poems, and other sorts of disparate notes. Apart from this clutter of fragmentary voices, however, there is also a more elaborate illness narrative labeled "pathography."[7] Works in this category are testimonies written solely for the purpose of turning the author's illness experience into a uniform and often carefully edited story. In pathographies, patients describe their illnesses in literary text, with a dramaturgy and a chronological setting similar to that of a novel or a short story. In contrast to the brief and often impersonal medical reports formulated by doctors, nurses, and other caregivers, pathography could rightly be regarded as "an extended narrative situating the illness experience within the author's life and the meaning of that life."[8]

Several scholars have written extensively on different aspects of the pathographical genre: its literary characteristics,[9] its position within the academic field of medical humanities,[10] its impact on the medical establishment, and the usefulness of pathographical testimonies for educational purposes.[11] In this chapter I do not attempt to comment on that broader discussion. Instead, I focus on the rise of the pathographical genre—or, rather, on the circumstances preceding that rise.

The Emergence of Pathography

Written testimonies of the experience of illness are not an exclusively modern phenomenon, but, as literary scholar Anne Hunsaker-Hawkins points out in her work *Reconstructing Illness: Studies in Pathography* (1999), the pathographical genre is not particularly old, either.[12] In our days, most pathographies are written by patients suffering from either stigmatized or debilitating diseases, such as cancer, multiple sclerosis, dementia, depression, and bipolar disorder.[13] Similarly, when the pathographical genre first appeared in the early twentieth century, these accounts, too, were written by patients with a diagnosis both debilitating and stigmatized, namely tuberculosis. Anne Hunsaker-Hawkins states that "with few exceptions, such as . . . sanatorium narratives from the 1920s and 1930s, pathography seems to belong exclusively to the second half of the twentieth century."[14]

Something in the sanatorium environment thus seems to have triggered a desire in its patients to create narratives. To fully understand the narrative of Harriet Löwenhjelm presented later in this chapter, I will shortly discuss three of the circumstances behind this momentum.

First among these was the widespread establishment of the sanatorium as an institution. During the decades around the turn of the twentieth century, large sanatoriums were built on the outskirts of almost every major city in the Western world. Within a few decades, residence in a sanatorium— with its fresh air, nourishing food, and balance between rest and physical activity—became the leading means of treating tuberculosis. At the sanatoriums, men, women, and children were isolated from their families and the rest of society for months, or even years, with endless amounts of time on their hands and an uncertain future ahead of them. Sheila Rothman has estimated that, in 1925, there were seven hundred thousand beds in North America alone.[15] This large-scale hospitalization, never before seen, detached the tuberculosis patient from the rest of society and turned his or her illness into a full-time existence.[16]

Second, the rapid progress in the medical sciences by this time led to an increasing objectification of the patient. In the course of a few decades at the turn of the century, tuberculosis became "a technologically based entity, grounded in bacteriology and identified by such tools as tuberculin skin tests, sputum examinations, the thermometer, and chest x-rays."[17] The progress of medical science entailed changes in medical practice, including the medical encounter.[18] At the turn of the twentieth century, physicians at sanatoriums, as well as in many other medical settings, could examine, diagnose, and even treat patients without interacting with them as individuals. A scientific and seemingly distant attitude toward the patient replaced the physician's earlier attentiveness to the patient's individual illness story.

Mike Bury argues that with the rise of "scientific bio-medicine" in the late nineteenth century, "subjective accounts of the patient were virtually irrelevant. As illness was increasingly sequestrated from everyday life by professional medicine, so the patient's suffering was effectively silenced."[19] It seems reasonable that these changes in doctor-patient relations triggered an urge among patients to make their voices heard in new ways. In that sense, it could be argued (and illustrated through the illness narrative of Harriet Löwenhjelm) that, rather than being silenced, as Mike Bury presumes, sanatorium patients gave vent to their personal stories of illness in a new forum, the written narrative.

Third, and finally, the stigmatization of tuberculosis, following the discovery in 1882 of its bacterial origin and contagious nature, also seems to have served as an incentive for pathographical writing. Historian Tim Boon writes that "to become a consumptive carried enormous stigma in the first half of the 20th century that set its sufferers apart, often spatially, by their dependence . . . on the sanatorium."[20] The formulation of illness narratives at sanatoriums thus became an act of protest against campaigns depicting tuberculosis patients as dangerous carriers of a deadly disease.

Proposing Pre-pathographical Testimony

Thus, at least three incentives drove the emergence of a pathographical writing at the sanatoriums in the first decades of the twentieth century. But, before full-length pathographical testimonies emerged, fragmentary or semiorganized narrative expressions seem to have taken form: narratives—letters, poems, diary entries, and other literary fragments—that already contained most of the basic elements of a true pathography, while lacking its uniform structure. As this chapter suggests, the first pathographies were in fact preceded by such "pre-pathographical testimonies," unedited, though not necessarily unpolished, testimonies created at a time when illness experience was not yet considered a matter of public interest.

An interesting question is whether it is possible to apply the theoretical framework of pathography to these pre-pathographical testimonies. Do they share the same characteristics? Do they orbit around the same major themes? Are they addressing the same problems as the full-length pathographies later would? To confront these questions, I present an analysis of the fragmentary illness narrative of the Swedish poet and painter Harriet Löwenhjelm. Three features characterizing pathography will be referred to, as identified by Anne Hunsaker-Hawkins in *Reconstructing Illness: Studies in Pathography* (1999): *alienation, restitution,* and *cultural themes.*

Alienation

According to Hunsaker-Hawkins, a pathography "restores the person ignored or cancelled out in the medical enterprise and it places that person at the very center."[21] Writing about illness often seems to be a response to a sense of alienation vis-à-vis the medical establishment, the rest of society, and, perhaps not least, the disease itself. Hunsaker-Hawkins describes pathography as a "counterpart"[22] to the medical chart that allows the patient to freely and fully express his or her perception of the events taking place. In that sense, a pathography is often triggered by alienation, and a sense of alienation seems to be a recurring theme in pathography.

Restitution

Second, according to Hunsaker-Hawkins, "The common denominator of all pathographies . . . is that the act of writing in some way seems to facilitate recovery: the healing of the whole person."[23] Through the writing process, the patient restores a sense of logic and meaning to the chaotic experience of illness and suffering. Several other scholars (e.g., Arthur Frank and Jeffrey Aronson) have similarly highlighted this restorative capacity of illness narratives, in which the act of formulation provides the afflicted individual with a sense of coherence.[24]

Cultural Themes

Third, Hunsaker-Hawkins states, "These very personal accounts of illness, though highly individualized, tend to be confined to certain repeated themes of an archetypal, mythic nature."[25] A number of different themes thus recur in most pathographies. Often, these metanarratives represent different ways of incorporating the illness into a familiar narrative setting by using metaphors or archetypes rooted in a common cultural heritage. Three of the most common themes noted by Hunsaker-Hawkins are attempts to understand the process of illness and recovery as either *a journey, a battle,* or *an aspiration toward rebirth.* Keeping these three characteristics of pathography in mind, we now turn to the illness narrative of Harriet Löwenhjelm.

Harriet Löwenhjelm: Biographical Background

Harriet Löwenhjelm was born on February 18, 1887, on the outskirts of Helsingborg, in southern Sweden. At the age of six, she moved north with her parents, her sister, and her three brothers to Örebro; they later moved to Stockholm, where the family settled in 1896. As a member of the Swedish aristocracy, Harriet Löwenhjelm was born into a world of strong norms and social duties. But within the sphere of the privileged upper class, there was also a certain freedom to shape one's own destiny. For Harriet, her destiny and desire were unmistakable: she wanted to become an artist.[26]

Beginning in childhood, Harriet Löwenhjelm devoted herself to poetry and painting. As a teenager, she invented a fairy-tale land named Klondike populated by some one hundred different characters, each ingeniously described in Löwenhjelm's poems and fictive newspaper articles.[27] After finishing school, Löwenhjelm took private lessons in painting until October 1908, when she enrolled in the Academy of Arts in Stockholm.[28] Her years as an art student, however, proved more difficult than she had imagined. Löwenhjelm had problems conforming to the school's disciplinary code, she constantly doubted her talent, and her painting and sculpture received only modest recognition from her teachers. Overall, she seems to have felt more discouraged than inspired by the Academy of Arts, and, in 1911, she decided to leave the school. Afterward, she engaged more actively in writing poetry instead and compiled her first collection of poems, which was rejected by the publishing house Norstedts in November 1913.[29] That same month, owing to her persistent fever and steady weight loss, Harriet's brother, Carl Löwenhjelm—a sanatorium physician at Löt's sanatorium, west of Stockholm—performed a medical examination on his sister, ultimately confirming active tuberculosis.[30]

The Illness Narrative of Harriet Löwenhjelm

From the moment Harriet Löwenhjelm entered the sanatorium world at the age of twenty-seven, until her death in 1918, she resided more or less continuously at various sanatoriums in Scandinavia: Vejlefjord in Denmark, Romanäs in Sweden, and Mesnalien, on the outskirts of Lillehammer, Norway. During these four years, she wrote numerous poems and diary entries and an endless number of letters to friends and family.[31] When reading them cohesively, her writings provide detailed accounts reflecting her changing states of physical, as well as spiritual, health.

Harriet Löwenhjelm's illness narrative actually began six months before she was diagnosed with active tuberculosis, with an x-ray performed on April 12, 1913, after a period of persistent coughing. A week later, in a letter to her cousin Marianne Mörner, Löwenhjelm wrote, "I was x-rayed on three different plates, and tubercles were found slumbering like fossils in my lungs, mostly in the right apex."[32] Exactly one year later, she was sent to the Vejlefjord sanatorium in Denmark. Surprisingly, her first reaction to her tuberculosis diagnosis was mostly enthusiasm. Löwenhjelm's diary entries refer to the illness as a "decent occupation" liberating her from the inactivity of daily life as an unsuccessful upper-class art student in Stockholm.[33] In Denmark, furthermore, Löwenhjelm found herself far from home for the first time, with no friends or family members watching over her. Excited by this newfound independence, she embarked on various escapades with her fellow patients: snake hunting, swimming, smoking, and singing. On a more-or-less daily basis, it seems, Löwenhjelm broke most of the strict regulations at the sanatorium. Rather soon, however, the monotony of the institutional routines began to enervate her. After one month, in May 1914, a slowly increasing sense of alienation clearly takes shape in Löwenhjelm's writing about her illness experience. In a letter from Vejlefjord to her friend Elsa Björkman, she writes, "I have found that in order to feel normal at a sanatorium you need to have at least 98 fellow patients under the same curse."[34]

And that sense of alienation it seems, related not only to the sanatorium but rather to a feeling of mismatch between body and mind, an incongruity between the tuberculosis diagnosis, delivered by the doctors, and her own internal sensation of physical health. In another letter to Elsa Björkman, this one penned in August 1914, Löwenhjelm wrote, "Staying at a sanatorium is boring. . . . At the moment I feel alone. It is a devilish disease this consumption. . . . I have never considered myself anything other than a healthy and fully capable human being."[35]

At the outbreak of World War I, Löwenhjelm left Denmark and returned to Sweden. After a short stay in Malmö, she continued northward, and on August 14, 1914, she entered the Romanäs sanatorium in southern Sweden. At Romanäs, her defiance of the strict regulations continued. She was described by her fellow patients as an enfant terrible,[36] and in his memoirs, Alfred von Rosen, who began his tenure as a physician at Romanäs in 1917, noted that as a patient Harriet Löwenhjelm was "difficult to manage and more than a little bit spoiled, and had been so during her entire illness period. Her artistic nature, her integrity, her demand and longing for independence violated the restraint of freedom so imperative at the sanatorium."[37] When comparing the diary notes from Vejlefjord and Romanäs, it seems as if with time Harriet Löwenhjelm's restlessness steadily intensified. During her first years accepting the medicalization and institutionalization of the sanatorium proved difficult for her impatient personality.

An interesting observation is the extent to which World War I influenced Löwenhjelm's mental state. Even though she was not personally affected by the war, it was being waged during her entire sanatorium stay. Perhaps this discrepancy between the tranquility and peacefulness at the sanatorium and the brutal reports from the front intensified her impression of living in the shadow of death. Repeatedly, Löwenhjelm refers in her writing to newspaper articles about the ongoing battles, and, as she became sicker, she even incorporated the terminology of the battlefield into her testimonies on her own situation. She wrote the following, for example, in a Christmas letter to her friend Hedda Björkman, in 1916, after spending several weeks in bed for repeated pulmonary hemorrhages: "I myself am also stuck in a war trench, fighting back the latest assault."[38] And in 1918, at the end of her life, Löwenhjelm again referred to ongoing battles in a note to Elsa Björkman: "I could always turn to God, but he seems so fully occupied with the European continent these days."[39]

In May 1915, Harriet Löwenhjelm was expelled from Romanäs because she had flouted the strict sanatorium routines. For a while she underwent outpatient treatment with tuberculin injections, but when she started losing weight in early 1916, she was transferred to the Mesnalien sanatorium in Norway. This is where she first recognized that something was wrong with her voice. Initially, it became hoarse and croaky, and then slowly she began experiencing pain in her throat. In a June 1916 letter to Elsa Björkman, she wrote, "I've been hoarse for one month, and it is not getting better. Do you think I will get tubercles in my throat?"[40] Later, it turned out that this was exactly what had occurred. Staying at the Mesnalien sanatorium did not improve her health particularly, and in September 1916 Löwenhjelm was allowed to return to Sweden. There, she became a permanent resident once more of Romanäs sanatorium, where she lived for the remaining two years of her life.

Harriet Löwenhjelm was now twenty-nine years old, and, even though she was physically marked by disease, her final two years constituted one of the most creative periods of her life. A number of her most beloved poems and paintings were written during 1916–18. The poetry from these years is to some extent despairing but is also characterized by joy, hopefulness, and rebirth. Consider, for example, the following short poem, written in the spring of 1917: "Look how spring has come out yonder. / Snow has melted, gone the strife. / Yet again we muse and ponder on the miracles of life."[41]

During the autumn of 1916, Harriet Löwenhjelm suffered from repeated pulmonary hemorrhages. Hoarse and feverish, she stayed in bed, and for the first time she began to express a growing sense of stigmatization due to her tuberculosis. In a letter to Elsa Björkman, she commented, "Only tell those I am fond of that I am poorly. . . . Being ill feels like a criminal act, like something to be ashamed of."[42] Even though death, day by day, was becoming the most likely outcome, Löwenhjelm still made an effort to remain positive. In a letter to her cousin, Marianne Mörner, she wrote, "I have lost count of how many friends I offered to let hold my hand while I'm dying. I guess they will have to encircle me holding one finger each."[43] And a letter from September 1917 describes the change in her voice due to the illness' spread with the same flash of humor: "My voice sounds just like Monte Cristo's after spending fourteen years in prison. I sometimes whisper and sometimes roar."[44]

Despite this humor, Löwenhjelm's attitude toward the world had changed. Her curiosity had faded; she no longer felt as if her true place was outside the sanatorium. In another letter from this period, she wrote, "I feel left out—or rather, left in. Landscapes used to be for walking; now they are merely for watching. The sense of belonging has disappeared."[45] Harriet Löwenhjelm's previous feelings of alienation from the sanatorium had now developed into feelings of alienation from everything *but* the sanatorium—alienation from life itself, as well as from her own physical body. In a spring 1917 letter to her mother, Margaret Löwenhjelm, she touched upon this dualism as she commented on her heightened artistic productivity: "I guess it means that I am getting better. At least my mind—as for my lungs, I do not know."[46]

In addition to the standardized sanatorium regimen of good food, fresh air, rest, and exercise, Harriet Löwenhjelm also underwent two surgical procedures. In January 1917, an unsuccessful treatment for a pneumothorax was attempted, and one year later a palliative operation was performed on her throat. By that time, her tuberculosis was medically out of control, and, in the last six months of her life, Löwenhjelm spent most of her time in bed.[47] In a diary entry on January 15, 1918, she laconically noted, "The temperature is rising outside, just as my own is rising inside."[48]

Later that spring of 1918 she rapidly lost weight, while the pains in her throat intensified. Still, she did her best to remain positive. In a letter to Honorine Hermelin dated April 25, 1918, she wrote, "You see, Honorine, I do not seem to be able to eat, and the fever has started all over again, so I might not be able to stay alive so much longer. . . . If I wasn't so agonized by my throat, life would be rather pleasant."[49]

One month later, on May 24, 1918, Harriet Löwenhjelm passed away at Romanäs sanatorium. She died aged thirty-one, after four years of more or less permanent residency at various sanatoriums throughout Scandinavia. She died an unknown, aspiring artist, leaving behind a failed career as an art student in Stockholm. And she died after handing over four volumes of unpublished poems to her good friend, Elsa Björkman, who had arrived by train a few days before Löwenhjelm's death. In the years to come, Elsa Björkman would play the same role for Harriet Löwenhjelm that Max Brod did later for Franz Kafka—editing and publishing her literary testimony, paving the way for Löwenhjelm's posthumous breakthrough in 1927.

Harriet Löwenhjelm's Illness Narrative in a Broadened Perspective

In this chapter a narrative stance on medical history has been taken in an attempt to trace the roots of the pathographical genre. Even though Harriet Löwenhjelm never wrote a pathography as such, the letters, poems, and diary notes she composed provide valuable insight into her years as a tuberculosis patient. Furthermore, it seems as if her fragmentary testimony includes many of the attributes (such as they have been described by Hunsaker-Hawkins) that would reach maturity in the pathographical genre emerging a few decades after Löwenhjelm's death. In her illness narrative, Löwenhjelm not only expresses explicit feelings of alienation, both from the sanatorium and, later, from life itself. She also uses at least two of the cultural patterns or archetypes, highlighted in Hunsaker-Hawkins's categorization of pathography: the battle and the sense of rebirth. It might be argued that feelings of alienation and metaphorical analogies have always characterized the way people relate to losing their good health. Still, I believe that this way of thinking has changed over time, becoming more distinct when illness narratives started to appear on the book market in the 1920s and 1930s. And some elements of that change had probably started earlier still. In the sanatoriums, the institutional melting pots for the first pathographies, patients such as Harriet Löwenhjelm contributed to making these formulas explicit, in a way that the narratives of illness experience could later take a more uniform and public shape. Less evident is whether Löwenhjelm's writing on her illness helped her to restore a sense of coherence. In her poems, letters, and diary notes, she never explicitly refers to her writing as filling the purpose of organizing thoughts and emotions on her illness. While some of the poems written during her time at the sanatorium clearly process and verbalize her ongoing thoughts on death and her hope for recovery, other poems are entirely detached from her illness. Rather than starting to write as a response to her illness, which often seems to be the case for writers of pathographies, Löwenhjelm had written ever since childhood. In that sense writing was a natural activity for her, and rather than writing in an attempt to restore a sense of logic and meaning to her illness in particular, the act of formulation had probably always provided her with a sense of coherence of the world at large.

This chapter has primarily focused on Harriet Löwenhjelm and the emergence of the pathographical genre. Analyzing accounts of sanatorium patients from the first half of the twentieth century is, however, equally interesting from a "circulation of knowledge" perspective. To a greater extent than most other patients of the early twentieth century, individuals diagnosed with tuberculosis traveled across national borders. Scandinavian patients such as Harriet Löwenhjelm, Edith Södergran, and Knut Hamsun traveled readily, between institutions in Norway, Denmark, and Sweden, but also farther afield. When choosing a suitable sanatorium, the similarities between the Nordic languages, as well as the widespread knowledge of German, made most parts of the Baltic Sea region accessible to patients from Scandinavia. Many of the most attractive sanatoriums were in fact meeting points for well-to-do people from the entire European continent. In these institutions, thoughts, and attitudes regarding all aspects of life—not least their experiences of illness—were exchanged, intermingled, shaped, and reshaped, before being transported back home or on to the next sanatorium. Similarly, doctors of different sanatoriums exchanged ideas and opinions with each other through visits and through the growing number of scientific journals appearing by this time. As a result, the regulations and routines at the sanatoriums of the early twentieth century were internationally rather uniform, even though national differences occurred. Probably as a result of this, despite writing from sanatoriums in three different countries, Löwenhjelm's illness narrative remains relatively intact. It is as if the cultural differences between Denmark, Norway, and Sweden were of minor importance for Löwenhjelm. What mattered was the symptoms she developed as the disease progressed, making national borders subordinate to the illness itself in the experiences described by Harriet Löwenhjelm.

The nomadic roaming of tuberculosis patients was, of course, in some sense a consequence of an ineffective medical establishment in which, as Flurin Condrau notes, treatment at sanatoriums predominantly "continued to rely on the self-healing proficiencies of the patients."[50] But the extensive travel of sanatorium patients was probably also driven by the scientific developments that began in the 1880s. Pulmonary surgery, tuberculin treatment, x-rays, and other technological advances fueled rumors of cures and instilled hope for a more effective treatment at the next sanatorium. When their health failed to improve, patients moved on. Furthermore, the sanatorium environment—or tuberculosis itself—seems to have triggered a restlessness among patients. Perhaps to feel less trapped, or to regain a sense of control, patients resorted to traveling as a "safety valve" in a dangerous and frustrating situation. Prior to her move from Romanäs to Mesnalien in 1916, Harriet Löwenhjelm noted in a letter that "changing location seems to be the only thing promoting my health."[51]

***

Among Harriet Löwenhjelm's diary entries is a sketch that depicts a man stretching for the moon from the top of a ladder. As an image symbolizing a person with high aspirations and a dreamlike imagination, the sketch is a suitable illustration of Löwenhjelm's own personality. In the spring of 1918, in room 14 at Romanäs sanatorium, suffering from an aching throat, a rising temperature, and steady weight loss, Harriet Löwenhjelm wrote one of her most beloved poems. It comprises a few sentences on her upcoming death, translated here into English by Anne-Charlotte Harvey:

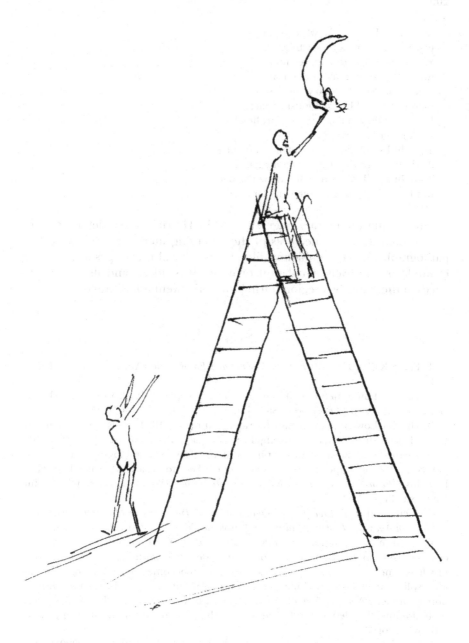

Figure 8.2. Sketch made by Harriet Löwenhjelm in her diary on May 23, 1911. Courtesy of the National Library of Sweden in Stockholm.

Take me. Hold me. Slowly caressing,
gently enfold me a little while.
Weep a tear for facts depressing,
watch me asleep and tender a smile.
O, do not leave, you do want to stay,
O, stay here till I myself must depart.
Lay your beloved hand on my forehead—
yet for a little while not apart.
Tonight I shall die. There flickers a flame.
A friend by my side is holding my hand.
Tonight I shall die. But who knows the name
of where I am going—unto what land?[52]

When reading the literary fragments left by Harriet Löwenhjelm, not only is it possible to trace the roots of the emerging literary genre now called pathography, but Löwenhjelm's illness narrative also emerges as a moving example of the lively circulation of individuals, ideas, and illness experiences in the Baltic Sea region during the early twentieth century.

Notes

1. Franz Kafka, *Letters to Friends, Family, and Editors* (New York: Schocken, 1977), 373.

2. Harriet Löwenhjelm to Marianne Mörner, April 29, 1914, in Elsa Björkman-Goldschmidt, *Harriet Löwenhjelm* (Stockholm: Pan/Norstedts, 1967), 181.

3. Harriet Löwenhjelm to Elsa Björkman, June 16, 1914, trans. Anne-Charlotte Hanes Harvey, http://harrietlowenhjelm.se/engelska.html, accessed June 18, 2018.

4. In this chapter, a "pathography" is defined as an autobiography or biography centering on a specific illness experience. See, for example, Anne Hunsaker-Hawkins, *Reconstructing Illness: Studies in Pathography* (West Lafayette, IN: Purdue University Press, 1999), 11.

5. Sheila Rothman, *Living in the Shadow of Death: Tuberculosis and the Social Experience of Illness in American History* (Baltimore: Johns Hopkins University Press, 1995).

6. It is interesting to note that Franz Kafka and Harriet Löwenhjelm shared many characteristics in addition to their premature deaths from tuberculosis. Both were privileged members of society with a strong urge to become artists. Each had a somewhat split personality in which a quirky sense of humor coexisted with a predisposition to anxiety. And neither of them achieved any major artistic breakthrough in their lifetimes but left behind manuscripts that would posthumously bring them artistic immortality.

7. Jeffrey Aronson, "Autopathography: The Patient's Tale," *BMJ* 321 (2000): 1599.

8. Hunsaker-Hawkins, *Reconstructing Illness*, 13.

9. Aronson, "Autopathography."

10. Katarina Bernhardsson, *Litterära besvär: Skildringar av sjukdom I samtida svensk prosa* (Lund: Ellerströms, 2010).

11. Rolf Ahlzén, *Why Should Physicians Read? Understanding Clinical Judgment and Its Relation to Literary Experience* (Karlstad: Universitetstryckeriet, 2010).

12. Hunsaker-Hawkins, *Reconstructing Illness*, 3.

13. Karl Häggblom and Per-Olof Mattson, "Patografin—den sjukes egen journal," *Läkartidningen* 104, no. 47 (2007): 3548–51. Similarly, the emergence of the highly stigmatized illness AIDS in the 1980s corresponded with a rapid increase in the number of published pathographies on this disease. See Anne Whitehead, "The Medical Humanities: A Literary Perspective," in *Medicine, Health, and the Arts: Approaches to the Medical Humanities*, ed. Victoria Bates et al. (New York: Routledge, 2014), 107–27.

14. Anne Hunsaker-Hawkins, "Pathography: Patient Narratives of Illness," *Western Journal of Medicine* 171, no. 2 (1999): 128.

15. Sheila Rothman, *Living in the Shadow of Death: Tuberculosis and the Social Experience of Illness in American History* (Baltimore: Johns Hopkins University Press, 1995), 198.

16. Hunsaker-Hawkins, *Reconstructing Illness*, 11.

17. Linda Bryder, Flurin Condrau, and Michael Worboys, "Tuberculosis and Its Histories: Then and Now," in *Tuberculosis Then and Now: Perspectives on the History of an Infectious Disease*, ed. Flurin Condrau and Michael Worboys (Quebec: McGill-Queen's University Press, 2010), 3–23.

18. Nicholas Jewson, "The Disappearance of the Sick-Man from Medical Cosmology, 1770–1870," *Sociology* 10 (1976): 225–44.

19. Mike Bury, "Illness Narratives: Fact or Fiction?," *Sociology of Health and Illness* 23, no. 3 (2001): 266.

20. Tim Boon, "Lay Disease Narratives, Tuberculosis, and Health Education Films," in *Tuberculosis Then and Now: Perspectives on the History of an Infectious Disease*, ed. Flurin Condrau and Michael Worboys (Quebec: McGill-Queen's University Press, 2010), 24–48, esp. 32.

21. Hunsaker-Hawkins, *Reconstructing Illness*, 12.

22. Ibid., 12.

23. Hunsaker-Hawkins, "Pathography," 129.

24. See, for example, Aronson, "Autopathography"; Arthur Frank, *The Wounded Storyteller* (Chicago: University of Chicago Press, 1995).

25. Hunsaker-Hawkins, *Reconstructing Illness*, 27.

26. Boel Hackman, *Att skjuta en dront: Harriet Löwenhjelm—dikt, bild, konstnärskap* (Stockholm: Albert Bonniers förlag, 2011), 37–46.

27. Ibid., 24.

28. Björkman-Goldschmidt, *Harriet Löwenhjelm*, 129.

29. Hackman, *Att skjuta en dront*, 163.

30. Ibid., 263.

31. Most of Löwenhjelm's preserved letters were addressed to her cousin, Marianne Mörner, her classmate, Honorine Hermelin, or her friend and posthumous editor, Elsa Björkman-Goldschmidt. Most of her diaries, and part of her correspondence to friends and family, are today kept at the National Library of Sweden (Kungliga Biblioteket) in Stockholm.

32. Björkman-Goldschmidt, *Harriet Löwenhjelm*, 166. Unless otherwise stated, all quotes by Harriet Löwenhjelm have been translated into English by Jonatan Wistrand.

33. Ibid., 169.

34. Ibid., 181.

35. Harriet Löwenhjelm, *Brev och dikter* (Stockholm: Norstedt & söners förlag, 1952), 160.

36. Hackman, *Att skjuta en dront*, 220.

37. Alfred von Rosen, *Människan, livet och döden: Utblickar och minnesbilder* (Uppsala: J. A. Lindblads förlag, 1954), 134. Quote translated into English by Jonatan Wistrand.

38. Harriet Löwenhjelm to Hedda Björkman, December 22, 1916, National Library of Sweden.

39. Björkman-Goldschmidt, *Harriet Löwenhjelm*, 218.

40. Löwenhjelm, *Brev och dikter*, 168.

41. Harriet Löwenhjelm, *Selected Poems*, trans. Mike McArthur (Wintringham: Oak Tree Press, 2007), 73.

42. Björkman-Goldschmidt, *Harriet Löwenhjelm*, 207.

43. Ibid., 186.

44. Hackman, *Att skjuta en dront*, 236.

45. Ibid., 232.

46. Björkman-Goldschmidt, *Harriet Löwenhjelm*, 210.

47. Von Rosen, *Människan, livet och döden*, 134.

48. Harriet Löwenhjelm, diary note, January 15, 1918, National Library of Sweden.

49. Björkman-Goldschmidt, *Harriet Löwenhjelm*, 226.

50. Flurin Condrau, "Beyond the Total Institution: Towards a Reinterpretation of the Tuberculosis Sanatorium," in *Tuberculosis Then and Now: Perspectives on the History of an Infectious Disease*, ed. Flurin Condrau and Michael Worboys (Quebec: McGill-Queen's University Press, 2010), 72–99, esp. 77.

51. Björkman-Goldschmidt, *Harriet Löwenhjelm*, 202. Similarly, after a few weeks in Graal-Müritz by the Baltic Sea, in August 1923, Franz Kafka wrote in a letter to his friend Tile Rössler, "I don't like it here as well as I did [at] first. . . . Perhaps I'm not allowed to remain too long in one place; there are people who can acquire a sense of home only when they are travelling." Franz Kafka, *Letters to Friends, Family, and Editors*, 375.

52. "Harriet Löwenhjelm: Swedish Poet and Artist," trans. Anne-Charlotte Hanes Harvey, http://harrietlowenhjelm.se/engelska.html, accessed June 18, 2018.

Chapter Nine

Biobanking at the Baltic Sea

An Analysis of the Swedish, Estonian, and German Approaches

KATHARINA BEIER

While the Baltic is ascribed a high potential for regional integration in Europe, in this chapter I look at a particular field of cooperation, biobank research. Given that recent discussions about the Baltic area "are no longer emphasizing unifying structures but are seeking for combining elements like the sea itself or the dynamics that create a zone,"[1] the practice of biobanking appears as a particularly interesting study subject to circumstantiate the notion of the Baltic as a vital contact zone.

What Is Biobanking?

Collections of human bodily materials have been kept in medicine for centuries. The crucial point about *modern* biobanking is thus not the mere storage of human body substances (e.g., tissue, blood, and DNA) but its large-scale collection together with a systematic and often ongoing linkage to donors' health records and lifestyle data. In addition, the advance of data information technologies involves the constant refinement of analytical tools. This allows for, in principal, an indefinite amount of information that can be consulted to answer newly emerging research questions. Besides clinical biobanks, which are mainly used for diagnostic purposes, there is an increasing number of population-based biobank projects world-wide.[2] As a research infrastructure, the latter provide a powerful resource to understand the causes of widespread diseases, unlock interactions between genetic and environmental factors, and detect candidate genes for certain diseases. In the long run, biobank-based research may thus generate pivotal knowledge for the invention of new therapies and prevention measures in health care. Moreover, biobanking plays an increasing role in the detection of biomarkers and the development of personalized medicine.[3]

Whether biobanks can deliver on these expectations, however, depends on the availability of large volumes of well-characterized specimens and data, the possibility of constant information updates through recontact of sample donors, cross-border exchange of samples and data, and the consolidation of biobanks. These requirements, however, also raise a range of ethical and legal questions at international level.[4] For example, modern biobanking has a prospective character, that is, it is directed at future research whose aims and scope cannot be foreseen at the time of sample taking. Obtaining the research participants' informed consent (IC), as it is the default in traditional human subject research, thus faces several limits in the context of biobanking. Consequently, alternative approaches have been suggested, for example, broad consent,[5] authorization,[6] or dynamic consent.[7] Another challenge results from rapidly developing information technologies. With the possibilities of linking biobank data with other databases and registries and sharing them with researchers in countries where potentially lower data-protection requirements apply, new threats to people's privacy emerge. Moreover, biobank research also raises questions with regard to participants' rights and entitlements. Given that biobanks are also subject to commercial interests, questions of ownership and donor involvement are increasingly discussed.[8] In addition, although biobanks, by nature, are a collective resource, it cannot be ignored that individually relevant health information (incidental findings) accrue. As this implies a merger of biobank research with health care, there are not only discussions about when the disclosure of information to donors would be morally required but also about the mode of resulting communication.[9] Not least, the need for biobank interoperability raises questions of biobank governance[10] and the harmonization of ethical and legal frameworks.[11]

The most important document for the regulation of research with human tissues at European level is the Council of Europe's *Recommendation 2016(6) on Research on Biological Materials of Human Origin*, which recently succeeded the *Recommendation 2006(4)*. However, the recommendation does not abolish regulatory heterogeneity, as it provides only for basic rules that leave considerable leeway for their transposition into national law by the member states. Despite this fact, there is some convergence among certain countries' approaches to human tissue and biobank research due to shared research traditions.[12] The countries in the Baltic Sea area have a long tradition in epidemiological research and are also on the cutting edge of setting up new population-based biobanks. Thus, the Baltic Sea region is an important contact zone for biobanking that builds bridges across the Baltic but also has a power of attraction beyond this region. This argument will be fleshed out by an exemplary analysis of Sweden's, Estonia's, and Germany's approaches to research biobanking and recent developments in this field. Sweden and Estonia are interesting insofar as population-based biobanks became an issue at the shift of the century, and regulatory efforts have been taken at a rather early stage. Moreover, though for different reasons, all three countries' biobank activities became subject to international debates. In what follows, I not only describe the three countries' approaches to biobanking but also analyze their commonalities as well as differences and provide some explanation for this.

There are also limitations to this analysis. First, biobanking is a global practice that is not unique to the Baltic Sea area. However, the northern countries' remote location renders them highly attractive for population-based research. In fact, there is strong awareness for the region's considerable potential in biobanking and a felt responsibility for pushing it further. While this is an attitude that is particularly present in the Nordic states of Denmark, Finland, Iceland, Norway, and Sweden,[13] cooperation in life sciences includes a broader range of Baltic Sea countries. The ScanBalt BioRegion, for example, is a network for cooperation in science and economy that connects eleven countries and regions in the Baltic Sea area. Second, I do not argue for clearly distinguishable lines of interaction between the biobanking discourses of Sweden, Estonia, and Germany. To make such a strong claim one would need to dig much deeper into the countries' public and expert discourses on biobanking. Therefore, the aim of this article is more modest. First, the focus on Sweden, Estonia, and Germany allows for an exemplary illustration of how the debate about certain issues in biobank research—for example, IC, privacy protection, and commercialization of human tissue research—unfolds at the turn of the twenty-first century. Second, the developments and debates in Sweden, Estonia, and Germany from a comparative perspective reveal common trends in biobanking but also highlight persisting differences due to diverging research traditions and specific path-dependencies in the regulation of research.

The Rise of Modern Biobanking and
the Role of Iceland's Health Sector Database

In 2009 the *New York Times* ranked biobanks as one of ten ideas changing the world.[14] At least for the Nordic countries, this news should not have come as a surprise. For example, Iceland, Sweden, Finland, Norway, and Denmark are on the cutting edge of the field of large-scale epidemiological research. Their competitive advantage rests on several pillars, for example, the existence of national health-care systems; the availability of comprehensive health registries, sometimes with obligatory participation; and the existence of a unique personal identification number for all citizens that allows for the matching of biobank information with entries in national registries on health, heredity, and sociodemographic factors, among others. Also, surveys indicate that Nordic people are mostly in favor of biobanks[15] and generally exhibit high levels of trust toward state and public authorities.[16]

While the collection of biomaterials for research has a long tradition, it is only at the turn of the twenty-first century that this practice becomes a matter of public concern. Inspired by the decoding of the human genome, the hope for innovation in health care became closely connected with prospects of economic profit. In this pioneer spirit, Iceland established a National Health Sector Database as the first country worldwide. To this end, the genetic data of almost all Icelanders is collected and linked with already existing health and genealogical data. In the eyes of the international research community, this turned Iceland into a gold mine. For making use of its unique national resource, the Icelandic parliament enacted a specific law in 1998. Under the terms of this law, the American enterprise deCODE was granted an exclusive license for the commercial use of the Icelanders' genetic information for twelve years, which was without precedence so far. While the project was greatly admired in the international research community, eventually it came under heavy criticism in Iceland, but also abroad. By referring to genetic information as a common good, critics argued that access to the Health Sector Database should not be restricted to just one company. Medical practitioners were hesitant to release medical information on the basis of the merely presumed consent of donors. By pointing to their duty of confidentiality, many hospitals and doctors declined to participate in a project that was also under attack for lacking data security measures.[17] However, this criticism was mainly coming from physicians and international scientists, while the lay public appeared extremely positive of the Health Sector Database, not least because of their trust in the country's regulatory systems. If they raised any concerns, they were about potential inequalities in the provision of health care rather than about privacy and confidentiality.[18]

However, in 2006 the Icelandic Supreme Court ruled that deCODE "could not create and mine a database of the entire country's medical records without getting consent from individuals."[19] As a consequence, the company resorted to building a research database that analyzes the DNA and clinical data of more than 120,000 Icelanders for selected single-nucleotide polymorphisms (SNPs). While deCODE succeeded in identifying specific genetic mutations that are associated with heart diseases, diabetes, and cancer and boasted of the "largest studies of whole-genome data ever published,"[20] it failed in the discovery of drugs and went bankrupt in 2009. In December 2012, the US biotechnology enterprise Amgen took over deCODE's drug discovery assets for $415 million. A more recent debate about deCODE came up in 2013. Given that whole genome sequencing is very costly, deCODE wanted to extend the data available so far from about 2,500 individuals to a larger population by using a so-called imputation approach. This means that when a variant of interest is found in the whole genome data, "the company can use the more limited SNP data that it has on thousands of volunteers to impute, or infer, with 99% accuracy whether these individuals also carry this mutation."[21] By combining the identified and estimated data with Iceland's genealogical database, it will also be possible to draw conclusions on the genotypes of family members of the SNP-chipped participants even posthumously. However, the Data Protection Authority blocked this initiative and required that deCODE first obtain the IC of the individuals concerned.[22] As the translation of genetic knowledge into clinical application turned out to be more difficult than expected, deCODE's focus is currently mainly on basic research.

At the beginning of the twenty-first century, the Icelandic venture clearly functioned as a trigger for international discussions on biobanking and staked out the "normative terrain" for future biobanking projects.[23] In several Baltic Sea countries, the establishment of population-based biobanks closely followed the Icelandic initiative, and the latter became a point of reference, mainly to distance one's own biobanking project from.

Sweden

Sweden provides a blueprint for a whole range of ethical and legal challenges in biobanking that came into focus at the beginning of the twenty-first century. Routine sample collection has been done in Swedish health care from the 1940s onward,[24] leading to huge amounts of samples stored in pathology labs and clinical care settings. According to conservative estimates, the countries' biobanks comprise about sixty million samples,[25] which comes up to seven samples per citizen.[26] Of the nearly six hundred registered biobanks in Sweden, the vast majority are used for medical purposes. In contrast to Iceland, where deCODE aimed at building a population-based biobank from scratch, Sweden has several large-scale biobanks already in place, for example the Umea Medical Biobank, the Malmö Preventive Project, and the newborn screening registry (PKU) that comprises about 2.7 million samples.

Public debates about biobanks were sparked for the first time in 1999 by a series of newspaper articles in *Aftonbladet*, a Swedish tabloid.[27] The two journalists, who were granted the Swedish Grand Journalism Award for their exposé, evoked the picture of huge sample collections secretly stored at the cellars of pathology labs and hospitals. Visibly inspired by the Icelandic case and ongoing commercial initiatives in Sweden,[28] the articles pointed to misuse and commercialization of samples and data and stressed the need for legal clarification.

As a result of these media-triggered debates, Sweden was among the first countries worldwide that released ethical guidelines on using biobanks for research[29] followed by a discrete biobank law (Biobanks in Medical Care Act) in 2002.[30] While samples obtained in the context of medical diagnostics were formerly used without patients' IC, the new law sets out IC as the default. Moreover, IC is required anew when samples will be used for another research project. By this Sweden established one of the strictest consent rules within Europe[31] or even the world.[32] For this reason, the law was criticized for hampering research by impeding the use and sharing of samples and data and imposing additional bureaucratic burden on healthcare providers, given that IC is also required for diagnostic and therapeutic purposes.[33]

Moreover, given the documented willingness of Swedish people to contribute research,[34] the law was criticized for undermining "the solidarity informing the willingness to donate"[35] and ignoring the autonomous rights of donors.[36] Requiring individual IC for every single use of samples was seen to fall short of the traditional close relationship between individuals as research subjects and their role as consumers of publicly financed health care to which they contribute in return.[37] According to anthropologist Klaus Hoeyer, "The encounters in the clinic provide a forum for expressing values central to the Folkhemmet and dominant in the social movements that brought the welfare state into existence (e.g. trust in scientific progress, solidarity, a special state-citizen relationship)."[38] However, the alliance between public health care and medical research in the Swedish welfare state is challenged not only by new legal requirements but also by the privatization and commercialization of research. According to Hoeyer, this creates a certain paradox: given that "Swedish donors hold many reservations toward commercial actors in the research infrastructure, it is ironic how policy changes during the past decade have facilitated a commercialization of the research infrastructure concomitantly with the increased emphasis on informed consent as a means for ensuring the right to self-determination."[39]

Commercialization in fact became an issue with regard to the Medical Biobank in Umea, though not from donors' but from researchers' side. The biobank contains blood samples of 60 percent of the geographically isolated population of Västerbotten county, which makes it highly attractive for epidemiological research. Conscious that academia alone cannot make effective use of biobanks, UmanGenomics was founded in 1999 as an independent clinical genomic company by Umea University and the County of Västerbotten. UmanGenomics received exclusive rights to sell genetic information derived from blood samples that are stored in the Medical Biobank to pharmaceutical companies. The foundation of a private gene-broking company raised high expectations internationally as well. In an effort to avoid popular outrage as in Iceland,[40] UmanGenomics developed an ethics policy by renaming the prior "donation act" as "informed consent."[41] The success of this strategy became most visible when *Nature* advertised the company's ethical approach as the "Swedish model."[42] Although there was nothing substantially new in its ethical framework, UmanGenomics was praised as forerunner of successful interaction between public biobanks and commercial actors.[43] In this regard, "ethics" was used as sales pitch, particularly for making the difference to Iceland clear from the outset.[44]

Irrespective of this optimistic (self-)presentation, UmanGenomics got into trouble.[45] Researchers at Umea University questioned the right of the company to make use of the blood samples that originally were collected for medical purposes but not research, let alone commercial ends. Moreover, it was argued that commercial users would need to submit the results of their analyses to the biobank. However, as private companies usually do not have an interest in sharing their results, at least not before patenting them, UmanGenomics did not succeed in attracting private investors.[46] As a consequence the company challenged the public-private partnership and required more exclusive rights for the samples' use. This, however, was not accepted by the county council. As a result of these struggles, UmanGenomics went bankrupt in 2006.[47] In 2007, the Umea Medical Biobank became reorganized and is based on public funding today.

Another issue that was prominently discussed in Sweden is the protection of biobank samples and data against access of third parties, for example, the state.[48] After the murder of Anna Lindh, the Swedish minister for foreign affairs, in 2003, the police opened the national newborn-screening biobank (PKU registry) to match the DNA of the suspect (which was collected at the crime scene) with the blood stored in the biobank. After this incident, which led to the apprehension of the murderer, almost 450 people requested the withdrawal of their samples.[49] This showed that trust in public authorities is not without limits in Sweden. In 2010, the Swedish government officially outlawed the forensic use of registries. Internationally, however, the case of Anna Lindh became exemplary for illustrating a new type of risk that sets biobank research apart from other human subject research.

The latest debate about biobanking was triggered by the LifeGene project, which aims at the collection of samples and health data from five hundred thousand Swedes between zero to forty-five years. Because the scope of research that the samples and data will be used for cannot be clearly defined at the time of enrollment, participants are asked for their broad consent.

However, in 2011 it became obvious that the setup of such large-scale biobanks fell into a legal limbo in Sweden. When the Ethical Review Board declared that it was not qualified to make any judgment because LifeGene would not be a specific research project but a research infrastructure, the Data Inspection Board concluded that there is no legal basis for the collection and processing of personal data. This made Swedish researchers once again worry about being faced with competitive disadvantages in medical research. The problem of LifeGene was finally solved by a new law that came into force by the end of 2013. The act addressing "health research on environmental and genetic causes of diseases" (SFS 2013:794)[50] allows Swedish universities to create research registries as long as data providers give their explicit consent.[51] This law is valid until the revision of the Biobanks in Medical Care Act comes into force.[52] Because of ongoing political debates,[53] the legal process is expected to last until the end of 2020.[54]

Estonia

Compared to Sweden and other Nordic countries, where biobank research is mainly driven by the goal of health improvement, the setup of the Estonian Genome Project followed a somewhat different narrative. From the beginning, the project received strong political and economic support. With its original aim to collect the genetic profiles and information on individual health status and lifestyle from 75 percent of the Estonian population, the database would be the world's largest. Given Estonia's varied history and its only recently regained independence from Russia, the establishment of a national database raised high expectations. Specifically, the Estonian Genome Project was hailed as the "Estonian Nokia" and a "bridge to Europe" that would bring Estonia back onto the world map[55] and provide the country with a unique advantage in the rapidly growing world of biotechnology. This was not a completely new vision for Estonia, as the country was already at the "forefront of molecular biology and genetics"[56] during Soviet times. Moreover, Estonia has traditionally close connections to Finland, whose success in biotechnology fueled Estonia's ambitions of taking on a similar role in the field of biobanking.

At the same time, the economic aspirations of the Estonian Genome Project were closely interwoven with promises to restructure the country's aging health-care system and to erase the traces of the former Soviet health-care system. For example, the Estonian Genome Project strengthened the newly introduced family doctor system[57] by entrusting it with the enrollment of participants. The modernization of health care was another reform goal that the Estonian Genome project supported. For example, an early version of the project's information brochure stressed its "unique potential to catapult Estonia's healthcare system into the forefront of personalized medicine."[58] As will be shown below, the realization of a genome-based and personalized medicine is currently at the center of research activities using the Estonian database.

Similar to Iceland, in Estonia the "introduction of the idea of a gene bank corresponds well with the dominating image of the country being or becoming an example case of a small, effective, knowledge-based economy."[59] The "nationalistic rhetoric" and the emphasis on "entrepreneurial dynamism"[60] are additional features that link the Estonian with the Icelandic Genome Project. This notwithstanding, the Estonian project was also eager to distinguish itself from the Icelandic Health Sector Database. Besides ethical reasons, this disassociation was also driven by the wish to stress the uniqueness of the Estonian biobank project. For example, while Iceland advertised the homogeneity of its population as an attractive feature for potential investors, Estonia stressed the heterogeneity of its people. Specifically, it was argued that the Estonian gene pool is more closely related to that of mainland Europe, and especially to that of the other Baltic countries, and would thus be particularly suitable for the transfer of results to other countries.[61]

Moreover, for avoiding critical debates about commercialization as they occurred in Iceland, the inventors of the Estonian biobank stressed its embedding into the national health-care system. For this reason, the Estonian Human Genes Research Act bans any cross-border transfer of samples and requires that all analyses must take place in Estonia, whereas data, services, and knowledge can be made available to collaborating partners abroad. In addition, donors are promised to receive individual feedback on their genetic data, which is without precedence so far. In contrast to the Swedish Life Gene Project and the Icelandic Health Sector Database, where participants benefit at a rather general level, the Estonian biobank's national framing builds on a direct personal benefit: the state asks donors for their health information and DNA, and, in return, donors will be allowed to access their genetic profiles. This provision distances the Estonian Genome Project noticeably from the medical traditions of the Soviet system in which the disclosure of medical information was not habitually practiced.[62] At the same time this approach remains sensitive to the legacy of the Soviet system. Given that abuses of medical power affected people's trust in the medical system, individual incentives for participation in the genome project may be more successful than appeals to the common good of a rather abstract collective whose contours became particularly doubtful with the collapse of the Eastern Bloc and its subsequent political changes.[63]

Another feature that distinguishes the Estonian Genome Project from Iceland's Health Sector Database is the requirement of the donor's informed (though open) consent. This is remarkable because the introduction of IC as a general rule is a more recent achievement in Estonia that can be seen as another sign of the country's emancipation from the former Soviet medical system. However, there may still be limits to voluntary participation, though for different reasons than in Iceland. For one thing, the relationship between patients and doctors in Estonia is—at least to some extent—still built on paternalism, which may impact the recruitment of donors by family doctors.[64] For another thing, doctors are paid between thirty-two and thirty-four euro per patient enrolled in the database. While this is meant to cover the costs incurred by filling in the questionnaires (taking between sixty to ninety minutes), the remuneration may also serve as a monetary incentive[65] given that the hourly wage of a general practitioner in Estonia was about two euro in 2001.[66] In this way, the reimbursement might also have helped to avoid the kind of resistance among practitioners that had occurred in Iceland.

Although public debates about the genome project hardly emerged in Estonia, it was not without challenges. For example, critics, mostly from the academic sector, complained about the lack of regulations on the communication of health-relevant findings to donors.[67] Moreover, because of regulatory focus on large-scale databases, small biobanks remain underregulated.[68] Also, it has been complained that "significant government funds would go into high-tech approaches with long term aims when Estonia needs to improve the basic standard of its all-public health care system."[69] In contrast to criticism from experts, the Estonian public—similar to the Icelandic one—appeared extremely optimistic about the population database's setup. In fact, more than 90 percent were convinced that it will improve medical care. In addition, the majority of Estonians perceived a link between the biobank's success and the country's economic development and international reputation.[70]

The Estonian Genome Project became internationally known for its legal framework. In 2001, scientists, doctors, and politicians established the Estonian Genome Project Foundation (EGPF) as a "quasi-autonomous non-governmental organization" that formally belongs to the state (i.e., the Ministry of Social Affairs).[71] This legal construction enabled the involvement of private funding while the state could remain the legal owner. To pave the way for the population biobank, the Estonian government adopted the Human Genes Research Act that went into force in 2001.[72] The law was perceived as a model regulation that could be used by other countries "intending to launch their own genome projects."[73]

Despite these legal provisions, however, the Estonian Genome Project also began to totter before it could fully start. From the very beginning and contrary to former agreements, public funding of the project remained mostly "symbolic" until 2007.[74] To overcome these problems, the EGPF founded a private company, EGeen Limited, in 2001 with a registered seat in Estonia to finance and also to commercialize the results of the database. EGeen

Limited, in turn, was founded by the private venture EGeen International Inc. from the United States.[75] Commercialization rights were granted to EGeen for twenty-five years. The company in return "was obliged to make the annual payment of about 300 thousand euros to the Foundation."[76] Additional payments became due depending on the company's financial success.[77] After these preliminary steps, the Estonian Genome Project started its pilot phase in 2002 and intensified its efforts for data collection in 2003.

However, at the end of 2003 disagreements between EGeen Ltd. and EGeen International arose. The latter became more interested in research on a few specific diseases in hope of achieving marketable results much sooner than by taking a broad approach to different diseases.[78] Given this clash between business and scientific values, which is also a conflict between short-term and long-term success,[79] the EGPF finally cancelled the contract with its main financier, EGeen Ltd. This, however, disrupted the funding of the Estonian Genome Project.[80] From 2004 until 2007 its future remained blurry. For the first time, a public debate about the project emerged. Given the pull-out of private venture capital, it was particularly contested whether the project should be bolstered by public money.[81]

Because of the project's prominent political status, however, the Estonian parliament finally decided on an amendment of the Human Genes Research Act in 2007 that guaranteed the continuation of the Genome Project as a structural unit of the University of Tartu with public funding. While the biobank originally aimed to collect samples and data of one million Estonians, the target was reduced to one hundred thousand samples by 2010. However, according to the project's website, the number is even smaller, with fifty-two thousand samples, representing 5 percent of the population. Though not the world's largest biobank, the Estonian database is at least the largest epidemiological cohort in the Baltic region today.[82]

Currently, research efforts have shifted from the recruitment of donors to the completion and in-depth analysis of related health data. In particular, genotyping of all fifty-two thousand participants of the Estonian database is foreseen. Moreover, implementation of the genetic data of the population biobank into medical practice is planned. [83] This is facilitated by the fact that the Estonian Human Genes Research Act allows for the linkage of the genetic database with the National Health Information System and other medical registries without recontacting participants.[84] In this way, continuously updated calculations of disease risks and potential drug responses can be performed.[85] These recent initiatives render Estonia a test case for the national implementation of personalized and genome-based medicine that is likely to impact other countries' approaches in this field.

The fate of the Estonian national biobank is instructive for two reasons. First, it exemplifies the need for stable funding. While venture capital financing is economically attractive, it implies restrictions for the scientific use of samples. In particular, researchers' interest in the sharing of samples and data is likely to contradict the interests of private investors. Or—as a German newspaper commented on the Estonian project, "Researchers' blessing is private stakeholders' curse."[86] Public ownership has thus been identified as an important determinant for the public's support of the Estonian database.[87] Consequently, as the case of Sweden also indicates, "there appears to be a clear tendency to bring genetic databases under the auspices of public universities and use direct public funding."[88]

Second, the Estonian Genome Project illustrates the limits of an approach that is mainly directed at commercial exploitation. Following Rainer Kattel and Margit Suurna, the Estonian biobank project "suffered from a misunderstanding about the nature of the undertaking: a project that was thought to have more or less immediate commercial success (i.e. innovative R&D results) turned out to be in fact a basic scientific venture with many open-ended questions."[89] Consequently, when the Estonian biobank was reorganized as a publicly owned institution, its focus shifted to international cooperation instead of building its own resources with mainly private funding. In this way, the Estonian Genome Project "was turned (back) into a basic scientific venture, where results will be available only in the long term."[90] Today, the Estonian biobank, among others, is part of the Public Population Project in Genomics alongside, for example, Sweden, Norway, Germany, and Canada. The aim of this project is to make the countries' national databases mutually accessible by harmonizing practical, ethical, and legal standards.

Germany

In Germany, there are many small-scale biobanks affiliated with hospitals and research institutions. Most of them are publicly financed and primarily used for research, also at an international scale.[91] In addition, some population-related projects exist, for example, in the PopGen project and the Study of Health in Pomerania in northern Germany, and the KORAgen database in southern Germany.[92] Surveys rank Germany among those countries where people are most reluctant to provide their tissue and data for research.[93] This attitude is also reflected in comments on other countries' biobanking projects, particularly Iceland's and Estonia's. For example, the Estonian Genome Project's commercial framing was viewed with suspicion in the German media. Newspaper headlines read, "About the Bad Luck of Being Born in Estonia,"[94] "The Sold Nation,"[95] and "A Symbol of the Genomic Age Is Tottering."[96] In contrast to Sweden, where media reports led to the enactment of the biobank law, and Estonia, where the national biobank project was solicited with national pride, biobanking received less public attention in Germany. However, at the expert level, researchers, ethicists, lawyers, and politicians have been involved in debates about the regulation of biobanking in Germany, too.

At least until 2012 Germany had no national biobank project in place whose scope was comparable to the Icelandic, Swedish, and Estonian databases. According to Ingrid Schneider, reasons for this can be found in both scientific conditions and historic experiences. Specifically, the availability of well-characterized data sets, which is regarded important by German researchers, can be limited in large-scale databases.[97] Researchers are also skeptical of the success of solo attempts in biobanking as in Iceland and Estonia.[98] Another challenge results from the fact that "biobanks symbolize repositories of the national population and its bio-social heritage." As Schneider explains, however, images of genetic homogeneity or representativeness are highly critical in Germany because they invoke "the historically tainted NS-ideology of a (unified) 'Volkskörper.'" In addition, the establishment of national genetic registries might spark new concerns about state surveillance and control.[99] According to Schneider, there is thus no trustworthy and innocuous metanarrative for the establishment of a *national* database in Germany. Given that any talk of national genes, resources, and data invokes rather problematic memories of the past, the focus on local biobank projects, which implies the depoliticization of biobank research, seems to be the most acceptable approach in Germany.[100] This is best illustrated by the PopGen biobank that was established in 2003 in the county of Schleswig-Holstein. The location for the biobank was chosen because the region's border with the Baltic Sea binds people closer to their local practitioners,[101] which resembles, at least to some extent, the favorable conditions in the Nordic countries. However, with its aim of providing evidence for the prevalence of certain diseases in the population,[102] PopGen clearly distinguishes itself from the more ambitious goals of the national databases in Iceland and Estonia.[103]

Although abusive or at least wrongful medical practices also occurred in Sweden and Estonia, these experiences seem to be less present in discussions about biobank research. In Sweden this might be explained by the long-standing tradition of national (health) registries, which is widely known and accepted. In Estonia, in the wake of profound political changes, the narrative of scientific and economic progress became particularly strong. In this way, the genome project became a means to emancipate the country from its communist past and was thus positively connoted from the outset.

The establishment of a National Cohort Study is the most recent development in Germany. While the aim of collecting medical, health, sociodemographic, and lifestyle data of two hundred thousand participants over about twenty-five years seems to speak against Schneider's thesis that there is no support for a national biobank in Germany, it is important to note, however, that the cohort study by design remains closely linked to local regions and study centers. This avoids the impression that a specific region or population is being singled out as a "national" resource.[104]

Debates about the ethical framing and legal regulation of biobanking were mainly sparked by the National Ethics Council in Germany. In 2004, it presented its first opinion as a result of several international expert consultations, which included the evaluation of other countries' biobanking activities. In its opinion, the council highlighted the Estonian biobank as example of the far-reaching consequences that the linkage of genetic and personal lifestyle data may have.[105] However, the council's recommendations showed less concerned with this type of large-scale research project but rather focused on the most pressing question in the German biobanking landscape, that is, the vast amount of minor sample collections scattered about hospitals and research facilities. The Ethics Council recommended that any future legislation should avoid unnecessary cumbersome regulations for their use.[106] Because of this, the council's opinion was internationally hailed as "an enlightened, pragmatic and practical" and, in ethical terms, a very "sensible" approach.[107] A commentary published in *Nature* even proclaimed that "practical wisdom has finally arrived in the world of 'ethical' biobanking."[108] Contrary to Sweden, for example, broad consent is regarded acceptable for research use of samples that have been lawfully obtained in the context of medical care and diagnostics (and also for samples that are directly obtained for research purposes). Moreover, the Ethics Council recommended a waiver of consent in the case of anonymized or coded samples, provided researchers have no access to the key for the donor's reidentification.[109] In addition, the council stressed that information about potential risks should be limited to those that are directly connected to the use of data and samples in biobank research. Consequently, researchers are not obliged to inform donors about potential misuse of their samples and data.[110] Contrary to all Nordic countries, there is no need for approval for setting up a biobank in Germany, as the collection and use of human biological samples is regarded as part of the normal routine in medical research. In contrast, for large-scale population-based biobanks a prior licensing has been suggested.[111]

In 2010, the German Ethics Council released another opinion on biobanks, which takes up new trends and challenges that result, for example, from increased networking between biobanks, their internationalization and commercialization, as well as third-party access to samples and data. In this latter context, the council explicitly mentions the use of the Swedish PKU registry for identifying the murderer of Anna Lindh. Against the background of these challenges, The Ethics Council outlines five pillars for the regulation of biobank research: the introduction of "biobank secrecy," purpose-restricted use of data, involvement of ethics commissions, quality assurance, and transparency.[112]

The introduction of a biobank secrecy, which involves the duty of confidentiality and discretion for all persons who deal with samples and data to prevent access by nonresearch third parties, including state authorities, became the most contested aspect among the council's recommendations. In its opinion the council justifies the biobank secrecy as compensation for the limits of IC: "Biobanks, as a resource for scientific research, cannot be narrowly limited to specific purposes in the use of samples and data. Nor is it usually possible to inform the donors in advance of the precise purposes of use and of the duration of storage and use. Both these deficiencies should be compensated for by legislation that use should be exclusively for scientific research, together with biobank secrecy."[113]

However, researchers and other experts in the field were concerned that a biobank secrecy will lead to a German *Sonderweg*. For example, the German Research Foundation worried that biobank secrecy would hamper international research, as no other country has such a strict regulation in place.[114] Moreover, a public hearing about the council's recommendation at the German Bundestag revealed that researchers, both in academia and industry, do not see the need for additional regulation. In their opinion, the recommendations have already sufficiently been taken into account in daily biobanking practices. In contrast, ethicists and data protection advocates called for stricter regulations.[115] In 2012, the majority coalition in the German Bundestag finally decided against a specific biobank law, with the main argument being that it would pose new obstacles to research. Instead of enacting a new law, it was argued that the recommendations of the German Ethical Council should be regarded as "gold standard" by all researchers on their own responsibility.[116]

The German debate allows for an interesting comparison regarding the ethical framing of biobank research. While the Baltic Sea neighbors in the North seek to align individual interests and the common good, the German debate stresses the balance of individual self-determination and freedom of research. In Germany, people are particularly concerned about the use of genetic data.[117] Given the risks that the linkage of genetic data entails, participants from the KORA cohort (Collaborative Health Research in the Region of Augsburg), for example, perceive the return of individual health information as a "fair deal."[118] In Estonia, the communication of individual genetic results is even perceived as the most important feature of the database by the general public. This is in striking contrast to the Swedish context, where the perception of biobanks as a collective endeavor is used as an argument to principally reject the disclosure of individual results. In particular, it is argued that "returning individual results fails to respect the premises under which the public health project of large-scale biobank research is undertaken and inevitably reduces the prospect of achieving advances by consuming resources that should be allocated to benefiting the public good."[119]

However, regarding the forensic use of biobanks, an interesting permutation of arguments can be observed for the three countries. German lawyers, for example, rather doubt that biobank privacy could be maintained toward public authorities. Given that state security is a matter of the common good, it may legitimately override individual interests in privacy protection.[120] This is in striking contrast to Sweden, where the forensic use of biobanks has been ruled out by law despite a traditionally high acceptance of common good arguments. Also, Estonia prohibits access to clinical genetic data by state authorities,[121] not least to distance itself from the former Soviet system. However, infringements of individuals' privacy might still occur in health care due to a lack of awareness for potential breaches of confidentiality. In Soviet times it was quite common among physicians "to discuss a patient's condition freely with others and without first obtaining the patient's consent."[122] Changes to this practice may only slowly win recognition. According to Margit Sutrop and Kadri Simm, "Most often the breaches [of confidentiality] are not caused by hackers or thieves but by malevolent or negligent employees of the relevant institutions."[123] This is particularly troubling in light of the fact that, for the Estonian e-health project, which started in 2007, patients' participation is mandatory and the requirement for consent has been abandoned altogether.[124]

However, Estonians seem hardly troubled by this. Besides their traditionally high trust in scientists and widespread digital literacy, people are very open minded toward information technologies and their constant improvement. Estonia is currently a forerunner of e-health systems worldwide, closely followed by the Nordic countries Sweden, Finland, and Denmark. In particular, Estonia has established a centralized system where all patient medical data are electronically stored. To avoid the image of a surveillance society, however, patients are allowed to access their data, and unauthorized access to a patient's records by doctors is penalized.[125]

Also, Sweden allows its citizens full access to electronic medical records. Moreover, health information can be shared by doctors across the country. Though patients may block this option, few do so. A survey shows that people not only accept but even expect that health-care professionals follow up on patient outcomes as long as this occurs for professional reasons.[126] Nevertheless, Swedish doctors have been sentenced for unauthorized access to patient data and even lost their license in several cases.

In contrast to Estonia and Sweden, in Germany the introduction of e-health still lags behind. Similar to biobank research, concerns about data protection are one reason for this. A survey of doctors' attitudes toward telemedicine revealed that, though the majority is optimistic about this development, there is a particular fear among practitioners about rising costs, detrimental effects on patients' privacy, and the doctor-patient-relationship.[127] However, with the passage of the e-health law in 2015, the introduction of nationwide electronic patient records is approaching. Among other things, the law foresees the storage of emergency and medication data as well as the electronic transmission of doctors' and hospitals' discharge letters. In the run-up to the law, the German Medical Association, among others, complained, for example, that patients' emergency data are not sufficiently protected, as they will be made available to a broad range of professional groups in the medical sector. Moreover, in contrast to Sweden and Estonia, where patients are explicitly granted access to their medical data, access facilities for German patients are still more restricted.

A Look into the Future: Harmonization through Cooperation

Without doubt, the Baltic Sea region is currently one of the most important areas of biobanking worldwide and takes on a leading role in telemedicine and e-health as well. While the Nordic countries traditionally cooperate on a broad range of political, economic, social, and scientific issues (e.g., in the Nordic Council), there is special awareness of collaboration in the field of biotechnology in general and biobank research in particular, which even comprises a wider range of countries bordering the Baltic (e.g., the ScanBelt BioRegion). Currently, there are several initiatives aiming at the consolidation of biobanking infrastructures in this region, for example, the Swedish Biobanking and Biomolecular Resource Research Infrastructure (BBMRI.se) and the Joint Nordic Biobank Research Infrastructure (BBMRI Nordic). As one of its long-term goals, the latter aims to "set an international standard on how to collaborate on biobank-based research."[128] Moreover, the BBMRI.se "is the first national BBMRI hub to implement the BBMRI minimum data set" that will pave the way towards a unified standard for sample and data management "connecting biobanks at the Nordic and European level."[129]

The importance of the Baltic Sea area in biobanking is not only the result of large sample numbers stored in this region. Given the region's early experience with large-scale biobanks, it can provide an instructive reference point for the regulation and organization of biobanking in other countries. For example, given the difficulties resulting from commercial-actor involvement in the Icelandic, Swedish, and Estonian databases, the commercialization of the Norwegian Nord-Trøndelag Health Study (HUNT) biobank by the HUNT Biosciences Ltd. in 2007 was organized as a "for-profit-for-public" model from the outset.[130] This implies that the biobank is publicly owned, and all profit is directly reinvested into medical research for the public good.

Moreover, as divergent legal approaches present an obstacle to research, a trend toward harmonization in the Baltic Sea region can be observed. For example, in 2013, Finland enacted the first all-purpose biobank law in Europe that applies to all biobanks in the country.[131] For research purposes, the donors' broad consent is accepted. In future, this might become the common rule in a broader range of countries. Cooperative exchange on biobanking and its regulation can also be observed in Sweden. In the run-up to the revision of the Swedish Biobank Act, the Ministry of Health and Social Affairs released a report that explicitly starts with an overview on the legal regulation of biobank research in the other Nordic countries.[132]

In light of different research traditions and historic experiences, however, it is rather unlikely that there will ever be a completely identic approach to biobanking, either in the Baltic Sea region or worldwide. In fact, as the exemplary analyses of Sweden, Estonia, and Germany show, research traditions and the countries' political and economic backgrounds matter to a considerable extent. This, however, must not be to the detriment of biobank research. Rather, different approaches may stimulate discussions and provide incentives for a harmonization through cooperation. Examples can be found at several levels in the Baltic Sea area. The development strategy for the Estonian Genome Project (2011–16) stipulates, for example, "Since the collaboration with the German National Cohort (genome bank) and the Nordic Biobank Consortium is considered to be of particular importance, the Estonian Genome Center of the University of Tartu (EGCUT) needs to study our gene donors in the coming period applying the same methods as these two groups." Moreover, it is stressed that "EGCUT is actively participating in the research conducted in Europe by being one of the connecting points to coordinate the biobanks in Baltic States."[133] Last but not least, Sweden with the LifeGene project, Estonia with its Genome Project, and Germany with the KORAgen cohort are active members in the Public Population Project in Genomics, which aims at the "creation of an open, public, and accessible knowledge database"[134] for future international collaborations. In light of this, it might not be an exaggeration to characterize the Baltic Sea region as an important contact zone for biobanking that builds bridges across the Baltic, but also beyond.

Notes

1. Marki Lethi, "Mapping the Study of the Baltic Sea Area: From Nation-Centric to Multinational History," *Journal of Baltic Studies* 33, no. 4 (2002): 436.

2. Karen J. Maschke, "Navigating an Ethical Patchwork—Human Gene Banks," *Nature Biotechnology* 23 (2005): 539–45.

3. Robert E. Hewitt, "Biobanking: The Foundation of Personalized Medicine," *Current Opinion in Oncology* 23, no. 1 (2011): 112–19.

4. Anne Cambon-Thomsen, Emmanuelle Rial-Sebbag, and Bartha M. Knoppers, "Trends in Ethical and Legal Frameworks for the Use of Human Biobanks," *European Respiratory Journal* 30, no. 2 (2007): 373–82. Katharina Beier, Christian Lenk, "Biobanking Strategies and Regulative Approaches in the EU: Recent Perspectives," *Journal of Biorepository Science and Applied Medicine* (2015): 69–81.

5. Mats G. Hansson, "Building on Relationships of Trust in Biobank Research," *Journal of Medical Ethics* (2004): 415–18.

6. Vilhjálmur Árnason, "Coding and Consent: Moral Challenges of the Database Project in Iceland," *Bioethics* 18, no. 1 (2004): 27–49.

7. Jane Kaye, Edgar A. Whitley, David Lund, Michael Morrison, Harriet Teare, and Karen Melham, "Dynamic Consent: A Patient Interface for Twenty-First Century Research Networks," *European Journal of Human Genetics* 23 (2015): 141–46.

8. K. O'Doherty, A. K. Hawkins, and M. M. Burges, "Involving Citizens in the Ethics of Biobank Research: Informing Institutional Policy through Structured Public Deliberation," *Social Science and Medicine* 75, no. 9 (2012): 1604–11.

9. M. H. Zawati and Bartha M. Knoppers, "International Normative Perspectives on the Return of Individual Research Results and Incidental Findings in Genomic Biobanks," *Genetics in Medicine* 14, no. 4 (2012): 484–89.

10. Herbert Gottweis and Alan Petersen, eds., *Biobanks: Governance in Comparative Perspective* (London: Routledge, 2008).

11. Andrea Boggio, Nikola Biller-Andorno, Bernice Elger, Alex Mauron, and Alexander M. Capron, "Comparing Guidelines on Biobanks: Emerging Consensus and Unresolved Controversies," 2005, http://www.ruig-gian.org/ressources/Boggio%20et%20al%20on%20Biobanks%20070827.pdf; Christian Lenk and Katharina Beier, "A Unified European Approach on Tissue Research and Biobanking? A Comparison," in *Biobanks and Tissue Research: The Public, the Patient and the Regulation,* ed. Christian Lenk, Judit Sándor, and Bert Gordijn (Dordrecht: Springer, 2011), 143–64; Elini Zika, Daniele Paci, Tobias Schulte in den Bäumen, Anette Braun, Sylvie Rijkers-Defrasne, Mylène Deschenênes, Isabel Fortier, Jens Laage-Hellman, Christian A. Scerri, and Dolores Ibarreta, "Biobanks in Europe: Prospects for Harmonisation and Networking," Joint Research Centre 2010.

12. Lenk and Beier, "A Unified European Approach on Tissue Research and Biobanking?"

13. Marie Sandberg, "Reinforced Nordic Collaboration on Data Resources: Challenges from Six Perspectives," Nordic Council of Ministers 2012; NordForsk, "Joint Nordic Registers and Biobanks: A Goldmine for Health and Welfare Research," policy paper 5, 2014.

14. Alice Park, "Biobanks," *New York Times*, March 12, 2009.

15. George Gaskell, Sally Stares, Agnes Allansdottir, Nick Allum, Paula Castro, Yilmaz Esmer, Claude Fischler, Jonathan Jackson, Nicole Kronberger, et al., "Europeans and Biotechnology in 2010: Winds of Change?," Directorate-General for Research October 2010.

16. George Gaskell and Herbert Gottweis, "Biobanks Need Publicity," *Nature* 471, no. 10 (2011): 159–60; Lars Ø. Ursin, Klaus Hoeyer, and John-Arne Skolbekken, "The Informed Consenters: Governing Biobanks in Scandinavia," in Gottweis and Petersen, *Biobanks*, 177–93.

17. Gísli Pálsson, "The Rise and Fall of a Biobank: The Case of Iceland," in Gottweis and Petersen, *Biobanks*, 41–55.

18. Janine M. Traulsen, Ingunn Björnsdóttir, and Anna Birna Almarsdóttir, "'I'm Happy If I Can Help': Public Views on Future Medicines and Gene-Based Therapy in Iceland," *Community Genetics* 11, no. 1 (2008): 2–10.

19. Jocelyne Kaiser, "Agency Nixes deCode's New Data-Mining Plan," *Science* 340 (2013): 1388–89.

20. "The Genomic Portrait of a Nation," deCode website, March 25, 2015, https://www.decode.com/the-genomic-portrait-of-a-nation/.

21. Kaiser, "Agency Nixes deCode's New Data-Mining Plan."

22. Ibid.

23. David E. Winickoff, "Genome and Nation: Iceland's Health Sector Database and Its Legacy," *Innovations: Technology, Governance, Globalization* 1, no. 2 (2006): 80–105.

24. Kjell E. Eriksson, "Sweden," in *The Ethics and Governance of Human Genetic Databases*, ed. Matti Häyry, Ruth Chadwick, Vilhjálmur Árnason, and Gardar Árnason (Cambridge: Cambridge University Press, 2007), 59–65.

25. According to other estimates, the Swedish national biobank program contains between fifty and one hundred million samples, while the number is said to increase by three or four million every year. Walter Pytlik, "Biobanks—Treasure Chests for Biomedical Research," *BIOPRO Biotechnology and LifeSciences in Baden-Württemberg*, June 18, 2012, https://www.gesundheitsindustrie-bw.de/en/article/dossier/biobanks-treasure-chests-for-biomedical-research/.

26. This even exceeds the relation between samples and populations in Denmark, Finland, or Norway. Ursin, Hoeyer, and Skolbekken, "The Informed Consenters," 179).

27. Maria Trägårdh and Magnus Ringman, "Ditt liv är till salu" [Your life is for sale], *Aftonbladet*, April 19, 1999, http://wwwc.aftonbladet.se/nyheter/9904/10/cell.html.

28. Ursin, Hoeyer, and Skolbekken, "The Informed Consenters," 181.

29. Swedish Medical Research Council, "Research Ethics Guidelines for Using Biobanks, Especially Projects Involving Genome Research," (Dnr 1999-570), Stockholm, 1999.

30. Ministry of Health and Social Affairs, "Biobanks in Medical Care Act (2002:297)" [Lag om biobanker i hälso- och sjukvården], http://biobanksverige.se/wp-content/uploads/Biobanks-in-medical-care-act-2002-297.pdf; Elisabeth Rynning, "Legal Challenges and Strategies in the Regulation of Research Biobanking," in *The Ethics of Research Biobanking*, ed. Jan Helge Solbakk, Sören Holm, and Björn Hofmann (Dordrecht: Springer, 2009), 277–314; Katharina Beier, "Between Individualism and Solidarity: Biobanking in Sweden," in *New Challenges for Biobanks: Ethics, Law and Governance*, ed. Kris Dierickx and Pascal Borry (Antwerp: Intersentia, 2009), 49–64.

31. Rynning, "Legal Challenges and Strategies," 119

32. Sven Ove Hansson and Barbro Björkman, "Bioethics in Sweden," *Cambridge Quarterly of Health Care Ethics* 15 (2006): 285.

33. Ursin, Hoeyer, and Skolbekken, "The Informed Consenters," 182.

34. Klaus L. Hoeyer, "Ambiguous Gifts: Public Anxiety, Informed Consent and Biobanks," in *Genetic Databases: Socio-ethical Issues in the Collection and Use of DNA*, ed. Richard Tutton and Oonagh Corrigan (London: Routledge, 2004), 97–116; Linus Johnsson, Mats G. Hansson, Stefan Eriksson, and Gert Helgesson, "Patients' Refusal to Consent to Storage and Use of Samples in Swedish Biobanks: Cross Sectional Study," *British Medical Journal* (2008): 337, a345 (online first); Åsa Kettis-Lindblad, Lena Ring, Eva Viberth, and Mats G. Hansson, "Genetic Research and Donation of Tissue Samples to Biobanks: What Do Potential Sample Donors in the Swedish General Public Think?," *European Journal of Public Health* 16 (2006): 433–40; Tore Nilstun and Göran Hermerén, "Human Tissue Samples and Ethics: Attitudes of the General Public in Sweden to Biobank Research," *Medicine, Health Care and Philosophy* 9 (2006): 81–86.

35. Klaus Hoeyer, "The Role of Privacy and Informed Consent in Danish and Swedish Biobank Practices," *Medical Law International* 10 (2010): 281.

36. Mats G. Hansson, "Building on Relationships of Trust in Biobank Research," *Journal of Medical Ethics* (2004): 415–18.

37. Ibid; Joanna Stjernschantz Forsberg, Mats G. Hansson, and Stefan Eriksson, "Changing Perspectives in Biobank Research: From Individual Rights to Concerns about Public Health regarding the Return of Results," *European Journal of Human Genetics* 17 (2009): 1544–49; Ursin, Hoeyer, and Skolbekken, "The Informed Consenters."

38. Klaus L. Hoeyer, "'Science Is Really Needed—That's All I Know': Informed Consent and the Non-verbal Practices of Collecting Blood for Genetic Research in Northern Sweden," *New Genetics and Society* 22, no. 3 (2003): 239.

39. Hoeyer, "The Role of Privacy and Informed Consent in Danish and Swedish Biobank Practices," 282.

40. That this is not an unrealistic concern can be explained by the fact that Sweden and Iceland are both welfare states with a tradition in register-based research that is expected to be used for the public good.

41. Klaus Hoeyer, "Studying Ethics as a Policy: The Naming and Framing of Moral Problems in Genetic Research," *Current Anthropology* 46 (2005): 74.

42. Alison Abbott, "Sweden Sets Ethical Standards for Use of Genetic 'Biobanks,'" *Nature* 400, no. 3 (1999): 3.

43. Hilary Rose, "An Ethical Dilemma," *Nature* 425 (2003): 123.

44. Ibid; Hoeyer, "Studying Ethics as a Policy," 74. Most interestingly, and in contrast to international perception, UmanGenomics had never released any official ethics document. The "Uman model," as it was punchy named by the company, "was never written down in a certified, official version, but it was widely discussed and several written descriptions of it had circulated" (72).

45. Rose, "An Ethical Dilemma," 123.

46. Jens Laage-Hellmann, "Clinical Genomics Companies and Biobanks: The Use of Biosamples in Commercial Research on the Genetics of Common Diseases," in *Biobanks as Resources for Health*, ed. Mats G. Hansson and Marianne Levin (Uppsala: Universitetstryckeriet Uppsala, 2003), 51–90.

47. Erik Lindenius, "Guldgruvan som försvann? En mediestudie av konflikten kring UmanGenomics och Mediciniska Biobanken 2001–2006" (PhD diss.,

Umeå University, 2009). Last but not least, critics complained about the fact that UmanGenomics did not even have to pay a fee for getting access to the biobank samples for the reason that the Swedish Biobanks Act rejects any kind of trade with human biological tissue. This had the paradoxical effect that the right of exploitation has been granted to UmanGenomics at a relatively low price compared to what the setup of a biobank and its maintenance would cost. Laage-Hellmann, "Clinical Genomics Companies and Biobanks."

48. Ricky Ansell and Birgitta Rasmusson, "A Swedish Perspective," *Biosocieties* 3, no. 1 (2008): 88–92.

49. Hansson and Björkman, "Bioethics in Sweden."

50. Svensk Författningssamling, "Lag om vissa register för forskning om vad arv och miljö betyder för människors hälsa (2013:794)," https://www.riksdagen.se/sv/dokument-lagar/dokument/svensk-forfattningssamling/lag-2013794-om-vissa-register-for-forskning-om_sfs-2013-794.

51. BBMRI.se, "Biobank Sweden. the newsletter of BBMRI.se," December 11, 2013.

52. Statens Offentliga Utredningar (SOU 2010:81), "En ny biobankslag. Betänkande av Biobanksutredningen," Stockholm 2010, http://vebook.org/en-ny-biobankslag-betnkande-sou-2010-81.pdf.

53. Kommittédirektiv: En ändamålsenlig reglering för biobanker (Dir. 2016:41), https://www.regeringen.se/49bde0/contentassets/edc21a8464e14db680829061357eec6f/en-andamalsenlig-reglering-for-biobanker.pdf.

54. Regeringens proposition 2016/17:204: Fortsatt giltighet av lagen om vissa register för forskning om vad arv och miljö betyder för människors hälsa, https://www.regeringen.se/rattsliga-dokument/proposition/2017/06/prop.-201617204/.

55. As Eensaar stresses, considerable efforts have been spent on "contextualizing the Estonian Biobank Project within policy narratives dominant in Estonia" at that time. Rainer Eensaar, "Estonia: Ups and Downs of a Biobank Project," in Gottweis and Petersen, *Biobanks*, 56–70, 56).

56. Frank Lone, "Biotechnology in the Baltic," *Nature Biotechnology* 19 (2001): 513–15.

57. Agris Koppel, Kersti Meiesaar, Hannu Valtonen, Andrus Metsa, and Margus Lember, "Evaluation of Primary Health Reform in Estonia," *Social Science & Medicine* 56 (2003): 2461–66.

58. The information brochure has been replaced by an updated version and is no longer available. The author, however, is in the possession of a hard copy of the cited version.

59. Külliki Korts, Sue Weldon, and Margrét Lilja Guðmundsdóttir, "Genetic Databases and Public Attitudes: A Comparison of Iceland, Estonia and the UK," *Trames* 8 (58/53), nos. 1/2 (2004): 146.

60. Pálsson, "The Rise and Fall of a Biobank," 53.

61. Amy L. Fletcher, "Fields of Genes: The Politics of Science and Identity in the Estonian Genome Project," *New Genetics and Society* 23, no. 1 (2004): 9; Eensaar, "Estonia"; Justine Petrone, "Q&A: Estonian Genome Center's Andres Metspalu on Biobanks, Arrays, and Personalized Medicine," December 29, 2014, https://www.genomeweb.com/microarrays-multiplexing/qa-estonian-genome-centers-andres-metspalu-biobanks-arrays-and-personalized#.W9MGMMSYSUk.

62. Donald A. Barr, "The Ethics of Soviet Medical Practice: Behaviors and Attitudes of Physicians in Soviet Estonia," *Journal of Medical Ethics* 22 (1996): 33–40.

63. In fact, surveys have shown that the promise of being granted a personal gene card is what most Estonians (86 percent) remembered about the biobank. Korts et al., "Genetic Databases and Public Attitudes," 142.

64. Jeffrey H. Barker, "Common-Pool Resources and Population Genomics in Iceland, Estonia, and Tonga," *Medicine, Health Care and Philosophy* 6 (2003): 139.

65. Deutscher Bundestag, "Bericht des Ausschusses für Bildung, Forschung und Technikfolgenabschätzung," Drucksache 16/5374, May 5, 2007, 37; http://dip21. bundestag.de/dip21/btd/16/053/1605374.pdf.

66. Uta Wagenmann, "Osteuropäische Ölfelder," *Gen-ethischer Informationsdienst* 175, (2006): 45–49, http://www.gen-ethisches-netzwerk.de/osteuropaische-olfelder.

67. Margit Sutrop and Kadri Simm, "The Estonian Healthcare System and the Genetic Database Project: From Limited Resources to Big Hopes," *Cambridge Quarterly of Healthcare Ethics* 13 (2004): 254–62.

68. Vilius Dranseika Eugenijus Gefenas, "Procurement, Storage and Transfer of Tissues and Cells for Non-Clinical Research Purposes," in *The Ethical and Legal Regulation of Human Tissue and Biobank Research in Europe*, ed. Katharina Beier, Silvia Schnorrer, Nils Hoppe, and Christian Lenk (Göttingen: Universitätsverlag Göttingen, 2011), 131–38, esp. 132.

69. Frank Lone, "Give and Take—Estonia's New Model for a National Gene Bank," *Genome News Network*, October 6, 2000, http://www.genomenewsnetwork.org/articles/10_00/Estonias_genebank.shtml.

70. Korts et al., "Genetic Databases and Public Attitudes," 140.

71. Judit Sándor and Petra Bárd, "The Legal Regulation of Biobanks. National Report: Estonia," CELAB Paper Series no. 5, 2009, 3.

72. Although the Estonian Genome Project was presented as distinct from the Icelandic database, its legal framework was clearly inspired by the Icelandic one. Susan M. C. Gibbons, "Governance of Population Genetic Databases: A Comparative Analysis of Legal Regulation in Estonia, Iceland, Sweden and the UK," in *The Ethics and Governance of Human Genetic Databases*, ed. Matti Häyry, Ruth Chadwick, Vilhjálmur Árnason, and Gardar Árnason, (Cambridge: Cambirgde University Press, 2007), 132–46, esp. 134.

73. Sándor and Bárd, "The Legal Regulation of Biobanks," 4.

74. Rainer Kattel and Margit Suurna, "The Rise and Fall of the Estonian Genome Project," *Studies in Ethics, Law, and Technology* 2, no. 2 (2008): 7.

75. The shares of EGeen Ltd were in coownership of EGeen Inc. (97,5%) and the EGPF (2,5%). Kattel and Suurna, "The Rise and Fall of the Estonian Genome Project," 10.

76. Sándor and Bárd, "The Legal Regulation of Biobanks," 4.

77. Ibid., 4.

78. Kattel and Suurna, "The Rise and Fall of the Estonian Genome Project," 8.

79. Ibid., 8.

80. Funding was provided only to an extent that allowed the maintaining of samples collected so far.

81. Eensaar, "Estonia," 64.

82. Liis Leitsalu, Helene Alavere, Mari-Liis Tammesoo, Erkki Leego, and Andres Metspalu. "Linking a Population Biobank with National Health Registries—the Estonian Experience." *Journal of Personalized Medicine* 5 (2015): 97.

83. A recent joint initiative by the Ministry of Social Affairs, the National Institute for Health Development, and the Estonian Genome Center, offers to provide information to one hundred thousand Estonians about their genetic risk. This initiative is backed not least by the wish to increase the number of biobank participants. See the Estonian Genome Center, University of Tartu (The Estonian Biobank), https://www.geenivaramu.ee/en/about-us, accessed May 3, 2018.

84. However, donors agree to this at least by giving their broad consent at the time of enrollment to the database.

85. Leitsalu et al., "Linking a Population Biobank with National Health Registries—The Estonian Experience," 97.

86. Author's translation (Des Forschers Freude, ist des Anlegers Leid).

87. Leitsalu et al., "Linking a Population Biobank with National Health Registries," 98.

88. Kattel and Suurna, "The Rise and Fall of the Estonian Genome Project," 12.

89. Ibid., 14.

90. Ibid.

91. Zika et al., "Biobanks in Europe," 69.

92. For a comprehensive overview on biobanks in Germany, see Deutscher Bundestag, "Bericht des Ausschusses für Bildung, Forschung und Technikfolgenabschätzung," 21.

93. Gaskell and Gottweis, "Biobanks Need Publicity."

94. Uta Wagenmann, "Vom Pech, in Estland geboren zu sein" [About the bad luck of being born in Estonia], *Freitag* no.12, March 23, 2006, 18.

95. Andreas Weber, "Das verkaufte Volk" [The sold nation], *SZ Magazin,* January 23, 2001.

96. Joachim Müller-Jung, "Estlands Gendatenbank: Ein Symbol des Genom-Zeitalters wankt" [Estonia's genetic database: A symbol of the genomic age is tottering], *Frankfurter Allgemeine Zeitung,* no. 77, March 31, 2004: N1.

97. Ingrid Schneider, "'This Is Not a National Biobank . . .': The Politics of Local Biobanks in Germany," in Gottweis and Petersen, *Biobanks,* 88–108, 90.

98. Stefan Schreiber, "Biobanken und Populationsgenetik im Deutschen Humangenomprojekt," *Biobanken: Chance für den wissenschaftlichen Fortschritt oder Ausverkauf der "Ressource" Mensch? Vorträge der Jahrestagung des Nationalen Ethikrates 2002* (Berlin: Nationaler Ethikrat, 2002): 10, https://www.ethikrat.org/fileadmin/Publikationen/Dokumentationen/Dokumentation_JT_2002_Biobanken.pdf.

99. Schneider, "'This Is Not a National Biobank,'" 93.

100. Ibid., 93.

101. Ibid., 90.

102. The focus is specifically on twelve lifestyle diseases that are followed up in 2.3 million people.

103. The director of PopGen thus describes the biobank as a "verification and validation machinery" that is not out for the detection of "new genes" but examines the penetration factor for certain diseases in the population (Schneider, "'This Is Not a National Biobank,'" 91).

104. However, the samples will be stored in a central biobank at the Helmholtz Association in Munich, while backup samples are kept in local study centers.

105. Rita Wellbrock, "Biobanken—Nutzung menschlicher Zellen und Gewebe: Information, Einwilligung und Datenschutz," *Biobanken: Chance für den wissenschaftlichen Fortschritt oder Ausverkauf der "Ressource" Mensch? Vorträge der Jahrestagung des Nationalen Ethikrates 2002* (Berlin: Nationaler Ethikrat, 2002): 21, https://www.ethikrat.org/fileadmin/Publikationen/Dokumentationen/Dokumentation_JT_2002_Biobanken.pdf.

106. Ibid., 47.

107. Bartha M. Knoppers, "Ethics Watch," *Nature Reviews Genetics* 5 (2004): 485.

108. Ibid.

109. Eva Marie Engels, "Biobanken für die medizinische Forschung—Zur Einführung," *Biobanken: Chance für den wissenschaftlichen Fortschritt oder Ausverkauf der "Ressource" Mensch? Vorträge der Jahrestagung des Nationalen Ethikrates 2002* (Berlin: Nationaler Ethikrat, 2002): 13, https://www.ethikrat.org/fileadmin/Publikationen/Dokumentationen/Dokumentation_JT_2002_Biobanken.pdf.

110. Ibid., 17.

111. Ibid.

112. Deutscher Ethikrat, *Human Biobanks for Research: Opinion* (Berlin: Deutscher Ethikrat, 2010), 27, https://www.ethikrat.org/fileadmin/Publikationen/Stellung nahmen/englisch/DER_StnBiob_Engl_Online_mitKennwort.pdf.

113. Ibid., 49.

114. Deutsche Forschungsgemeinschaft (DFG), "Biomaterialbanken für die Forschung—Klare Konzepte und Empfehlungen notwendig," Pressemitteilung no. 12 (2011), http://www.dfg.de/service/presse/pressemitteilungen/2011/pressemitteilung_nr_12/.

115. Pytlik, "Biobanks."

116. Deutscher Bundestag, "Beschlussempfehlung und Bericht des Ausschusses für Bildung, Forschung und Technikfolgenabschätzung," Drucksache 17/8873, March 6, 2012, http://dip21.bundestag.de/dip21/btd/17/088/1708873.pdf.

117. George Gaskell, Herbert Gottweis, Johannes Starkbaum, Jacqueline E. W. Broerse, Monica Gerber, Ursula Gottweis, Abbi Hobbs, Helén Ilpo, Maria Pashou, Karoliina Snell, et al., "Publics and Biobanks in Europe: Explaining Heterogeneity," LSG Working Papers no. 2, October 5, 2011, 6, http://www.univie.ac.at/LSG/papers2011/LSG%20Working%20Paper.pdf.

118. A. Hobbs, Johannes Starkbaum, Ursula Gottweis, H.-Erich Wichmann, and Herbert Gottweis, "The Privacy-Reciprocity Connection in Biobanking: Comparing German with UK Strategies," *Public Health Genomics,* June 20, 2012, 279. Though the communication of individual results is not excluded by the German Ethics Council, it calls for precautionary measures in the context of biobank research. Nationaler Ethikrat, "Biobanken für die Forschung," 68; Deutscher Ethikrat, "Human Biobanks for Research." The recently established National Cohort Study in Germany also advertises participation by promising individual feedback of results. See Wichman et al., "Die Nationale Kohorte," 784.

119. Stjernschantz Forsberg, Hansson, and Eriksson, "Changing Perspectives in Biobank Research," 1548.

120. Jochen Taupitz, "Rechtliche Vorgaben für ein Biobankgesetz," in *Regelungsbedarf für Forschung mit Humanbiobanken? Expertengespräch in Zusammenarbeit mit der TMF*, 2011, 67, https://www.ethikrat.org/fileadmin/PDF-Dateien/Veranstaltungen/expertenge spraech-biobanken-simultanmitschrift.pdf.

121. Lotta Wendel, "Third Parties' Interest in Population Genetic Databases: Some Comparative Notes Regarding the Law in Estonia, Iceland, Sweden and the UK," in *The Ethics and Governance of Human Genetic Databases*, ed. Matti Häyry, Ruth Chadwick, Vilhjálmur Árnason, and Gardar Árnason (Cambridge: Cambridge University Press, 2007), 119.

122. Barr, "The Ethics of Soviet Medical Practice," 37.

123. Sutrop and Simm, "The Estonian Healthcare System and the Genetic Database Project," 261.

124. Petra Bárd and Judit Sándor, "Anonymisation and Pseudonymisation as a Means of Privacy Protection," in *The Ethical and Legal Regulation of Human Tissue and Biobank Research in Europe*, ed. Katharina Beier, Silvia Schnorrer, Nils Hoppe, and Christian Lenk (Göttingen: Universitätsverlag Göttingen, 2011), 27.

125. Ralf Leonard, "Das Rezept kommt per Email" [Prescription comes by email], *TAZ*, October 19, 2014, http://www.taz.de/!5030777/.

126. Elin C. Lehnbohn, Andrew J. McLachlan, and Jo-Anne E. Brien, "A Qualitative Study of Swedes' Opinions about Shared Electronic Health Records," MEDINFO (2013), https://doi.org/10.3233/978-1-61499-289-9-3, 6.

127. Institut für Demoskopie Allensbach, "Der Einsatz von Telematik und Telemedizin im Gesundheitswesen aus Sicht der Ärzteschaft," April/May 2010, 5–7, http://www.bundesaerztekammer.de/fileadmin/user_upload/downloads/eHealth_ Bericht_kurz_final.pdf.

128. *Present Status and Future Potential for Research in the Nordic Countries*, Nordic White Paper on Medical Research, Helsinki 2011, http://www.nordforsk.org/files/ present-status-and-future-potential-for-medical-research-in-the-nordic-countries, 13.

129. Loreana Norlin, Martin Fransson, S. Eaker, G. Elinder, and Jan-Eric Litton, "Adapting Research to the 21st Century—the Swedish Biobank Register," *Norsk Epidemiology* 21, no. 2 (2012): 153. In addition, the website of the Swedish national biobank program is the first in the EU to provide a list of all European biobanks grouped according to human and nonhuman resources (see Pytlik, "Biobanks").

130. Kristin Solum Steinsbekk, Berge Solberg, and Bjørn Kåre Myskja, "From Idealism to Realism: Commercial Ventures in Publicly Funded Biobanks," in *New Challenges for Biobanks: Ethics, Law and Governance*, ed. Kris Dierickx and Pascal Borry (Antwerp: Intersentia, 2009), 137–51.

131. Sirpa Soini, "Finland on a Road towards a Modern Legal Biobanking Infrastructure," *European Journal of Health Law* 3 (2013), 289–94, access through: http://www.julkari.fi/bitstream/handle/10024/110331/Soini%20EjHL%20 2013_3%20biobankact%20preprint%20version%20.pdf;sequence=2.

132. Statens Offentliga Utredningar (SOU 2010: 81).

133. University of Tartu, Estonian Genome Center, "Estonian Genome Center of the University of Tartu Development Plan for 2011–2016" (private copy, in the author's possession).

134. Zika et al., "Biobanks in Europe," 137.

Chapter Ten

The Simultaneous Embedment and Disembedment of Biomedicine

Intercorporeality and Patient Interaction at Hemodialysis Units in Riga and Stockholm

Martin Gunnarson

Local and Global Biomedicine

Biomedicine has today gained global reach. Although access to biomedical therapies varies greatly across the globe, the faith in their ability not only to explain but also to cure human suffering is almost universal. Increasingly, however, concerns are being raised, within academia and elsewhere, about the universalization of the human body and the application of standardized therapies and methods of measurement taking place in biomedical practice. Since the human body as a biological entity cannot be separated from and is never unaffected by the person embodying it and his or her embedment within particular social, historical, cultural, and political contexts, biomedicine has to take such contingencies into account, it is argued.[1] Moreover, since the practice of experimental and clinical biomedicine is itself always already located within a specific spatiotemporal context and thereby deeply "embedded within a complex cultural world with historical depth,"[2] so are the very universal body and standardized therapies it purports to enact.[3] Yet the transnationalism of biomedicine is unmistakable. By incessantly transferring knowledge, therapies, people, and technologies across societal and national borders, an increasing number of people worldwide are today diagnosed, treated, and cured by means of the application of standardized biomedical interventions.[4]

Taken together, the claims above paint a complex picture, suggesting that contemporary biomedicine is simultaneously embedded in and disembedded from the particular contexts in which it is practiced.[5] The present chapter sets out to underscore and explore this complexity by means of a study of the intricate interplay between biomedicine as a transnational culture of its own, on the one hand, and a scientific and clinical practice fundamentally shaped by local and national material, cultural, and historical conditions, on the other. Offering a historically informed ethnographic exploration of the practice of hemodialysis in two national contexts, the chapter shows how this particular biomedical therapy both exceeds and relies on the conditions engendered by the local and national contexts in which it is practiced. More specifically, in this chapter I look at the interaction between patients taking place at four hemodialysis units, one in Riga, Latvia, and three in Stockholm, Sweden.

The empirical basis of this chapter is taken from a study on the practice of renal replacement therapies in Stockholm, Sweden, and Riga, Latvia.[6] My decision to locate the study in Latvia and Sweden, or more specifically, Riga and Stockholm, was motivated mainly by my desire to study how the divergent histories of these two countries and the similarities of their development in the present—toward, for example, an increased neoliberalization—have affected the provision and practice of renal replacement therapies. In this chapter I situate my study of the current practice of hemodialysis in the context of previous research on the twentieth-century history of health care and patienthood in Sweden and Latvia. To date, there are few studies with a similar theme, approach, and geographical scope. Worth mentioning are Jenny Gunnarsson Payne's[7] work on the reproductive travel of Swedish couples to Latvia and Katarzyna Wolanik Boström's and Magnus Öhlander's[8] work on the mobility of medical knowledge in the case of Polish doctors' migration to Sweden.

The Sociomedical Setting

In need of hemodialysis are persons whose chronic kidney disease has progressed to the fifth and final stage, what in everyday care situations is referred to as kidney failure.[9] At this stage, the kidneys no longer function and are therefore incapable of removing toxins and excess fluid from the body. When left untreated, the condition is fatal.[10] In hemodialysis the patient's blood is circulated through a machine that rids the blood of toxins. This typically takes place in a hospital setting. Generally, patients undergo the treatment three times a week, three to five hours at a time. That this is considered an adequate treatment dose internationally is reflected in the *European Best Practice Guidelines on Haemodialysis,* according to which "[hemo]dialysis should be delivered at least 3 times per week and the total duration should be at least 12h per week, unless supported by significant renal function."[11]

This tells us that hemodialysis can be seen as a fundamentally standardized biomedical therapy, one founded on the notion of the universality of the human body and applied similarly across the globe. This applies at least to the form of treatment practiced at three of the four hemodialysis units explored in this chapter, a form of treatment that I, in accordance with the medical literature, term "conventional" hemodialysis.[12] At the fourth unit, which is a so-called self-care unit, patients manage their own treatment and therefore have the opportunity to determine the frequency and duration with which they undergo it.

Yet the treatment practiced at the self-care unit largely remains standardized, not least because the scientific foundation on which it is based and the technologies that are applied are the same as in conventional hemodialysis. This standardization is reflected also in the very spatiality of the units. At all four of them, the hemodialysis machines and the beds or chairs in which the patients lie or sit during the treatment take center stage. Moreover, at all units, patients undergo the treatment in the same room as other patients.[13] Lying, sitting, or reclining in their bed or chair, the patients are placed in such a way that they are oriented inward, toward the center of the room and toward one another. Adding to the spatial standardization is the existence at all four units of waiting rooms, dressing rooms, and corridors in which patients frequently come into contact with one another before and after the treatment. Thus, by means not only of a universalization of the human body but also of a spatio-temporal standardization, hemodialysis orients patients to regularly see and meet each other. It is the nature of and patients' views on this interaction that I analyze in the present chapter. But before doing so I will account briefly for the methodological and theoretical approach that guides this analysis.

Methodological Approach and Theoretical Points of Departure

Between the fall of 2009 and the spring of 2011, I conducted ethnographic fieldwork at four hemodialysis units, one in Riga and three in Stockholm. The empirical material thus gathered consists of audio-recorded and transcribed in-depth interviews with patients and medical professionals and notes taken during observations of the care practices. This chapter devotes particular attention to the interview data, more specifically to the interviews with patients. What I am interested in is the patients' descriptions of and views on their interaction with their fellow patients. In total I interviewed twenty-five patients, ten women and fifteen men, with ages ranging from twenty-two to seventy-three years old. Since I speak neither Latvian nor Russian, I relied on an interpreter for the majority of the interviews in Riga. These interviews were subsequently transcribed and translated by the interpreter. To ensure patient privacy, all interviewees have been assigned pseudonyms. The study received ethical approval from the regional ethical committee in Stockholm and from the ethical board of the hospital in Riga where the study took place.

Theoretically, I draw on writings rooted in the phenomenological tradition, especially on writings thematizing the concept of the lived body. The body is lived, phenomenologists argue, because it is as bodies that we have access to and project ourselves into the world. If it were not for the "sensorimotor powers" of our body, there would not be a world for us.[14] It is through our perceptual organs and our ability to move that we come into contact with the objects and others around us, phenomenologists contend. However, our being-in-the-world is not a causal effect of these bodily functions but the result of a meaningful encounter between body and world. Perception is not a "primitive function," Maurice Merleau-Ponty argues, but a "system of meanings which makes the concrete essence of the object immediately recognizable, and allows its 'sensible properties' to appear only through that essence."[15] When we perceive an object, we do not understand it by attending to its "sensible properties" but rather through the immediate process by which these properties are filtered through a "system of meaning." But how does such a system of meaning come about?

To answer this question Merleau-Ponty uses a modified version of the psychological concept of "body schema." For him, this concept denotes the simultaneous process by which the body coordinates its different parts and comes to have a world.[16] "The body schema, as Merleau-Ponty understands it," Erik Malmqvist and Kristin Zeiler write, "is an implicit awareness that is rooted in motility, and by virtue of which the lived body simultaneously forms a whole and aligns itself with its surroundings."[17] It is this synthesis of the body and its inextricable entwinement with the world that gives rise to the system of meaning on which every act of perception relies. The meaning is therefore neither in the world nor in the body, but in their encounter.[18] Consequently, our embodied being-in-the-world cannot be separated from, but is rather inextricably intertwined with, the historical, social, cultural, and political context that we inhabit in any given situation.

As Malmqvist and Zeiler point out, furthermore, our lived body and the system of meaning it maintains tend to be practical and prereflective rather than intellectual and thematized.[19] This idea informs what Drew Leder identifies as the absence of the lived body.[20] Insofar as the body is our lived connection with the world, he argues, it necessarily recedes from our attention. When we look at something, for instance, what we see is not our own seeing, but a certain meaningful object. The same applies to all our perceptual and motor organs. When we hear, we hear *something*, when we walk, we walk *somewhere*, when we touch, we touch *something*, and so on. Our attention is thus generally directed *from* our body *to* the surrounding world, according to Leder.[21]

However, neither the world nor the body are static. The lived body, Merleau-Ponty argues, should be viewed as a fundamentally dynamic structure capable of habitually incorporating new objects and abilities into its prereflective and practical being-in-the-world. When Merleau-Ponty develops the concept of incorporation, he gives the famous example of the blind man's stick. For the blind man, he argues, the stick is no longer an object. It is a part of the perceptual and motor powers with which he, as an embodied being, extends into and becomes engaged with the world. When he perceives things with it, he does not have to make explicit the length of the stick, he is immediately aware of the positions of objects through it.[22] Incorporation, thus, transforms a person's body schema, creating new "perceptual and motor possibilities" for the person's engagement with the world and comprises the disappearance of the incorporated object from his or her attention.[23]

But the lived body is also itself an object, a thing of flesh and blood, an entity that can be seen and touched and might break down. Without this simultaneous subjectivity and objectivity of the body, phenomenologists argue, our active inhabitance of and existence in the world would not be possible. Nor would it be possible for others to be with us. It is essentially by means of our bodily appearance and movements that we are recognized by others. But the body's materiality also allows us to attend to our own bodies. Although we are ordinarily outwardly directed, the thingness of our own body allows us to orient ourselves toward it, to attend to it as an object. And we sometimes do so, Leder points out, "in the interest of enjoyment, self-monitoring, cultivating sensitivity, satisfying curiosity, or for no particular reason at all."[24]

But there are instances when the body-as-object forces itself upon us and demands our attention. This is evident, for example, in illness, where our body tends to emerge for us as a problematic and painful thing beyond our control.[25] Today, in order to regain a sense of control over it, we often seek medical assistance, an assistance, however, that also orients us to view our own body as an object, but as a *medical* body-as-object.[26] As I have demonstrated elsewhere, for chronically ill persons—who tend to be in constant contact with medicine—the challenge is to successfully incorporate one's own body as a medical object into one's body schema, in order to make it absent.[27]

In the following sections, I draw on the phenomenological foundation that I have outlined here to explore the interaction between patients
that takes place at the four hemodialysis units that I visited. In doing so,
I elaborate further on this theoretical approach by adding the concept of
intercorporeality.

Intercorporeality in Hemodialysis

When I ask Veronica, who undergoes hemodialysis at one of the conventional
units in Stockholm, how she thinks spending so much time at the treatment
unit has affected her as a person, she says, "I think it has made me more
attentive to and appreciative of what's good, what I have that is good. . . .
Because you see that some [patients] suffer a lot and struggle a lot." Lidija,
who receives her treatment at the unit in Riga, describes it similarly: "I see
that there are people in a worse state than I, who have no arms, have no feet.
But I am able to walk, even crawl. I am able to crawl ahead at least."

What these two short empirical examples illustrate is that there exists an
intercorporeal connection between patients in hemodialysis. Merleau-Ponty
uses the concept of intercorporeality to denote the fundamental coexistence
or compresence of our bodies in the world.[28] Referring to the famous phenomenological example of the right hand touching the left hand, he writes,
"My two hands 'coexist' or are 'compresent' because they are one single
body's hands. The other person appears through an extension of that compresence; he and I are like organs of one single intercorporeality."[29] What
Merleau-Ponty wants to get at here, and what is peculiar about the relationship we have to our own body, is that we can experience ourselves simultaneously as touching and being touched or seeing and being seen. It is this
experience, he argues, that prepares us "for understanding that there are
other *animalia* and possibly other men."[30] In other words, it is through the
"schism" between "seeing one's body 'from the outside'" and "being intro-
ceptively aware of one's body 'from the inside,'" as Gail Weiss puts it, that we
understand that we can be seen and touched by others and that the other
person seeing or touching us is an embodied self just as we are.[31] We experience the other not as an inert object but as another embodied self who has a
particular situated perspective on us and who also experiences him- or herself as simultaneously touching and being touched or seeing and being seen.

According to Merleau-Ponty, our compresence with other bodies in intercorporeality is fundamentally prereflective. This is so because, in being
directed toward the world and its objects, "intercorporeality goes beyond
itself and ends up unconscious of itself as intercorporeality."[32] In fact, it is
only through this process that there are objects for us in the first place. "The
things it [the body] perceives would really be being only if I learned that

they are seen by others, that they are presumptively visible to every viewer who warrants the name," Merleau-Ponty writes.[33] Since, due to the limitations of our own perceptual organs, we only have a limited perspective on things, we need the totality of perspectives offered to us in intercorporeality to accomplish objectivity. Without prereflectively incorporating the perspectives of others, we would not be able to understand a table as a table or a car as a car. Then we would only have "half-disclosed things" around us.[34]

The thing central to the practice of hemodialysis is the medical body-as-object or, more specifically, the dysfunctional kidneys, the kidney failure. It is because they have all been diagnosed with kidney failure that the patients I met share the space of the hemodialysis unit several hours every week. Clearly, this is something that they are all aware of. But, as Veronica and Lidija's words indicate, by repeatedly seeing others and experiencing oneself as being seen by others undergoing the same treatment, this awareness eventually becomes incorporated into one's body schema. When Veronica and Lidija see "that there are people in a worse state" than they who "suffer a lot and struggle a lot," they immediately and prereflectively understand that they could be the ones experiencing this rather than their fellow patients. As Weiss points out, through the intercorporeal connection one establishes with another, one may incorporate "the perspective of the other towards one's own body."[35] Since the perspectives of the other persons at the unit—patients, doctors, nurses—on the thing—the kidney failure—is inseparable from how Veronica and Lidija themselves understand it, this is what they do. They immediately and unreflectively relate what their fellow patients go through to their own embodied existence. In Veronica's and Lidija's case, the experiences that they thereby have of themselves cause them to conclude that they should be happy about the relative health they currently enjoy.

But this is not always the case. When Marianne fell ill with kidney failure, she was only twenty-five years old and was assigned to a hemodialysis unit in Stockholm where many of the patients were old and suffered from multiple conditions. She describes this experience as follows: "There were many who were waiting to die and people who, you know, were screaming, and diabetics with amputated legs and so on. So, for me it was a horrific experience. 'Will I survive this year?' I wondered." Because of the intercorporeal connection Marianne had established with her fellow patients at this unit, their suffering and poor condition immediately translated into the question "Will *I* survive this year?" Since she had incorporated the perspective of the others on the disease that she herself embodied, she experienced their suffering as her own. The intercorporeal bond we have with other human beings, thus, is not always beneficial for us. As Weiss so convincingly illustrates, our intercorporeal exchanges with others often reproduce the power relations through which we are placed in oppressive categories.[36] To a great degree this is also what happens in hemodialysis. At the treatment units, and elsewhere, patients are lumped together in a category—sufferers of kidney failure—and forced to experience themselves as similar to the others who are a part of this category.

But, according to Weiss, the differences that such categories create and rely on are unstable, characterized by a fluidity with the potential to afford intercorporeal exchanges a "diversity and richness."[37] What Weiss wants to get at here, I believe, is the dynamic nature of embodiment and intercorporeality, a dynamism that may allow persons to habitually incorporate the categories they embody in a way that enables them to extend beyond these categories. That this might be the case in hemodialysis care is evident in the following quote from my interview with Boris, who undergoes the treatment at the unit in Riga.

> We [the patients] communicate like all people communicate. What's the difference? [He's] a patient, but first of all he's human. We don't suggest during our conversations that we are patients, we communicate like persons who know each other well. And the communication is founded on this premise. But you don't talk about very private things with everybody. But we share the information that is possible to speak about, of course.

As Boris's words indicate, because the treatment—and thereby also the intercorporeal exchanges between the patients—is repeated so often, Boris and his fellow patients are able to extend beyond the thing—the disease—that initially was the only thing binding them together. Since they have habitually incorporated the disease into the prereflective and practical absence of their body schema, the patients are able to meet each other as persons, as individuals, rather than as people belonging to the patient category.

Different Intercorporealities in Riga and Stockholm

It is telling that the words above were uttered by a patient who undergoes hemodialysis at the unit in Riga, since the patient interaction was more intense there than at the conventional units in Stockholm, and since the Latvian patients themselves tended to value this interaction more than their fellow Swedish patients do. As an outsider visiting the units for the first time, this difference was striking. At the unit in Riga, patients not only interacted before and after the treatment in the lunchroom and waiting room, but many of them also engaged in lively conversations during the treatment. At the conventional units in Stockholm, however, I was struck by the fact that several patients who undoubtedly recognized each other did not even greet one another. There was of course some interaction taking place—mainly in the waiting rooms or corridors before and after the treatment—but not as extensively and intensely as at the unit in Riga.

What was also striking for me as an outsider, which partly explains the difference I detected, was how rather minor differences in the spatial environment and the temporal organization of the treatment between the unit in Riga and the two conventional units in Stockholm affected the conditions for patient interaction. While at the unit in Riga all patients belonging to the same treatment session started their treatment at the same time, many patients in Stockholm had a so called "individual dialysis time," which meant that they, even though they belonged to the same session, arrived at the unit at a few minutes' interval. Moreover, patients in Riga ate together in a lunchroom before or after the treatment. At the two conventional units in Stockholm, patients were served a light meal during the treatment. Finally, and perhaps most importantly, the distance between the beds in which the patients lay during the treatment varied. At the unit in Riga, not more than one meter separated the beds, a proximity made possible by the fact that the hemodialysis machines had been placed behind the head of the beds. At the conventional units in Stockholm, conversely, the machines were placed between the beds, making the space between them at least three meters.

This is how Bengt, who undergoes hemodialysis at one of the conventional units in Stockholm, describes how this fairly significant gap between the beds affects the possibility of interacting with other patients during the treatment. I ask him if he engages in such interaction.

> No, that's not possible. Because, I mean, you have a bed that's three meters away. Who . . . what am I going to speak to there? A nose protruding? That doesn't work. That's a bit boring. You have no one, that's the downside of this place. They lie in their bed and then there's nothing more than that. You go out [into the corridor] afterwards and if you're lucky you find someone to talk to for a while before they go away in their taxi. . . . So I can't say that you talk to anyone at all.

As is evident in this quote, Bengt regrets the absence of interaction between patients at the unit. It is clear that he would favor a spatiotemporal reorganization of the treatment practice that made it easier to communicate. However, several of his fellow patients at the conventional units in Stockholm would not. This is how Tomas describes his experience:

> MARTIN: Do you feel that you would like to have more contact with the others here?
> TOMAS: No, I don't [laughs a little].
> MARTIN: Why not?
> TOMAS: No, we're so different.

There is one patient with whom Tomas communicates more than the others, who lives in the same part of Stockholm as he. But with the other patients, he says, the exchange is limited to the illness—and inquiries such as, "Do you feel as bad as I do after dialysis?" or "Do you get as many blood pressure drops as I?"—themes that Tomas is not overly interested in. Likewise, the reason Eva does not want to extend her contact with her fellow patients is the difference between them and her. But what matters the most to her is the varying severity of their conditions. She says, "They are all pretty ill. I'm quite . . . I'm one of those who are pretty well actually [laughs a little]."

Tomas's and Eva's accounts demonstrate that the disease category within which patients are placed when they begin to undergo hemodialysis does not necessarily create an intercorporeal bond strong enough to relegate other, differing personal traits to the background. Instead of being experienced as an extension of me, the other patients emerge as different personalities with their own bodily reactions to the disease. Consequently, Tomas and Eva do not feel that they have enough in common with their fellow patients to motivate an extended interaction. But it is also possible to see Tomas's and Eva's renunciation of a deepened interaction and their emphasis on difference as strategies to escape the category they have been placed in and the danger of intercorporeally experiencing themselves through other patients who are in a worse condition. Rather than transcending the intercorporeality based on the disease by building a deepened personal relationship with their fellow patients, Tomas and Eva try to avoid it completely. It is also worth recalling Bengt's words above, which indicated that, even if Tomas and Eva wanted to, the spatiotemporality of the treatment would likely prevent them from deepening their relationship with their fellow patients.

There are examples of similar ways of reasoning at the unit in Riga, such as Yevgeniy, who argues that, since "everyone has his own organism, . . . you can't share your experience," and Stanislav, who says, "I try not to have personal relationships with them [his fellow patients], because they are all going to die soon, just like me, so why should I stuff my head with that?" More often, however, the Latvian patients describe their interaction with other patients as important and valuable. Here is Liouba:

LIOUBA: When I came to my senses last year, I thought, "You need the other people [meaning her fellow patients] who are nearly family already." We spend three times a week together. So I brought coffee before dialysis, treated everyone. We got to talking . . . and now we have a get-together before dialysis.
MARTIN: So would you say that this feeling of community is important to you?
LIOUBA: Yes, yes, yes, we have the same illness, so we are one with another in that way.

Here, Liouba really accentuates the "need" she felt the year before to expand and deepen her relationship with the other patients beyond sheer patient-hood. As she points out, this was not a big leap, since the repetitiveness of hemodialysis had made them "nearly family already." Moreover, although quite implicitly, Liouba's words indicate that the need she felt was not just a need for get-togethers but for support of a deeper kind. Having just regained her senses, after falling ill the year before, she realizes that she needs her fellow patients to help her deal with and understand her new situation.

That developing such a relationship with one's fellow patients, besides generating emotional support, may serve as a source of information is evident among the patients at the unit in Riga. Ivan, for instance, says, "I learned all the necessary information [about the disease and treatments] from people [fellow patients] I know." While the doctors tend to provide only "half the information" and not infrequently "beautify the situation," he may learn "what the reality is" from his fellow patients. Liouba describes it similarly: "What can doctors say? We do not have conversations in a comfortable atmosphere, face-to-face with them. But we [the patients] have time and we discuss everything in detail." The patients in Stockholm do not advance the same criticism of their doctors. But, on a few occasions, the exceptional character of the information one may get from fellow patients is contrasted with the information one may get from doctors—as when Hans says, "You get information from doctors too, but not in the same way as from a treated patient"—but on the whole the patients at the conventional units in Stockholm describe the doctors as providing sufficient information.

Two Interrelated Causes for
the Intercorporeal Difference

There is a lot to indicate that the differences between the unit in Riga and the two conventional hemodialysis units in Stockholm have two interrelated causes. The first may be found by turning to the twentieth-century history of the practice of medicine in the two countries, the second by taking into account the minor spatiotemporal differences between the units.

On a general level, the ideas that governed the policies in the health-care sector during the twentieth century were similar in the Swedish welfare state and the Soviet Union—to which Latvia belonged until it gained independence in 1991. Health care was supposed to be free and universally accessible for all citizens. While these ideals to a large extent became a reality in Sweden, because of a constant lack of resources and a fundamentally hierarchical and centralized system, the goal of equal access for all was never reached in the Soviet Union, nor was health care completely free. Corruption was widespread; patients' access to care often hinged on their ability to make payments under the table. Once inside the system, however, Soviet socialized medicine took over all responsibility for the patient's health.[38] There is an overwhelming consensus among scholars studying the Soviet medical system that health care during communist rule was profoundly paternalistic.[39] "At that time," Latvian physician Guntis Kilkuts writes, "the ideology was that the health care system took over the patient's disease."[40] Once within the confines of a medical facility, patients were no longer responsible for their own health and were neither permitted to participate in nor influence the decision-making. According to anthropologist Aivita Putnina, patients were predominately viewed as a passive collective whose well-being could be ensured only by means of an undisturbed implementation of biomedical knowledge. Putnina contends that this view caused a vast rift between how patients and professionals perceived the events that unfolded within the boundaries of medical facilities.[41] But this "estrangement between doctors and patients" was also to a great extent political in nature.[42] While patients often understood their illnesses as caused by political oppression, medical professionals not infrequently dismissed them as malingerers.

During the 1970s and 1980s the public grew increasingly dissatisfied with the way health care was organized and practiced in Sweden. During the previous two decades, the provision of care had become increasingly bureaucratized. Inspired by industrial corporations, the organization of services was centralized in so-called district health authorities, and much of the care was performed in large hospitals. The criticism that was now being heard turned against this bureaucratization and industrialization; "the big hospitals were compared with factories, and the organization of healthcare was accused of being too complex and bureaucratic."[43] But the quality of the care itself was also criticized as being dehumanizing, non–service-minded, and incapable of meeting patients' needs.[44]

This criticism sparked the beginning of a process of radical and thoroughgoing organizational changes in the Swedish health-care system. Starting in the 1980s, a process of decentralization began through which the responsibility for the provision and financing of health care was delegated to the county councils, while the local municipalities became responsible for the care of the elderly and the disabled.[45] This process was accompanied by an orientation toward the market.[46] At this time, a system of family doctors, in which patients were allowed to choose their caregiver and health-care facility, was also implemented. The introduction of this system was very much in line with a process on a more general and international level where the perspectives of patients were increasingly taken into account.[47] Patients were to a growing degree viewed as unique individuals and active participants in their care practices and were given the right to receive information about and choose between treatment alternatives. In line with the market orientation of the health-care sector, patients were also increasingly viewed as consumers shopping around for the medical therapies best suited to their particular needs.[48]

Since its independence from the Soviet Union in 1991, the Latvian health-care system has also been subject to extensive reforms. These have, as in Sweden, primarily been oriented toward decentralization and market orientation. In Latvia, however, health care is financed by the state, while the responsibility for the provision of care is delegated to the providers themselves. Many of the health-care facilities are privately run, especially those in primary care. As in Sweden, family doctors, whom patients actively register with, provide the primary care. These are trained as general practitioners and often "work independently, either as self-employed individuals or as private sector agents."[49]

Despite these processes of decentralization and market orientation, patients' rights in Latvia are still weak. According to the World Health Organization, Latvian patients are not provided with a satisfactory legal protection. There are, for instance, deficiencies in the confidentiality, privacy, and complaint procedures. Patient associations are, furthermore, unable to exert significant influence. They are often chronically underfinanced and overseen by medical professionals. But, just as in Sweden, patients have the right to choose between caregivers and health-care facilities and receive clear and unbiased information.[50]

As this brief account demonstrates, the two national contexts provide different conditions for doctor-patient interaction, on the one hand, and patient-patient interaction, on the other. While, in the Swedish context, there has been a development toward an increased patient-centeredness since the 1970s, a similar development only began in the early 1990s in Latvia. Moreover, the profound paternalism that characterized health care during communist rule to some extent still influences the doctor-patient relationship in Latvia.[51] While the increased patient-centeredness has led to an accentuation of the patient as an individual in Sweden, this is less the case in Latvia, where patients to a larger extent are viewed as a collective.

As we saw above, in the context of hemodialysis, this is reflected in the spatiotemporal organization of the treatment practice itself. Even if the patients at the two conventional units in Stockholm wanted to deepen their relationships with their fellow patients, the spatiotemporal organization of the treatment made this next to impossible, while, at the unit in Riga, the space in which the treatment took place together with its temporal structuring allowed patients to deepen their interaction. There is much to indicate that these spatiotemporal differences are not just arbitrarily related to but rather deeply intertwined with the historical processes described above. While the distinctly delimited treatment places found at the two conventional units in Stockholm coincides nicely with the view of patients as individuals with unique needs and desires, the proximity of the patients at the unit in Riga illustrates the lingering view of them as a group categorically estranged from the doctors. But neither are the spatiotemporal circumstances just an outcome of historical processes. The reverse is also true. In order to persist, historical and cultural processes have to gain a foothold somewhere, and they do so in the materiality of objects, spaces, and moving bodies.[52] In summation, one can contend that the spatiotemporal differences that I have detected are both cause and effect of the differing doctor-patient and patient-patient relationships discernible at the unit in Riga as compared to the conventional units in Stockholm.[53]

Self-Care as a Way of Minimizing the Risks Associated with Intercorporeality

Another conclusion that can be drawn concerns the patients' perception of the risks built into the intercorporeal connection established in hemodialysis. As we saw above, this risk consists in intercorporeally experiencing oneself through others who are in a worse condition than oneself. This may have the adverse effect of bringing the fragility of one's own state into attention. However, the patients at the unit in Riga have no choice but to take this risk. In the absence of sufficient information from doctors, they have to rely on their fellow patients to learn about their condition and find out how to deal with it. Interestingly, this seems to allow them to go beyond an affinity based only on the disease, on the body-as-object. As they deepen their relationship, they exceed their patienthood and begin to interact as persons who know each other well and who talk about other things than disease and illness. This is not just considered less desirable, it is also more difficult at the conventional units in Stockholm, not least because of the spatiotemporal conditions but also because the risks of doing so seem to outweigh the benefits. If one may get all the necessary information from doctors and other medical professionals, why would one need to consult a fellow patient?

However, as I mentioned above, the idea that one's fellow patients may provide a form of information and support that doctors are unable to deliver is present also among the Swedish patients. But because of the historical and spatiotemporal conditions, the patients undergoing conventional hemodialysis at the units in Stockholm to a great degree miss out on this form of information and support. At the self-care unit in Stockholm, though, which I discuss below, an interaction between patients comparable to what takes place in Riga. One reason for this is that the risk mentioned above is perceived to be lower, a fact that is clearly illustrated by the following quote, in which Carlos answers my question concerning how he has experienced his move from one of the conventional units in Stockholm to the self-care unit.

> CARLOS: Positively, enormously.
> MARTIN: In what way?
> CARLOS: Well, to lie in a room with three other persons who are old and sick and who you know are just waiting to die, because many are in that situation. And in addition, they have trouble with the sugar [diabetes]; their fingers fall off and their feet fall off and, you know, it's a hospital. . . . It's a sick environment. But now, when I'm at the self-care unit, I meet relatively healthy people who look good and who are nice. Well, it's like you just have a small defect [laughs]. "I have to charge my batteries," something like that.

During my fieldwork at the self-care unit, several patients gave similar accounts. Rather than being potentially harmful, the presence of the other patients was generally seen as beneficial. According to Camilla, it was her short stay at the self-care unit before she began performing the treatment at home that made her realize that being dependent on hemodialysis is not the end of the world. She saw that "he can do that, despite the fact that he undergoes dialysis. Then I'll be able to do that too."

I believe this change in the benefit-risk ratio, as compared to the conventional units, ought to be viewed with an eye to the fact that patients are not only less sick at the self-care unit, but they also appear to be less sick.[54] Health, as several scholars have pointed out, is inextricably bound up today with pervasive ideals such as activity, control, and independence.[55] A chronically ill person who, despite suffering from a disease, exhibits an active lifestyle and exercises a degree of control will be perceived as less sick than a person who depends on others and who engages in few activities. Consequently, Carlos's and Camilla's fellow patients at the self-care unit are not only healthier than the patients at the conventional units, but they also appear to be so, on account of their active engagement with and the amount of control they exercise over the treatment.

But there are also details in the spatial arrangement of the unit that facilitate a deepening of the intercorporeal exchange. At the self-care unit patients undergo hemodialysis in small rooms with only two or three treatment places in each. During the treatment, they sit in leather chairs, which means that they are in an upright position and may easily orient themselves toward the patients with whom they share the ward.

In summation, although the historical processes accounted for above affects to what extent patients *need* to extend their interaction with fellow patients, they are not decisive in determining the extent to which patients actually do this. If the risks can be lowered and the spatial arrangements can be made more permissive, as at the self-care unit, patients will interact at Swedish hemodialysis units too.

The Complex Contingencies of the Intercorporeal Bond

In this chapter I have highlighted and explored the simultaneous embedment and disembedment of biomedicine through the example of patient interaction in hemodialysis. I began by outlining the fundamental bodily and spatiotemporal standardization of hemodialysis. I showed how its provision is based on a scientific foundation that presupposes the existence of a universal body, a body that is the same everywhere, and how this, in turn, constitutes the basis for a transnational standardization of its temporality and, to a great degree, spatiality. When patients become aligned with this universalized body and standardized spatiotemporality, they invariably become oriented toward each other, to the extent that an intercorporeal bond is created between them. Since the patients come to incorporate their embodiment of the disease—kidney failure—and live from it rather than toward it, they prereflectively begin to see themselves through the other patients. As such, the intercorporeal bond created between them is an effect both of their prereflective embodiment of a universal body and their inhabitance of the same standardized spatiotemporality.

Yet, the nature of and patients' views on their interaction with each other differed between the two national contexts studied. While the patients at the unit in Riga tended to interact a lot and assign this interaction great value, the patients at the two conventional units in Stockholm neither interacted a lot nor assigned it great value. This difference, I argued, had two interrelated causes. On the one hand, it had to do with the differing historical roots of the provision and practice of biomedicine in the two countries. On the other hand, it had to do with minor differences in the spatiotemporal organization between the two conventional units in Stockholm and the unit in Riga. Taken together, these differing historical, cultural, and spatiotemporal conditions oriented the patients to engage the intercorporeal bond in different ways.

The self-care unit in Stockholm was an interesting exception. At this unit, there was an interest among the patients to interact with each other, which was possible given the different spatial organization of the conventional units and perception among the patients of the interaction between them being less risky. This led me to conclude that, while Latvian hemodialysis patients, in the absence of sufficient information and support from doctors, may need to interact more with each other, Swedish patients would also interact with each other if they thought that the risks and benefits associated with it were balanced. This suggests that, even though the universalization of the body and the standardization of space and time associated with contemporary biomedicine penetrates deep into the everyday actions and relations enacted and experienced in the treatment practice, these actions and relations are inextricably intertwined with the conditions provided by particular historical, cultural, and highly local spatiotemporal circumstances. Contemporary biomedicine is thus always simultaneously embedded and disembedded.

Notes

1. See, e.g., Margaret Lock and Vinh-Kim Nguyen, *An Anthropology of Biomedicine* (Malden: Wiley-Blackwell, 2010); Arthur Kleinman, *The Illness Narratives: Suffering Healing and the Human Condition* (New York: Basic Books, 1988); Lisbeth Sachs, *Tillit som bot: Placebo i tid och rum* (Lund: Studentlitteratur, 2004).

2. Emily Martin, *Flexible Bodies: Tracking Immunity in American Culture—from the Days of Polio to the Age of AIDS* (Boston: Beacon Press, 1994), 7.

3. Sarah Franklin, *Embodied Progress: A Cultural Account of Assisted Conception* (London: Routledge, 1997).

4 Stefan Beck, "Biomedical Mobilities: Transnational Lab-Benches and Other Space-Effects," in *Reproductive Technologies as Global Form: Ethnographies of Knowledge, Practices, and Transnational Encounters*, ed. Michi Knecht, Maren Klotz, and Stefan Beck (Frankfurt: Campus, 2012), 357–74.

5. See Anthony Giddens, *Modernity and Self-Identity: Self and the Society in the Late Modern Age* (Stanford: Stanford University Press, 1991), 18. In this book, Giddens uses the term "disembedding mechanisms" to denote "the 'lifting out' of social relations from local contexts and their rearticulation across indefinite tracts of time-space." It is to capture such processes that I use the term "disembedded" here.

6. See Martin Gunnarson, *Please Be Patient: A Cultural Phenomenological Study of Haemodialysis and Kidney Transplantation Care* (Lund: Lund Studies in Arts and Cultural Sciences, 2016). This study was a part of the multidisciplinary research project The Body as Gift, Resource and Commodity: Organ Transplantation in the Baltic Region, funded by the Baltic Sea Foundation. See Martin Gunnarson and Fredrik Svenaeus, *The Body as Gift, Resource, and Commodity: Exchanging Organs, Tissues, and Cells in the 21st Century* (Huddinge: Södertörn Studies in Practical Knowledge, 2012).

7. See, e.g., Jenny Gunnarsson Payne, "Reproduction in Transition: Cross-Border Egg Donation, Biodesirability and New Reproductive Subjectivities on the European Fertility Market," *Gender, Place & Culture* 22, no. 1 (2015): 107–22.

8 See, e.g., Katarzyna Wolanik Boström and Magnus Öhlander, "A Doctor's Life-Story: On Professional Mobility, Occupational Sub-cultures and Personal Gains," in *Selling One's Favourite Piano to Emigrate: Mobility Patterns in Central Europe at the Beginning of the 21st Century*, ed. Jakub Isanski and Piotr Luczys (Newcastle upon Tyne: Cambridge Scholars, 2011), 205–22.

9. There are two types of dialysis treatment: hemodialysis and peritoneal dialysis. Hemodialysis is by far the more common. In peritoneal dialysis, patients manage the treatment by themselves. Three to five times a day they infuse a dialysis solution into their abdomen and let it set for a while, before draining it along with the excess fluid and toxic waste products it has attracted.

10. Patients with kidney failure may also undergo transplantation, which is generally viewed as the superior treatment option. However, the wait time for a donor kidney is ordinarily long, while waiting patients have to undergo dialysis.

11. James Tatterstal et al., "EBPG Guideline on Dialysis Strategies," *Nephrology Dialysis Transplantation* 22, no. 2 (2007): ii5.

12 See, e.g., Robert P. Pauly et al., "Survival among Nocturnal Home Haemodialysis Patients Compared to Kidney Transplant Recipients," *Nephrology Dialysis Transplantation* 24, no. 9 (2009): 2915.

13. At all units there are a number of private treatment rooms, which are generally intended for patients with particularly severe conditions or, as at the self-care unit, for patients who are learning to manage the treatment by themselves.

14. Drew Leder, *The Absent Body* (Chicago: University of Chicago Press, 1990), 5.

15. Maurice Merleau-Ponty, *The Phenomenology of Perception* (New York: Routledge, 2002), 13, 151.

16. Ibid., 273.

17. Erik Malmqvist and Kristin Zeiler, "Cultural Norms, the Phenomenology of Incorporation, and the Experience of Having a Child Born with Ambiguous Sex," *Social Theory and Practice* 36, no. 1 (2010): 137.

18. Merleau-Ponty, *The Phenomenology of Perception*, 157.

19. Malmqvist and Zeiler, "Cultural Norms, the Phenomenology of Incorporation, and the Experience of Having a Child Born with Ambiguous Sex," 137.

20. Leder, *The Absent Body*.

21. Ibid., 15.

22. Merleau-Ponty, *The Phenomenology of Perception*, 163–70.

23. Malmqvist and Zeiler, "Cultural Norms, the Phenomenology of Incorporation, and the Experience of Having a Child Born with Ambiguous Sex," 140.

24. Leder, *The Absent Body*, 91.

25. Ibid., 84.

26. See Katharine Young, *Presence in the Flesh: The Body in Medicine* (Cambridge, MA: Harvard University Press, 1997).

27. Gunnarson, *Please Be Patient*.

28. Maurice Merleau-Ponty, *Signs* (Evanston, IL: Northwestern University Press, 1964).

29. Ibid., 168.

30. Ibid.

31. Gail Weiss, *Body Images: Embodiment as Intercorporeality* (New York: Routledge, 1999), 12–13.

32. Merleau-Ponty, *Signs*, 173.

33. Ibid., 168.

34. Ibid., 170.

35 Weiss, *Body Images*, 13.

36. Weiss, *Body Images*.

37. Ibid., 85.

38. Mark G. Field, "The Soviet Legacy: The Past as Prologue," in *Health Care in Central Asia*, ed. Martin McKee, Judith Healy, and Jane Falkingham (Buckingham: Open University Press, 2002), 67–75.

39. Agita Luse and Lelde Kapina, "Intimacy and Control, Reciprocity and Paternalism: Madness and the Ambivalence of Caring Relationships in a Post-Soviet Country," in *Probing Madness*, ed. Katarzyna Szmigiero (Oxford: Inter-Disciplinary Press, 2011), 67–80; Christopher McKevitt, Agita Luse, and Charles Wolfe, "The

Unfortunate Generation: Stroke Survivors in Riga, Latvia," *Social Science & Medicine* 56, no. 10 (2002): 2097–108.

40. Öivind Larsen and Guntis Kilkuts, "Health in Latvia 1991–2004: Years of Conflicting Values," *Michael* 2, no. 1 (2005), 55.

41. Aivita Putnina, "Maternity Services and Agency in Post-Soviet Latvia" (PhD diss, University of Cambridge, 1999).

42. Vieda Skultans, *The Testimony of Lives: Narrative and Memory in Post-Soviet Latvia* (London: Routledge, 1998), 21.

43. Runo Axelsson, "The Organizational Pendulum: Healthcare Management in Sweden 1865–1998," *Scandinavian Journal of Public Health* 28, no. 1 (2000): 49.

44. Axelsson, "The Organizational Pendulum," 48–49.

45. Björn Lindgren, "Landstingens skyldigheter och individens rättigheter," in *Etiska utmaningar i hälso- och sjukvården*, ed. Kristofer Hansson (Lund: Studentlitteratur, 2006), 125–60, esp. 126.

46. Axelsson, "The Organizational Pendulum," 49.

47. Ibid., 50. Carl May and Nicola Mead, "Patient-Centredness: A History," in *General Practice and Ethics: Uncertainty and Responsibility*, ed. Christopher Dowrick and Lucy Frith (London: Routledge, 1999), 76–90; Stanley Joel Reiser, *Technological Medicine: The Changing World of Doctors and Patients* (New York: Cambridge University Press, 2009).

48. Kristofer Hansson, "Introduktion: Etiska utmaningar i en föränderlig hälso- och sjukvård," in *Etiska utmaningar i en föränderlig hälso- och sjukvård*, ed. Kristofer Hansson (Lund: Studentlitteratur, 2006), 11–26, esp. 16–17; Nikolas Rose, *The Politics of Life Itself: Biomedicine, Power, and Subjectivity in the Twenty-First Century* (Princeton, NJ: Princeton University Press, 2007); Annemarie Mol, *The Logic of Care: Health and the Problem of Patient Choice* (London: Routledge, 2008).

49. E. Tragakes et al., "Latvia: Health System Review," *Health Systems in Transition* 10, no. 2 (2008): 1–253.

50. Ibid., 54–60.

51. See, e.g., Luse and Kapina, "Intimacy and Control, Reciprocity and Paternalism."

52. Sara Ahmed, *Queer Phenomenology: Orientations, Objects, Others* (Durham, NC: Duke University Press, 2006).

53. Martin Gunnarson, "Delade erfarenheter eller egen expertis: att vara dialyspatient i Riga och Stockholm," *Socialmedicinsk tidskrift* 88, no. 3 (2011): 257–65.

54. The very old and sick patients are generally not given the option of self-care.

55. See, e.g., Ingrid Fioretos, *Möten med motstånd: kultur, klass, kropp på vårdcentralen* (Lund: Avdelningen för etnologi, Institutionen för kulturvetenskaper, Lunds universitet, 2009); Rose, *The Politics of Life Itself.*

Contributors

KATHARINA BEIER, PhD, is a medical ethicist and associate researcher in the Department of Medical Ethics and History of Medicine at the Göttingen University Medical Center, Germany. Her research is focused on research ethics, particularly in the field of biobanking and big data-based research, and the ethics of reproductive medicine.

MOTZI EKLÖF, PhD, is an associate professor in health and society. Her research area is the social and cultural history of medicine and health, including its ethical aspects. Eklöf has published works on topics such as the Swedish medical profession, the Swiss physician Bircher-Benner and his patients, homeopathy as a conflict zone, and early Swedish bacteriology.

FRANK GRÜNER, PhD, is a research fellow in the Cluster of Excellence "Asia and Europe in a Global Context" program at the University of Heidelberg.

MARTIN GUNNARSON completed his PhD in ethnology at Lund University and Södertörn University, Sweden, in 2016. His PhD project explored patients' experiences and the practice of hemodialysis and kidney transplantation.

NILS HANSSON, PhD, is an associate professor and lecturer in the Department of the History, Theory, and Ethics of Medicine at the University of Dusseldorf. His scholarly interests include the history of medicine around the Baltic Sea, the history of surgery, the Nobel Prize, and the enactment of excellence in medicine.

AXEL C. HÜNTELMANN, PhD, MA, MBA, is research fellow at the Institute for the History of Medicine, Charité – University Hospital Berlin. His scholarly interests include European public health institutions, history of growth, and laboratory animals. He has written a biography on Paul Ehrlich and is currently finishing a book on accounting and medicine.

KEN KALLING is a lecturer in the history of medicine at the Institute of Family Medicine and Public Health at the University of Tartu, Estonia. His fields of interest in scientific history include the history of eugenics, the history of race studies, and medicine and the natural sciences under totalitarianism.

MICHAELA MALMBERG completed her master's degree in history at the University of Göteborg in 2014, with a thesis entitled "Livmodersmassagens försvinnande, en nedtystad historia om medicin, kön och makt." Her areas of interest include the history of medicine, gender, professionalism, and power.

JOANNA NIEZNANOWSKA, MD, PhD, is an assistant professor in the Department of the History of Medicine and Medical Ethics, Pomeranian Medical University. Her main research interests are the German-Polish transfer of knowledge in gynecology and obstetrics in the nineteenth century, the changing concepts of the moral status of the fetus in the nineteenth and twentieth centuries, and, most recently, the medical history of Stettin, 1800–1945.

ANDERS OTTOSSON is senior fellow at the Department of Historical Studies, University of Gothenburg, Sweden. He has published widely on the history of Swedish physiotherapy and orthopedics and is currently running a project analyzing female interest (national and international) in becoming woodcraft teachers between 1885 and 1930. He is also completing a monograph that explores the historical and sociological origins of North American professions specializing in osteopathic and chiropractic manipulation.

MAIKE ROTZOLL, MD, is an associate professor in the Department of the History of Medicine and Medical Ethics at the University of Heidelberg.

ERKI TAMMIKSAAR is the director of the Karl Ernst von Baer House in Tartu (now the Centre for Science Studies at the University of Life Sciences) and senior research associate in the Department of Geography at the University of Tartu. His scholarly interests include the scientific activities of K. E. v. Baer, the history of the natural sciences at the University of Tartu in the nineteenth century, the role of the St. Petersburg Academy of Sciences in the Russian Empire, and the political activities of Baltic-German scientists in the Russian Empire.

JONATAN WISTRAND, MD, is a PhD student in the Department of Medical History, Lund University, Sweden. Illness narratives play a central role in his research, especially testimonies from the early twentieth century. He also teaches medical history and medical humanities at the medical school in Lund.

Index

Printed in the United States
By Bookmasters